C. von BÖNNINGHAUSEN'S

HOMŒOPATHIC THERAPEIA

OF

INTERMITTENT AND OTHER FEVERS.

121535

TRANSLATED, WITH THE ADDITION OF NEW REMEDIES,

BY

A. KORNDŒRFER, M.D.

BOERICKE & TAFEL.

NEW YORK: 145 GRAND ST.
PHILADELPHIA: 635 ARCH ST.

LONDON AND MANCHESTER:
HENRY TURNER & CO.

W. Hering & Co., Printers.

CONTENTS.

PART III. RELATION OF THE FEVER STAGES.

PART IV.

LIST OF REMEDIES.

Acon. Aconitum napellus.
Act. rac. Actæa racemosa.
Æsc. hip. Æsculus hippocastanum.
Agar. Agaricus muscarius.
Agn. cast. Agnus castus.
Alum. Alumina.
Ambra. Ambra grisea.
Amm. carb. Ammonium carbonicum.
Amm. mur. Ammonium muriaticum.
Anac. Anacardium orientale.
Angust. Angustura.
Ant. crud. Antimonium crudum.
Ant. tart. Antimonium tartaricum.
Apis. Apis mellifica.
Argent. Argentum metallicum.
Argent. nit. Argentum nitricum.*
Arnic. Arnica montana.
Arsen. Arsenicum album.
Arum tr. Arum triphyllum.
Asaf. Asa fœtida.
Asar. Asarum europæum.
Aurum. Aurum metallicum. (Formerly Foliatum.)
Baptis. Baptisia tinctoria.
Baryt. Baryta carbonica.
Bellad. Belladonna.
Bismuth. Bismuthum.
Borax. Borax veneta.
Bovist. Bovista.
Brom. Bromium.
Bryon. Bryonia alba.
Cact. grand. Cactus grandiflorus.
Calad. Caladium seguinum.
Calc. carb. Calcarea carbonica. (ostrearum, C.Hg.)
Camphor. Camphora.
Cann. sat. Cannabis sativa.
Canthar. Cantharis.
Capsic. Capsicum annuum.
Carb. an. Carbo animalis.
Carb. veg. Carbo vegetabilis.
Caustic. Causticum.
Chamom. Chamomilla.
Chelid. Chelidonium majus.
Chin. sulph. Chininum sulphuricum.
Cicut. Cicuta virosa.
Cimex. Cimex lectularius.
Cina. Cina.
Cinchon. Cinchona.
Cist. can. Cistus canadensis.
Clemat. Clematis erecta.
Coccul. Cocculus.
Coffea. Coffea cruda.
Colchic. Colchicum autumnale.
Coloc. Colocynthis.
Conium. Conium maculatum.
Corn. cir. Cornus circinata.
Corn. flor. Cornus florida.
Crocus. Crocus sativus.
Crotal. Crotalus horridus.*
Cuprum. Cuprum metallicum.
Cyclam. Cyclamen europæum.
Diadem. Diadema aranea.
Digit. Digitalis purpurea.
Droser. Drosera rotundifolia.
Dulcam. Dulcamara solanum.
Elaps. Elaps corallinus.*
Eup. perf. Eupatorium perfoliatum.
Eup. purp. Eupatorium purpureum.
Euphorb. Euphorbium officinarum.
Euphras. Euphrasia officinalis.
Ferr. Ferrum metallicum.
Fluor. ac. Fluoricum acidum.
Gelsem. Gelseminum sempervirens.
Glon. Glonoine.*
Graphit. Graphites.
Guaiac. Guaiacum officinale.
Helleb. Helleborus niger.
Hepar. Hepar sulphuris calcareum.
Hydrast. Hydrastis canadensis.
Hydr. ac. Hydrocyanicum acidum.
Hyosc. Hyoscyamus niger.
Hyperic. Hypericum perforatum.*
Ignat. Ignatia amara.
Iod. Iodium.
Ipecac. Ipecacuanha.
Kali bichr. Kali bichromicum.
Kali carb. Kali carbonicum.

Kali hydr. Kali hydriodicum.
Kreos. Kreosotum.
Laches. Lachesis trigonocephalus.
Lachnanth. Lachnanthes tinctoria.
Lauroc. Laurocerasus.
Ledum. Ledum palustre.
Leptand. Leptandra virginica.
Lobel. inf. Lobelia inflata.
Lycop. Lycopodium clavatum.
Magn. carb. Magnesia carbonica.
Magn. mur. Magnesia muriatica.
Mangan. Manganum.
Mar. ver. Marum verum.
Menyanth. Menyanthes trifoliata.
Merc. corr. Mercurius corrosivus.
Merc. viv. Mercurius vivus.
Mezer. Mezereum.
Mosch. Moschus.
Mur. ac. Muriaticum acidum.
Natr. carb. Natrum carbonicum.
Natr. mur. Natrum muriaticum.
Natr. sulph. Natrum sulphuricum.
Nitr. ac. Nitri acidum.
Nitrum. Nitrum ; Kali nitricum.
Nux mosch. Nux moschata.
Nux vom. Nux vomica.
Oleand. Oleander.
Opium. Opium.
Oxal. ac. Oxalicum acidum.
Paris. Paris quadrifolia.
Petrol. Petroleum.
Phosphor. Phosphorus.
Phosph. ac. Phosphori acidum.
Platin. Platina.
Plumbum. Plumbum.
Podophyl. Podophyllum peltatum.
Psorin. Psorinum.
Pulsat. Pulsatilla pratensis.
Ran. bulb. Ranunculus bulbosus.
Ran. scel. Ranunculus sceleratus.
Rheum. Rheum palmatum.
Rhodod. Rhododendron chrysanthemum.
Rhus tox. Rhus toxicodendron.
Ruta. Ruta graveolens.
Sabad. Sabadilla.
Sabin. Sabina.
Sambuc. Sambucus nigra.
Sanguin. Sanguinaria canadensis.
Sarsap. Sarsaparilla.
Scilla. Scilla maritima.
Secal. Secale cornutum.
Selen. Selenium.
Seneg. Senega.
Sepia. Sepia.
Silic. Silicea.
Spigel. Spigelia anthelmintica.
Spong. Spongia.
Stann. Stannum.
Staphis. Staphisagria.
Stramon. Stramonium.
Strontia. Strontia carbonica.
Sulphur. Sulphur.
Sulph. ac. Sulphuris acidum.
Tarax. Taraxicum.
Therid. Theridion curassavicum.
Thuya. Thuya occidentalis.
Valer. Valeriana officinalis.
Veratr. Veratrum album.
Verbas. Verbascum thapsus.
Viol. od. Viola odorata.
Viol. tr. Viola tricolor.
Zinc. Zincum.

N. B. During the progress of the work through the press it was thought desirable to change the typography of the highest degree from *small caps.*, the original design, to *caps.* Attention should also be called to the fact that the following remedies, viz., Argent. nitr., Crotal., Elaps, Glon., Hyperic., have been noticed in the repertory though not incorporated in the text.

A. K.

TRANSLATOR'S PREFACE.

In placing a work of this character before the profession, but little need be said by way of introduction; the intrinsic merit of the original speaks for itself. The arrangement adopted by the author has been followed in the present edition, as closely as possible. But few alterations have been made in the original text, and these only where the author has given in an obscure phraseology, some well known symptom; in such cases, which were but few, the translator has preferred the more lucid expression, as found in the original of Hahnemann's Chronic Diseases, or in the Materia Medica Pura. The typographical arrangement of the repertory has however, been changed; the highest degree is herein given in small caps.; the next lower degree in italics; while the two degrees still lower (as given by Bönninghausen), owing to the slight practical benefit to be derived from their distinction, have been given in roman type. The alterations here referred to have been necessitated, through the great difficulty and expense of the composition as found in the original. Many symptoms have been added to the repertory, some of which are recent observations, but all are from the best authorities.

Regarding part IV., we would remark: the additions thereto have been made with care; yet we would most earnestly commend the careful selection of the remedy, according to the individual symptoms, rather than place any dependence on such a pathological classification, which if relied upon, we will find a stumbling block to success.

Twenty-six remedies have been added to the text and arranged in the repertory; the text for these has been carefully excerpted from the most reliable sources, and in addition has received the sanction of

Dr. C. Hering, to whom the translator would here return sincere thanks, for the kind assistance rendered in the completion of this work.

With these remarks and explanations, the work is now submitted to the profession, with the hope that it may prove as useful to the English reader, as the original has to the

TRANSLATOR.

PREFACE

TO THE SECOND GERMAN EDITION.

Within the past ten years, the author of the "Essay on the homœopathic treatment of intermittent fever," published in the year 1833, (at Münster by Fried. Regensberg), has been frequently requested to publish a new edition of the same, the former being out of print. This request, coming as it does, from a distance as well as from nearer home, and renewed, always more earnestly, every year at the meeting of the homœopathic physicians of the Rheinlands and Westphalia, lays upon the author the duty to again take up a work, which through thirty years of accumulated observations and experiences, has not only decidedly increased its scope, but also its difficulties.

Although the first edition received sufficient approbation to afford gratification, and even received honorable mention from the founder of homœopathy, in the last (fifth) edition of his Organon (p. 251); yet we must in truth, admit the demand of to-day to be so widely different from what it was at that time, that an entire remodeling in an increased and more comprehensive form, must be looked upon as a prerequisite, in order to meet it.

This revision and remodeling has long kept the author from the work, the time requisite being great, while his advanced age, 79 years. with impaired vigor and power of endurance, together with diminished hours of leisure in which to write, render the conditions far different from thirty years ago. On the other hand is brought to bear, not only the long years of experience, but especially the important accumulation of 115 quarto volumes of the most carefully kept Case books, "Kranken Journal," which contain a great treasure of material gathered by himself, on which he can fully rely.

If therefore, through this last mentioned fact, the author is encouraged to again take up the work, that he may fulfill his involuntary promise, by laying before his honored friends and colleagues this work in a new and more complete form; he has on the other hand a duty towards himself to perform, viz: to explain and justify his mode of treating the subject. With this especial purpose the following lines have been written.

1. A limitation of the therapeutics to intermittent fever alone, as in the first edition of this work, could not properly receive unqualified favor, for the most cogent reason, that nowhere between intermittent fever in the broadest sense of the term, and the numerous other fevers, can a sufficiently sharp line be drawn. The title "Intermittent fever" should therefore be set aside, and the general term "Fever," as related to the various diseased states of Circulation, Chill (including coldness and shivering), Heat and Sweat, be used in its stead. As one or more of these conditions can, in general, indicate and characterize a fever, it is therefore not only advisable, but necessary, to treat each of these stages in a separate chapter.

2. Most fevers, not only intermittent and remittent, but even the continued fevers, have periods during which the fever, with its concomitants, is ameliorated; and others during which the condition of the patient is more or less aggravated. Herein lie sufficiently forcible reasons for distinguishing the so-called Pyrexia (the actual fever period), from the Apyrexia (during which the actual fever has for a time abated, and given place to this changed condition). Therefore it seems quite appropriate that this first volume should especially treat of the Pyrexia, and that the complaints of the Apyrexia should be reserved for a second volume. In the mean time every other homœopathic therapeia, can take the place of this last mentioned part, until the author is able to prepare it. *Si qua fata sinunt!*

3. For the first volume, which will therefore treat exclusively of the Pyrexia, it seems of paramount importance, that a short extract of the characteristic symptoms, relative to fever, of the drugs mentioned in the repertory, should be given. This constitutes the first principal part of this work. These symptoms will be found under four divisions. 1. The Circulation and pulse; 2. The Chill, including coldness and shivering; 3. Heat; and 4. Sweat. The author believes that this arrangement, in which he has confined himself to the most important symptoms, will in a great degree lessen the difficulties, in the study and comparison of the peculiarities and differences of the remedies; and that through it, a more sharply defined picture of each remedy

may be drawn. This first part is therefore especially adapted to, and set apart for, the study of the true genius of each remedy, in regard to its power to excite fever, and to the adaptability of the same to individual cases; while the following chapters will decide in regard to points still remaining in doubt. It may here be remarked, that the abbreviation adopted for each remedy will be found in parenthesis to the right of its respective name.

4. The second part is composed of a repertory, which has been made as complete as possible, as regards the four stages: 1. Circulation; 2. Chill, including coldness and shivering; 3. Heat; 4. Sweat. The subdivisions for each stage are set forth in the index; the symptoms under each are arranged, as much as possible, in systematic alphabetical order; first the essential varieties therewith connected, in general; then in regard to single parts and organs. Next follow aggravations as regards time, location and circumstance; then ameliorating circumstances and conditions; and finally (for the last three stages), the concomitant complaints, which latter are all of more or less importance, according to the fundamental principles of homœopathy, in deciding the adaptability of a given remedy, to the greatest possible certainty, for the individual case.

5. The third part gives a view of the compound fevers, that is, of such as are composed of more than one of the afore-mentioned stages, from which many combinations are formed. It is evident that this part will not only allow, but will actually require, considerable enlargement and improvement in the future. For the more ready review of this part, the headings are given with reference to the first stage, and arranged according to the transition from one to the other.

6. The fourth and last part, which treats only of the pathological names, as applied to the various forms of fever, and of the remedies which to the present have been used more or less frequently, in the treatment of the same; is given only at the request of a number of my colleagues, who hope thereby to facilitate the task of searching for the remedy. It need scarcely be said that here less than anywhere can anything determinate be given, and the author would especially protest against the misuse of this "Name Therapeia," a part, to which every true homœopath will attach but slight importance, and which in no case can supplant the careful valuation of the symptoms, in the selection of the remedy. The cause of the numerous complaints, which of late have become so loud, in regard to the difficulties in the treat-

ment of fevers, is no doubt the censurable practice of generalization and name prescribing "*Namen Unfug.*"

7. With great diligence and especial care the author has endeavored, through different type and setting of the same, in the repertory, to mark the degree of importance of each remedy. He has retained the distinguishing points, which were employed in his repertory (of 1833 and 1835) and in his therapeutic pocket-book (of 1846); these having been recognized by competent judges, as conformable to the object in view. According to this arrangement, as for instance on the last, therefore readily found page, under the heading Hectic fever, we find, in spread italics, *A r s. C a l c. K a l. L y c. &c.*; these hold the highest degree, being remedies most frequently useful and employed. Next in order the common set italics *Bry. Chin. Iod. Ipec. &c.* In still lower degree the spread roman, as B a r. C u p r. D r o s. F e r r. &c., and in the lowest degree the common set roman type, as Bell. Carb. veg. Con. Dig. &c. Those in brackets, which but seldom appear, require confirmation.

The author trusts that the friendly reader will at least recognize the labor and care, which has been bestowed on the preparation of this small, yet comprehensive work. He also hopes that even the experienced homœopath, may find many useful things therein, which in other books would be sought for in vain; as much of a not unimportant character has been taken from the records in the case books, "Kranken Journal" kept during a not insignificant practice of thirty-five years.

Whether the author will be spared to prepare a second volume, treating of the Apyrexia exclusively, remains in the hands of Him who rules over both health and life. In the mean time the want can, though with less convenience, be supplied by any good Homœopathic Therapeia, so that the necessity may be looked upon as of less imperative nature. Nevertheless it would without doubt, be a useful, and for many a welcome work, if some colleague, having the necessary experience with the peculiar conditions, which frequently manifest themselves both before and after fevers, would prepare and publish such a treatise. The author expresses this wish, which is also his own, unreservedly, and with the guarantee that it would in no case occur to his mind to prepare a work to compete therewith.

C. v. BÖNNINGHAUSEN.

Münster, Jan. 1, 1863.

PART I.

GENERAL FEVER SYMPTOMS.

ACONITUM NAPELLUS. (Acon.)

1. Pulse generally very full, hard and accelerated, sometimes intermittent; seldom small and thread-like, or imperceptible. Sensation of coldness in the blood-vessels.

2. Chill at the beginning of the attack, most severe in the evening after lying down, often with one hot cheek and contracted pupils. Chill from uncovering and from being touched. With the chill, frequently, internal heat with anxiety and redness of the cheeks. Shivering ascending from the feet to the chest.

3. Dry burning heat, generally extending from the head and face, with much thirst for cold drink. With the heat, great excitability, restlessness, and agonized tossing about. Continued external heat with inclination to uncover. Burning heat with chilly shiverings at the same time.

4. Long continued sweat over the whole body, of somewhat sour odor. The covered parts sweat the most.

ACTÆA RACEMOSA. (Act. rac.)

1. Pulse weak and irregular; or, quick and weak. Pulse feeble in the morning, with weakness and trembling. Pulse slow, intermitting.

2. Creeping chills upon the back, during the evening, followed by frequent waking during the night, and desire to throw off the bed clothes, although the room was very cold.

3. Heat, especially of the face.

4. Disposition to sweat at night (3 A. M.), commencing while asleep, disappearing after awaking. Sweat inclined to be cold.

ÆSCULUS HIPPOCASTANUM. (Æsc. hip.)

1. Pulse (66) soft and weak. Pulse accelerated (130).
2. Severe chilliness in the afternoon. Chilliness and goose-flesh.
3. Heat in the whole body. Hands hot and dry. Disposition to stretch and yawn all the time. Head aches as if it would burst.
4. Profuse hot sweat with the fever.

AGARICUS MUSCARIUS. (Agar.)

1. Pulse somewhat accelerated, in the morning; later in the day always slower; very unequal and at times intermittent.
2. Chill and chilliness predominating particularly in the cold open air, and from raising the bed clothes. Shiverings over the body, running from above downwards.
3. Heat slight, and principally on the upper part of the body.
4. Greasy, but not offensive smelling sweat, the whole night, during sleep. Sweat from slight exercise.

AGNUS CASTUS. (Agn. cast.)

1. Pulse weak and slow, often imperceptible.
2. Internal chill with trembling, with external warmth of the skin. Chill and heat alternating. Much chilliness with cold hands. Chill predominating.
3. Flushes of burning heat, mostly in the face, with coldness of the knees in the evening in bed.
4. Sweat, almost exclusively on the hands, when walking in the open air.

ALUMINA. (Alum.)

1. Pulse full and somewhat accelerated.
2. Chill predominating, and principally toward evening, even in bed, and by the warm stove; also after eating a warm soup; frequently with heat of the face. Chill during the day, heat at night.

3. In the evening, following the chill, heat commencing in and spreading from, the face, at times however taking in only the the right side of the body.

4. Sweat at night, especially toward morning in bed, with anxiety; most profuse in the face, and frequently only on the right side of the face. Entire inability to sweat.

AMBRA GRISEA. (Ambra.)

1. Pulse accelerated and circulation excited.

2. Chill in the forenoon, with lassitude and sleepiness, relieved by eating. Chill at night, preventing sleep. Chill of single parts of the body, with heat of the face.

3. Anxious flushes of heat, returning every quarter hour, most violent toward evening.

4. Profuse sweat at night, worse after midnight and most on the affected side. Profuse sweat, particularly on the abdomen and thighs, during exercise.

AMMONIUM CARBONICUM. (Amm. carb.)

1. Pulse hard, tense and quick.

2. Chill in the evening, frequently alternating with heat, till toward midnight. Chill in the open air.

3. Heat principally in the evening, particularly in the face, with cold feet.

4. Sweat in the morning, mostly at the joints. Continuous day or night sweat.

AMMONIUM MURIATICUM. (Amm. mur.)

1. Pulse accelerated, day and night continuously.

2. Chill with external coldness in the evening, and from uncovering at night. Chill alternating every half hour with heat. Chill running up the back.

3. Heat with red, puffed up face, particularly in the warm room and after bodily exertion. Flushes of heat, in frequent attacks, ending each time with sweat, which is most profuse in the face, palms of the hands and on the soles of the feet.

4. Sweat day and night, following heat. Profuse night-sweat over the whole body, most copious after midnight and early in the morning, in bed.

ANACARDIUM ORIENTALE. (Anac,)

1. Pulse accelerated, with beating in the blood-vessels.

2. Chill and chilliness with trembling, particularly in the open air, passing off in the sun. Shivering over the back, as if cold water was poured over it, with heat of the face. Internal chill even in the warm room.

3. External heat with internal chill. Heat of the upper body, with cold feet, internal shiverings and hot breath. Heat, from 4 P. M. till evening, daily, passing off after supper.

4. Evening sweat on the head, abdomen and back, even when sitting quiet. Night sweat on the abdomen and back. Clammy sweat in the palms, particularly the left. Cool sweat with internal heat.

ANGUSTURA. (Angust.)

1. Pulse accelerated, spasmodic, irregular and at times intermitting.

2. Chill, in the morning in bed, and in the forenoon, preceeded by thirst. Severe internal chill every afternoon (3 P. M.). Repeated shiverings over the affected part. Shivering in the back 9 A. M.

3. Heat in the evening, most in the face, after coming into the room and after supper. Heat after midnight (3 A. M.) which disturbs sleep, soon followed by shivering.

4. Sweat only in the morning, and only on the forehead.

ANTIMONIUM CRUDUM. (Ant. crud.)

1. Pulse extremely irregular, now accelerated and again slow, changing every few beats.

2. Chill predominating during the day, even in the warm room Violent shaking chill toward noon, with thirst (for beer). Sensitive cold feeling in the nose, during inspiration through the same. Shivering over the back; feet cold as ice, with sweat on the rest of the body. C. HG.

3. Heat at night predominant, but until midnight with cold feet. Great heat from the least exercise, particularly in the sun.

4. Sweat in the morning when awaking, which causes a shriveling of the tips of the fingers. Sweat which returns precisely at the same hour, usually every other (third) morning.

ANTIMONIUM TARTARICUM. (Ant. tart.)

1. Pulse full, strong and accelerated, at times trembling. Strong beating in the blood-vessels. As the fever passes off, the pulse frequently grows slow and imperceptible. Pulse uncommonly accelerated from the slightest motion.

2. Chill with external coldness, coming on at all times of the day, with somnolancy; mostly with trembling and shaking; frequently as if cold water was poured over one. Chill and heat alternating during the day.

3. Violent, but not long lasting heat, succeeding a long chill, aggravated by every motion. Long lasting heat after a short chill, with somnolency, and sweat on the forehead.

4. Profuse sweat all over, also at night. Sweat is frequently cold and clammy. The affected parts sweat most profusely.

APIS MELLIFICA. (Apis.)

1. Pulse full and accelerated; less frequently small and thread-like; at times intermittent and imperceptible.

2. Chill most severe toward evening. Shivering in the afternoon (3 to 4 P. M.) aggravated in the warmth. Chilliness from the slightest motion, particularly toward evening, with heat of the face and hands.

3. Dry heat towards evening. The sensation of heat is most severe on the chest and epigastric region.

4. Sweat alternating with dryness of the skin.

ARGENTUM METALLICUM. (Argent.)

1. Pulse accelerated in the evening, after lying down.

2. Chill in the afternoon and evening until going to sleep, also before midnight, every time the bed clothes are raised. Chill spreads from the back.

3. Heat in the forenoon, over the whole body, but less on the head.

4. Sweat only on the abdomen and on the chest.

ARNICA MONTANA. (Arnic.)

1. Pulse very changeable, mostly hard, full and accelerated. Pulse at times very weak and slow. Strong pulsations through the whole body in the evening.

2. Internal chill with external warmth. Chill, as if cold water was poured over him, mostly in the evening, attended with much thirst, which commences before the chill. Chill and coldness of the lower part of the body, with heat of the upper part, particularly of the head. General chill with heat and redness of one cheek. Chill after every sleep. Chill from the slightest lifting of the bed clothes. Chill alternating with heat. Sensation of coldness on the side on which he lies.

3. Dry heat which is either general; or, running only over the face or back. Burning in one spot which was cold to the touch. Heat or coldness now here and again there. Heat in the evening with pain in the limbs.

4. Sweat mostly sour or offensive smelling; at times cold sweat.

ARSENICUM ALBUM. (Arsen.)

1. Pulse weak and small but much accelerated, often imperceptible, or intermitting. Pulse frequent in the morning, slow in the evening. Burning or cold feeling in the blood-vessels.

2. Undefined development of chill (and heat); either simultaneously or in alternation. Chill in the forenoon not relieved by anything. Internal chill with external heat. Chill and shivering after every drink. External coldness with cold, clammy sweat. During the chill (and during the heat), aggravation of symptoms which existed previously, but were of slight importance. Nursing children have no distinct chill; must be covered; very thirsty.

3. Internal burning dry heat. Dry heat, evening and night, with thirst, and frequent drinking of but a small quantity at a time. Heat at night as if hot water was poured over one.

4. Sweat at the end of the fever, with cessation of all the pre-

vious symptoms. Sweat in the first sleep or through the whole night. Cold, clammy, or sour and offensive smelling sweat. During the sweat, unquenchable thirst.

ARUM TRIPHYLLUM. (Arum tr.)

1. Pulse accelerated.
2. Chill?
3. Dry heat of the skin, redness of the tongue with elevated papillæ; soreness of the mouth; cracked corners of the mouth and lips; stoppage of the nose, with or without profuse yellow discharge filling the whole nasal cavity and throat; putrid sore throat; submaxillary glands swollen; urine abundant and pale; itching eruption.
4. Sweat?

ASA FŒTIDA. (Asaf.)

1. Pulse small, but very frequent and unequal.
2. Chill, coldness and dryness of the skin. Shiverings, particularly over the back, in the afternoon.
3. Heat in the face, after dinner, with anxiety and sleepiness, but without thirst.
4. Sweat wanting; only occasionally cold, moist skin.

ASARUM EUROPÆUM. (Asar.)

1. Pulse quick and strong.
2. Chill and cold feeling in the forenoon, after eating or drinking, and in the open air, generally with heat of the head. Much chilliness during the day.
3. Heat, in the evening after lying down, particularly in the face and palms of hands. Alternate flushes of burning heat and coldness.
4. Sweat, increased at night, of a sour smell; most profuse in the axillæ; also when sitting quiet. In general sweats easily, particularly on the upper body.

AURUM FOLIATUM. (Aurum.)

1. Pulse small but accelerated. Orgasm of blood in the whole body, with stronger congestion to the head and chest.

2. Chill predominating. Chill and coldness of the hands and feet, also in bed, frequently lasting the entire night. General shivering in the evening in bed. Coldness of the whole body with nausea.

3. Heat principally in the face, alternating with chill.

4. Sweat in the morning hours, most profuse on and around the genitals.

BAPTISIA TINCTORIA. (Baptis.)

1. Pulse accelerated (190), full and soft; or, slow, round and soft; or, first accelerated, afterwards very slow and faint. The pulsations of the heart seem to fill the chest.

2. Chilliness all day. Chilliness with soreness of the whole body.

3. Heat at night.

4. Fetid sweat.

Accompaniments.—Dull, stupefying headache; confusion of ideas; she cannot go to sleep because she cannot get herself together; delirious stupor; dark red face with a besotted expression; injected eyes; coated tongue, brown and dry, particularly in the centre, or, dry and red; sordes on the teeth; fetid breath; fetid discharges from the bowels; fetid urine; debility and nervous prostration; ulcerations.

BARYTA CARBONICA. (Baryt.)

1. Pulse accelerated but weak; seldom full and hard.

2. Chill and chilliness predominating, often as if cold water was poured over one, relieved by external warmth. Chill alternating with heat, in the evening and at night. Chill extending from the face or from the pit of the stomach (Plexus solaris?), down the body. Chill beginning in the feet.

3. Frequent flushes of heat during the day. Nightly attacks of flushes of heat, with great anxiety and restlessness.

4. Debilitating night-sweat. Sweat of one (mostly left,) side. Sweat returning every other (third) evening.

BELLADONNA. (Bellad.)

1. Pulse generally quick, frequently full, hard and tense, yet

also at times small and soft, seldom slow, and then it is full. Throbbing of the carotids and temporal arteries.

2. Chill in the evening, particularly on the extremites; mostly on the arms, with heat of the head. Internal chill with external burning heat. Chill and heat alternating. Shaking chill in the evening. Coldness of the limbs, with heat of the head. Shiverings running down the back.

3. Continuous dry burning heat, with sweat only on the head. Internal heat with anxiety and restlessness. Heat of the forehead, with cold cheeks. Internal or external heat, or both at the same time. Heat of the head, with redness of the face and delirium. Heat predominating.

4. Sweat exclusively on the covered parts. Sweat with, or immediately after the heat, mostly in the face. Sweat staining the clothing, and of empyreumatic smell. Sweat during sleep, by day as well as by night. Entire want of sweat. Sweat ascending from the feet to the head.

BISMUTHUM. (Bismuth.)

1. Pulse generally contracted, somewhat spasmodic and at times intermittent.

2. Chill with deathly coldness of the whole body.

3. In the morning after arising, flushes of heat over the whole body, especially over the head and chest. External dry, burning heat.

4. Sweat wanting.

BORAX VENETA. (Borax.)

1. Pulse somewhat accelerated.

2. Chill and chilliness mostly during sleep. Chill predominating, especially in the afternoon and evening. Chill and heat alternating. Chill from uncovering.

3. Flushes of heat morning and evening.

4. Sweat during the morning sleep.

BOVISTA. (Bovist)

1. Pulse excited, with orgasm of the blood and palpitation of the heart.

2. Chill predominating, even near a warm stove, morning and evening, and even at night, generally with thirst. Chill with the pains. Shivering in the evening, spreading from the back.

3. Fever in the evening, daily (7 P. M.), preceeded by chill with thirst.

4. Sweat every morning (5 to 6 A. M.) most profuse on the chest.

BROMIUM. (Brom.)

1. Pulse much accelerated.

2. Chill every other (third) day, with shaking, yawning and stretching, and with cold feet.

3. Internal burning heat, like, between the skin and flesh.

4. Sweat from the least exertion or exercise.

BRYONIA ALBA. (Bryon.)

1. Pulse very full, hard, quick and tense; at times also intermittent, with strong orgasm of the blood.

2. Chill and chilliness predominating, frequently with heat of the head, red cheeks and thirst. Chill with external coldness of the body. Chill and coldness mostly in the evening, and frequently only of the right side. Chill worse in the room than in the open air.

3. Dry, burning heat, mostly only internal, and as if the blood in the veins was burning. Great aggravation of sufferings during the heat.

4. Profuse and very easily excited sweat, even from slow walking in the open cold air. Profuse night- and morning-sweat. Sour or oily sweat.

CACTUS GRANDIFLORUS. (Cact. grand.)

1. Pulse quick, tense and hard. Intermitting. Loss of pulse.

2. Chill, regular paroxysm at 11 A. M. and P. M.

3. Heat after the chill, with dyspnœa, headache, thirst, coma, stupefaction, insensibility till midnight, then unquenchable thirst, shortness of breath, inability to remain lying and very profuse sweat.

4. Sweat very profuse.

CALADIUM SEGUINUM. (Calad.)

1. Pulse hard and bounding.

2. Chill in the evening, with coldness, going from the abdomen to the feet and fingers. Chill after midnight.

3. Heat only internal, with throbbing in the body. Heat before midnight, during sleep, passing off quickly on awaking.

4. Sickly sweat, which attracts the flies very much. With the breaking out of the sweat, amelioration of all complaints.

CALCAREA CARBONICA. (Calc. carb.)

1. Pulse full and accelerated, often tremulous. Much beating in the blood vessels, and palpitation of the heart.

2. Chill with shivering, mostly in the evening, yet also in the forenoon. Internal chilliness in the morning, after arising. Chill alternating with heat.

3. Frequent attacks of flushes of heat, with anxious palpitation of the heart. Heat, followed by chill and cold hands. External heat with internal chilliness, in the evening in bed. Heat after eating.

4. Sweat from the slightest exercise, even in the cold open air. Sweat during the first sleep. Morning-sweat. Sweat most profuse on the head and chest. Clammy night-sweat, only on the legs.

CAMPHORA. (Camphor.)

1. Pulse small, weak and slow, often imperceptible. Diminished flow of blood, to those parts remote from the heart.

2. Chill, chilliness and sensitiveness to the cold air. Chill with shivering and shaking. General icy-coldness of the whole body, with deathlike paleness of the face.

3. Heat, with distention of the veins, increased by every motion.

4. Cold sweat, which is often clammy, and always exhausting.

CANNABIS SATIVA. (Cann. sat.)

1. Pulse very weak, slow, and frequently almost imperceptible.

2. Chill predominating, with thirst and shaking. Shivering

over the whole body. External coldness of the whole body, with the exception of the face.

3. Heat only in the face, and but slight. Nightly burning heat.

4. Sweat wanting.

CANTHARIS. (Canthar.)

1. Pulse very variable, mostly hard, full and accelerated, at times also intermitting; less frequently weak, slow and almost imperceptible. Pulsations through the trembling limbs.

2. Chill with general coldness, mostly in evening attacks, not relieved by external warmth. Fever consisting almost exclusively of the chill, succeeded by thirst, without heat. Chill running up the back. (Nursing children. Chill, passing urine very frequently.)

3. Heat during the night, only external, without one's self being able to feel it. Burning heat, with anxiety and thirst.

4. Sweat from every movement. Cold sweat, especially on the hands and feet. Sweat around the genitals. Sweat smells like urine.

CAPSICUM ANNUUM. (Capsic.)

1. Pulse very irregular and often intermitting.

2. Chill predominating and almost always with violent thirst. Chill with shivering, after drinking. Chill in the cold air, particularly in a draught. Evening chill. Diminution of the natural bodily warmth. Sensation, like from cold sweat, on the thighs.

3. Heat with simultaneous sweat and thirst. Internal heat, with cold swèat on the forehead. First heat and sweat, then chill with shivering, and chattering of the teeth.

4. Sweat with the heat. Sweat after the chill, without preceeding heat.

CARBO ANIMALIS. (Carb. an.)

1. Pulse excited and accelerated, with beating in the blood-vessels, mostly toward evening.

2. Chill especially in the afternoon, after eating, and in the evening. In the evening of every third day, shivering, continuing also in bed. Chill in the evening followed by sweat during sleep.

3. Heat always after a chill, mostly at night in bed.

4. Sweat after the heat, generally toward morning. Sweat during the day, from slight exercise, even when eating. Debilitating night sweat, of offensive odor and staining the clothes yellow. Sweat most profuse on the thighs.

CARBO VEGETABILIS. (Carb. veg.)

1. Pulse weak and languid, often imperceptible. Intermitting pulse. Irregular pulse, at one time much accelerated, then again as if quite suppressed. Small pulse with thirst and rapid sinking.

2. Chill and chilliness, mostly in the evening, at times of the left side only, generally with thirst. With the chill unusual lassitude. Chill with icy coldness of the body. Cold breath.

3. Heat after the chill, but also independent of chill; or, at night in bed, with many concomitants. Flushes of burning heat, in evening attacks, generally without thirst.

4. Profuse sweat, mostly of a putrid, or sour odor. Great disposition to sweat, even when eating. Night-sweat. Sour smelling morning-sweat.

CAUSTICUM, (Caustic.)

1. Pulse excited only toward evening, from orgasm of blood.

2. Chill and chilliness predominating, frequently with coldness of the whole left side. Much internal chilliness, immediately followed by sweat, without preceeding heat. Severe internal chill about midnight. Shivering beginning in and spreading from the face.

3. Heat from 6 to 8 P. M. Flushes of heat, followed by chill.

4. Sweat immediately after the chill, without preceeding heat. Profuse sweat when walking in the open air. Sour smelling night-sweat. Morning-sweat toward 4 A. M.

CHAMOMILLA. (Chamom.)

1. Pulse small, but tense and accelerated, frequently very unequal, and then for a time weak.

2. Chill and shivering, generally only of single parts, with heat of others. Shiverings, with internal heat. Chill and coldness of the whole body, with burning hot face and hot breath. Alternation of shivering and coldness of one part with heat of others. Chill of the posterior part, with heat of the anterior of the body, or vice versa. Shivering when uncovering, and from exposure to the cold air.

3. Heat and shivering intermingled, mostly with one red and one pale cheek. Anxious heat with sweat of the face and scalp. Long lasting heat, with violent thirst, and frequent starting in sleep.

4. Sweat during sleep, most profuse on the head, mostly of sour odor, and with smarting sensation in the skin. Revulsion of, and therefrom, entire want of sweat.

CHELIDONIUM MAJUS. (Chelid.)

1. Pulse small and quick. Toward evening pulse more full and hard, and but slightly accelerated.

2. Chill and chilliness, only internal, with severe shaking, in the evening in bed. Internal chill when walking in the open air, passing off in the room. Chill and coldness of the whole body, but worse on the hands and feet, with distention of the veins. Chill of one (right) leg. Shivering without external coldness. Shivering running down the back.

3. Internal heat without thirst, in the evening after lying down.

4. Sweat during sleep, after midnight and toward morning, passing off soon after awaking.

CINCHONA. (Cinchon.)

1. Pulse small, but hard and quick, calmer after eating. Pulse irregular, and at times intermitting. Uncommon distention of the blood-vessels.

2. Chill over the whole body, increased by drinking, thirst before or after, but not during the chill. Internal violent chill,

with ice-cold hands and feet, and congestion of blood to the head. Chill and heat alternating, in the afternoon. In the evening, in bed, he cannot get warm. (Nursing children. Bloated or tympanitic abdomen and hard spleen or liver).

3. Heat over the whole body, with distended veins. During the heat (as during the chill) thirstlessness, or thirst for cold drink only. After the heat, violent thirst. Long lasting heat, which frequently sets in late after the chill. During the heat, desire to uncover.

4. Very profuse and debilitating sweat. Sweats easily during sleep and when moving in the open air. Very debilitating night, or morning-sweat. The sweat is frequently greasy or cold. During the sweat, increased thirst. Revulsion of sweat, and therefrom want of sweat. Sweat on the side on which one lies.

CHININUM SULPHURICUM. (Chin. sulph.)

1. Pulse slow, particularly after eating, or during periodic diseases; full or small, but weak and slow; frequent during the heat.

2. Chill, regular paroxysms at the same hour; during the chill, blue lips and nails, ringing in the ears, pale face. During the paroxysm, pain in dorsal vertebræ on pressure; pain in the region of the liver and spleen, on bending, taking a deep breath, or coughing; urine gives a brick-dust like, or fatty sediment, or contains crystals of urates.

3. Heat, with red face.

4. Sweat, easily excited through the least exertion. Debilitating sweat.

CICUTA VIROSA. (Cicut.)

1. Pulse weak, slow and trembling, at times quite imperceptible.

2. Chill and chilliness, with desire for warmth and the warm stove. The chill starts in the chest and runs down the legs, and in the arms, with staring look.

3. Heat slight and only internal.

4. Sweat at night and in the morning hours, principally on the abdomen.

CIMEX LECTULARIUS. (Cimex.)

1. Pulse feeble, intermitting.

2. Before the chill, thirst and heaviness in the legs. Chill commencing with clenching of the hands and violent raging. Chill attended with pains in all the joints. Sensation as if the tendons were too short; the knee joints are usually contracted so that the legs cannot be stretched; the chest feels oppressed, obliging one to take a long breath frequently; irresistible sleepiness. Chill terminates with a tired feeling in the legs, obliging one to change position constantly; with thirst, drinking however, causes violent headache; continuous dry cough, oppression of breathing, heaviness in the middle of the chest, anxiety. Abstaining from drinking ameliorates all this.

3. Heat with gagging, the œsophagus feels constricted, and the water drank goes down only at intervals; no thirst.

4. Sweat mostly on the head and chest, accompanied by hunger.

CINA. (Cina.)

1. Pulse small, but hard and accelerated.

2. Chill with shivering and shaking, even when near a warm stove; the chill ascends from the upper part of the body to the head. Chill, with coldness of the pale face, and warmth of the hands. Chill not relieved by external warmth, mostly in the evening, and with great paleness of the face. (Nursing children. Chill in the evening and fever all night.)

3. Heat, most severe of the head and face, but with paleness of the face. Nightly heat with thirst.

4. Sweat generally cold, on the forehead, around the nose and on the hands. After the sweat (frequently also before the beginning of the chill), vomiting of food, with canine hunger at the same time.

CISTUS CANADENSIS. (Cist. can.)

1. Pulse?

2. Chilliness. Chill succeeded by heat. Cold feeling in the abdomen and larynx. Cold feet. Violent chill succeeded by

fever heat, with trembling, accompanied by a quick swelling and great redness of the glands below the ear and in the throat.

3. Heat with thirst, causing to drink frequently. Heat in the face.

4. Skin moist in a very warm room, forehead cold and sensation of coolness inside the forehead.

CLEMATIS ERECTA. (Clemat.)

1. Pulse excited, with throbbing through all the blood-vessels.

2. Chill with shivering, followed by sweat without intervening heat. Shivering from every uncovering.

3. Dry heat, with general hot sensation, only at night.

4. Profuse sweat at night, most toward morning, with aversion to uncovering.

COCCULUS. (Coccul.)

1. Pulse small and spasmodic, often imperceptible, seldom hard, and somewhat accelerated.

2. Chills frequently alternating with heat. Internal chill in the afternoon and evening; attended with shivering through the whole body, but more in the back and on the legs; not relieved by external warmth. Continuous chilliness with hot skin.

3. Dry heat the whole night through. Flushes of heat, with burning heat of the cheeks, and cold feet.

4. Sweat of the body from evening till morning, attended with cold sweat of the face. Morning-sweat, principally on the chest. Debilitating sweat over the whole body, from the least exertion. Sweat of the affected parts.

COFFEA CRUDA. (Coffea.)

1. Pulse scarcely changed, very slightly accelerated.

2. Chill increased through every (beginning) motion. Frequently recurring internal shiverings, with external heat of the face or whole body. Chilly feelings with internal and external warmth. Great sensitiveness to external cold. Chills running down the back.

3. External dry heat with shivering in the back, in the even-

ing after lying down. Dry heat at night with delirium. Great heat of the face. Hot breath.

4. Sweat occasionally follows the heat. Slight morning-sweat. Sweat in the face with internal shivering.

COLCHICUM ANTUMNALE. (Colchic.)

1. Pulse accelerated, hard and full.
2. Chill and shivering, running through all the limbs. Frequent chilly shiverings, running down the back.
3. Only external dry heat of the skin. External dry heat the whole night, with violent unquenchable thirst.
4. Sweat entirely suppressed and wanting.

COLOCYNTHIS. (Coloc.)

1. Pulse generally full, hard and accelerated; less frequently small and weak. Strong throbbing in all the blood-vessels.
2. Chill and coldness of the whole body, frequently with heat of the face. Coldness of the hands, or soles of the feet, while the rest of the body is warm. With the pains, chill and shivering.
3. External dry heat. Internal sensation of heat, with attacks of external flushes of heat.
4. Sweat at night, smelling like urine, causing itching of the skin. Sweat principally on the head and extremities.

CONIUM MACULATUM. (Conium.)

1. Pulse extremely irregular, principally slow and large, but with intervening small and quick beats. Sensible beating of the arteries through the whole body. Entirely pulseless.
2. Chill and coldness in the morning and afternoon (from 3 to 5 o'clock). Chill with continuous desire for warmth, particularly that of the sun. In the morning only internal chill; in the afternoon attended with shivering.
3. Great heat, internal as well as external, with great nervousness. Heat with profuse sweat at the same time.
4. Sweat day and night as soon as one sleeps, or even when

closing the eyes. Night and morning-sweat with offensive odor, and smarting in the skin.

CORNUS CIRCINATA. (Corn. cir.)

1. Pulse?

2. Coldness, followed by flushes of heat and perspiration. Chilly sensation, succeeded by transient flushes of heat.

3. Flushes of heat and coldness in alternation. Flushes of heat, followed by easy general perspiration. Transient flushes of heat, pervading the whole body, with shooting pains through the brain. Throbbing pains in the temples and vertex.

4. Copious general clammy sweat, succeeded by general chilliness.

CORNUS FLORIDA. (Corn. flor.)

1. Increased strength and frequency of the pulse, with fever heat. Pulse quick and hard.

2. Chill with cold, clammy skin; nausea, vomiting and violent pains in the bowels. Paroxysm preceeded for days by sleepiness, sluggish flow of ideas, dull headache, nausea, vomiting, loss of appetite and sometimes bilious or watery diarrhœa. Chill, followed by heat with thirst, drinks often, but not much at a time, then sweat; giddy all the time; hungry soon after eating; desire for sour things, later for sweet cakes.

3. Heat with violent headache. Heat with thirst. Hot, but moist skin; stupor.

4. Sweat.

CROCUS SATIVUS. (Crocus.)

1. Pulse feverish, accelerated. Anxious palpitation of the heart.

2. Chill in the afternoon, growing worse toward evening, with shivering, going from the back down the legs, attended with trembling. Thirst with the chill, as well as with the heat. Shivering only on the back of the body.

3. Flushes of internal heat, with prickling and crawling in the skin. Heat principally of the head and face, with paleness of

the cheeks, and thirst. Heat with intense redness of the face, and distention of the blood-vessels.

4. Sweat scant, only at night, and then cold and debilitating. Sweat only on the lower half of the body.

CUPRUM. (Cuprum.)

1. Pulse generally small, almost imperceptible, weak and very slow; less frequently full, hard and accelerated.

2. Chill over the whole body, most severe on the extremities. Chill after every attack of indisposition (also after an epileptic attack). Icy coldness of the whole body.

3. Flushes of heat. Debilitating, exhausting, internal heat.

4. Cold sweat at night. Many attacks (of epilepsy and mania) end with (cold) sweat.

CYCLAMEN EUROPÆUM. (Cyclam.)

1. Pulse not perceptibly changed.

2. Chill in the forenoon or evening. Morning or evening attacks of chilliness, over the whole body. With the evening chill, great sensitiveness to cold air and uncovering.

3. Heat, principally of the face, but without thirst, succeeds the chill, the hands continuing cold for a long time. Sensation of heat through the whole body, particularly in the face and on the hands. Heat of various parts, but not of the face. General heat after eating.

4. Sweat at night during sleep, moderate, but of offensive odor.

DIADEMA ARANEA. (Diadem.)

1. Pulse accelerated.

2. Chill every day or every other day, at precisely the same hour. Chill predominating. Constant chilly feeling; always worse on rainy cold days. Menses too early and too profuse. Enlargement of the spleen. Much exhaustion. Long lasting chill (24 hours.)

3. Slight heat preceeded by chill, no sweat; or, chill, *without* heat, sweat with thirst. Heat in the evening with heaviness in

the hypogastrium, qualmishness in the pit of the stomach and heaviness of the limbs.

4. Sweat with thirst.

DIGITALIS PURPUREA. (Digit.)

1. Pulse extremely slow, particularly when at rest. Pulse irregular and at times intermitting. The pulse becomes much accelerated, full and hard, from every motion, but soon returns to its former slowness when at rest.

2. Chill more internal, with warmth of the face, but beginning with coldness of the extremities, from thence spreading over the whole body. Chilliness and shivering over the whole back. Internal chill with external warmth. General chill, with heat and redness of the face. Chill and heat in alternation. Excessive coldness of the hands and feet, with cold sweat. Great sensitiveness to cold.

3. Heat, generally setting in late, after the chill. Sudden flushes of heat with subsequent weakness. Increased warmth over the body, with cold sweat of the face. Heat of one hand, with coldness of the other.

4. Sweat during the night, generally cold and somewhat clammy. Sweat immediately after the chill, without preceeding heat.

DROSERA ROTUNDIFOLIA. (Droser.)

1. Pulse unaltered.

2. Chill with coldness and paleness of the face, and cold extremities. Chill in the forenoon. Internal chill, at night in bed and during rest. During the morning hours, one (left) side of the face cold, the other (right) hot. Chill and shivering when at rest, it seems to him to be too cold everywhere, even in bed. Chill during the day, heat at night.

3. Heat almost exclusively in the face and on the head. Increased warmth of the upper body, in the evening.

4. Warm sweat at night, particularly after midnight, and in the morning hours, most profuse in the face.

DULCAMARA SOLANUM. (Dulcam.)

1. Pulse small, hard and tense, particularly at night.

2. Chill commencing in and spreading from the back, not relieved by external warmth; mostly toward evening. Chill with the pains. Chill with violent thirst.

3. General dry burning heat over the whole body. Heat and burning in the back. Heat with delirium, without thirst.

4. Offensive smelling sweat, at night and in the morning over the whole body; during the day more on the back, in the axillæ and in the palms of the hands. Sweat suppressed and entirely wanting.

EUPATORIUM PERFOLIATUM. (Eup. perf.)

1. Pulse?

2. Chill usually in the morning (7 to 9 A. M.), thirst long before the chill, continuing through the chill and heat. Chill after drinking water. Vomiting after drinking. During the chill intense aching in the bones, also a number of gastric or so-called bilious symptoms. A greater amount of shivering during the chill than is warranted by the coldness. Alternate chilliness and flushes of heat. Throbbing headache during the chill and heat. Vomiting at the conclusion of the chill. Very thirsty during the chill and heat; took only a little sip of water at a time.

3. Heat during the day. Headache increased but thirst diminished, during the heat. Great weakness and prostration during the fever with faintness from motion.

4. Sweat slight. Pungent heat attending the sweat at night. The intermission after the sweat is sometimes marked by a loose cough.

EUPATORIUM PURPUREUM. (Eup. purp.)

1. Pulse accelerated and full.

2. Chill commences at the small of the back and then spreads over the body. Lips and nails blue. Violent shaking with comparatively little coldness. The paroxysm comes on at different

times of the day; every other day. Violent bone pains during the chill and heat.

3. Heat after the chill, with thirst and pains in the bones.

4. Sweat after the heat may be profuse, or only a slight moisture.

EUPHORBIUM OFFICINARUM. (Euphorb.)

1. Pulse?

2. Chill and chilliness predominating. Chill when beginning to eat, and when walking in the open, not cold, air. Chill with sweat at the same time. Shivering chill over the whole upper part of the body, with heat of the cheeks. Want of natural external warmth of the body, with internal burning heat.

3. Heat with intolerance of clothing, they seem too heavy. Heat only on the head.

4. Sweat in the morning in bed. Cold sweat on the legs. Sweat only on the thighs.

EUPHRASIA OFFICINALIS. (Euphras.)

1. Pulse unaltered.

2. Chill and internal chilliness in the forenoon, which becomes an external chill and coldness, particularly on the arms, in the afternoon. Chill predominating.

3. Attacks of heat during the day, with redness of the face and cold hands.

4. Sweat during sleep at night, of very strong offensive odor, most profuse on the chest.

FERRUM METALLICUM, (Ferr.)

1. Pulse full and hard. Severe orgasm of the blood.

2. Frequent short attacks of chilly shivering. Chill with hot and red face, attended with thirst. General coldness in the evening in bed, frequently lasting the whole night. Chilliness with want of natural animal heat.

3. Dry heat over the whole body, especially toward evening, with great redness of the face and inclination to uncover.

4. Profuse and long lasting sweat, as well by day with every motion, as at night and in the morning in bed. Clammy and

generally very debilitating sweat. Every other (third) day, sweat from morning till noon. Strong smelling night-sweat. At times anxious cold sweat (with cramp of different parts).

FLUORICUM ACIDUM. (Fluor. ac.)

1. Pulse somewhat accelerated, only during exercise.
2. Chill entirely wanting.
3. General heat, with nausea from the slightest motion, with inclination to uncover, but mostly to wash with cold water.
4. Clammy, sour and unpleasant smelling sweat, mostly on the upper body, particularly during exercise in the afternoon and evening. The sweat promotes, to a great degree, excoriation of the skin and decubitus.

GELSEMIUM SEMPERVIRENS. (Gelsem.)

1. Pulse slow, accelerated by motion.
2. Chill commencing in the hands. Chilliness in the upper part of the body, back. Chilliness every day at the same hour. Chill mostly during the morning. Coldness of the feet, as if they were in cold water, with heat of the head and face, and headache.
3. Heat after the chill, principally of the head and face. Heat with nervous restlessness.
4. Sweat after the heat. Profuse sweat, relieving the pains. Sweats freely from slight exertion.

GRAPHITES. (Graphit.)

1. Pulse full and hard, but not perceptibly accelerated.
2. Chill and chilliness mostly in the evening. Chilliness day and night, particularly in the evening after 4 P. M.
3. General dry heat, in the evening and through the night, after the chill. Heat when riding in a carriage.
4. Sweat from the slightest motion. Profuse night-sweat. The sweat stains yellow, is sour and offensive smelling and frequently also cold. Entire inability to sweat.

GUAIACUM OFFICINALE. (Guaiac.)

1. Pulse small, weak and soft, but accelerated.
2. Internal chill through the whole body, even when near a warm stove, mostly in the afternoon and evening.
3. Evening heat, particularly in the face.
4. Sweat mostly on the head and forehead, also when walking in the open air. Night-sweat of very offensive odor.

HELLEBORUS NIGER. (Helleb.)

1. Pulse generally small, slow and almost imperceptible.
2. Chill predominating during the day, as long as he is out of bed, with heat of the face. Chill in alternation with pain in the joints. Shaking chill, with goose-flesh and pains in the joints. The shivering begins in, and spreads from the arms.
3. Heat in the evening and through the day, as soon as he lies down, generally with sweat at the same time. Burning heat over the whole body, with internal shivering and aversion to drinking, in the evening in bed. Repeated attacks of, first heat, then chill with pains in the abdomen.
4. Sweat with the heat, in bed, increased toward morning. Cold, at times clammy sweat.

HEPAR SULPHURIS CALCAREUM. (Hepar.)

1. Pulse hard, full and accelerated; at times intermitting, with excited circulation and beating in the blood-vessels.
2. Chill regularly every evening about 6, 7 o'clock. Chill, during the day, in alternation with heat and photophobia. Nightly chill in bed, with aggravation of all complaints. Great chilliness in the open air.
3. Dry burning heat with redness of the face and violent thirst, the whole night. Flushes of heat with sweat.
4. Continuous profuse sweat, day and night. Sweats very easily, during the day, particularly with every exertion of the mind. Night- and morning-sweat, with thirst. Cold, clammy, frequently sour or offensive smelling sweat.

HYDRASTIS CANADENSIS. (Hydrast.)

1. Pulse slow during the chill.
2. Chill either morning or evening; chilliness especially in the back and thighs.
3. Flushes of heat. Great heat of the whole body. Constant dull, burning pains all the evening.
4. Sweat?

HYDROCYANICUM ACIDUM. (Hydr. ac.)

1. Pulse rapid and feeble, (in scarlatina).
2. Coldness internal and external. Marble coldness of the whole body.
3. Heat in the head with coldness of the extremities. Heat and sweat, over the whole body.
4. Sweat over the whole body, with heat.

HYOSCYAMUS NIGER. (Hyosc.)

1. Pulse accelerated, full, hard and strong; less frequently weak, slow and intermitting. Great distention of the blood-vessels.
2. Chill ascending from the feet, with shivering over the whole body, attended with heat of the face. Nightly coldness ascending the back, from the small of the back. He cannot get warm in bed, during the night. General coldness of the body, with burning redness of the face. Chill alternating with heat.
3. Burning heat over the whole body, every evening. During the heat, unusual congestion to the head and putrid taste in the mouth.
4. Continuous debilitating sweat during sleep. Very profuse sweat. Cold, at times also, sour smelling sweat. He sweats most on the legs.

IGNATIA AMARÂ. (Ignat.)

1. Pulse generally hard, full and frequent, with throbbing in the blood-vessels; less frequently small or slow; on the whole very variable.

2. Chill and chilliness with increased pain. Chill always accompanied by thirst, and relieved through external warmth. Chill, frequently, of only the posterior half of the body. External coldness with internal heat. Internal chill with external heat.

3. External heat only, without thirst, with intolerance of external warmth. External heat with redness, attended with internal shivering. Flushes of external heat. Continuous quick alternations from heat to cold. One-sided burning heat of the face.

4. Slight sweat, often, only in the face. Sensation as if sweat would break out, which however does not follow. Sweat when eating. Sweat, at times cold, but generally warm and somewhat sour smelling.

IODIUM. (Iod.)

1. Pulse large, hard and accelerated, with orgasm of the blood and beating in the blood-vessels. Pulse rapid, but weak and thread-like. With every exertion the pulse becomes more rapid.

2. Chill, frequently alternating with heat. Cold feet the whole night. Chill with shaking, also in the warm room.

3. General flushes of heat, over the whole body. Internal dry heat with external coldness of the skin.

4. Very profuse sweat in the night. Very debilitating sweat, in the morning hours, of sour odor and with much thirst.

IPECACUANHA. (Ipecac.)

1. Pulse much accelerated, but frequently imperceptible.

2. Chill generally of short duration, soon passing over into heat. Internal chill as if under the skin, aggravated in the warmth. Chill with thirst. Moist coldness of the hands and feet. Chill mostly with thirst.

3. Continuous general heat, with dry, parchment-like skin, after a short chill. Anxious dry heat in the evening. Sudden attacks of general heat; with cold hands and feet. Heat, generally without thirst.

4. Very profuse sweat, mostly during the night. Pungent, mostly sour smelling sweat; frequently cold. Frequent attacks of hot sweat, in the room.

KALI BICHROMICUM. (Kali bichr.)

1. Pulse accelerated; irregular, small, contracted.

2. Chilliness in the back, with sleepiness; seeks a warm place. Great inclination to yawn and stretch. Chilliness alternating with flushes of heat. Chilliness with giddiness and nausea, followed by heat, with sensation of coldness and trembling, and periodical pains in the temples; without thirst. Attacks of chilliness extending from the feet upwards, and sensation as if the skull on the vertex became contracted, in frequently returning paroxysms. Chill followed in an hour by heat, with dryness of the mouth and lips, which have to be moistened all the time; followed in the morning by great thirst, but no sweat. Chilliness, especially on the extremities, and flushes of heat alternating with general sweat.

3. Flushes of heat. Heat of the hands and feet; nausea; pain in the upper part of the abdomen; dryness of the mouth; sleeplessness; followed by sweat of the hands, feet and thighs. Burning heat of the upper part of the body and face, with internal chilliness and violent thirst.

4. Sweat of the hands feet and thighs after the heat. Flushes of heat alternating with general sweat. Sweat on the back, during effort to stool.

KALI CARBONICUM. (Kali carb.)

1. Pulse very variable; often weak and slow frequently however, considerably accelerated and hard. At times the pulse is more rapid in the morning, and slower in the evening; seldom the opposite. Strong throbbing in the blood-vessels.

2. Chill mostly in the evening. Shivering at times during the day. Evening chilliness, soon relieved by the warmth of the stove, or after lying down. Chill frequently succeeds the pains.

3. Heat during the morning hours, already in bed. Internal heat with external shiverings.

4. Sweat every night. Morning sweat. Sweat easily excited during the day by motion and from exertion of the mind. Sweat especially on the upper body, also increased by warm drinks. Offensive or sour smelling sweat. Entire want of perspiration and inability to sweat.

KALI HYDRIODICUM. (Kali hydr.)

1. Pulse accelerated.
2. Chill in the afternoon; or lasting till morning; or from 4 to 7 P. M. (with thirst; chill not relieved by the stove, but is ameliorated when in bed.) Chill beginning in the back and from thence spreading over the whole body, (with sleepiness.) Chilliness in the evening, with thirst.
3. Flushes of heat, with dulness of the head and general discomfort of the body. Heat and then sweat, in the afternoon.
4. Sweat in the afternoon. Skin at times dry, and at other times profuse sweat.

KREOSOTUM. (Kreos.)

1. Pulse small and weak, with orgasm of the blood. Pulsations in all the blood-vessels when at rest.
2. Chill predominating, principally when at rest. Shaking chill, with severe flushes of heat, in the face, red cheeks and ice cold feet. Chill with great bodily restlessness. Chill alternating with heat.
3. Heat mostly in the face. Flushes of heat with circumscribed redness of the cheeks.
4. Sweat scant and only during the morning, with heat and redness of the cheeks.

LACHESIS. (Laches.)

1. Pulse small and weak, but accelerated, frequently alternating with full and strong beats; in general very unequal and intermitting.
2. General chill, with chattering of the teeth and desire for external warmth. Numbing coldness. Shivering chill, ascending the back, frequently every other (third) day. Chill and heat

alternating, and changing from place to place. Chill every other (third) day. After ice cold calves, shaking chill, with warm sweat; then a strumming through all the limbs, intermingled with flushes of heat. (Nursing children: Spasms during every paroxysm.)

3. Heat particularly of the hands and feet, in the evening. Burning in the palms of hands and soles of the feet, during the evening and night. Heat at night, like from orgasm of the blood, with great sensitiveness of the throat. Internal sensation of heat with cold feet.

4. Profuse sweat attends most complaints. Great inclination to sweat. Sweat cold, staining yellow, or bloody and staining red.

LACHNANTHES TINCTORIA. (Lachnanth.)

1. Pulse during the coldness 74, some beats fast, some beats slow. Pulse ranges from 58 to 68. Pulse 110 only in pneumonia.

2. Continuous chilliness. Sensation as if a piece of ice was lying on the back, between the shoulders, then a shock, followed by coldness over the whole body with gooseflesh; these attacks recur on moving and pass off after going to bed. Icy coldness of the body. External heat applied by heated flat-irons, ameliorates the coldness.

3. Flushes of heat alternating with chilliness. Evening fever, worse from 6 P. M. to midnight with redness of the face, more of the upper part. Feverish with somnolency. Dry heat with burning feet, rumbling in the bowels and tossing about. Burning heat with red face (right side) followed by circumscribed redness. Fever with delirium, circumscribed redness of the cheeks and brilliant eyes (in pneumonia.)

4. Slight perspiration all over. Sweat after restless sleep; much sweat after midnight. Morning sweat. Sweat with dizziness of the head, and boiling and bubbling, in the chest and region of the heart. Skin is cold, damp and clammy.

LAUROCERASUS. (Lauroc.)

1. Pulse extremely irregular; at times small and slow, often imperceptible; at others somewhat accelerated; seldom full and hard.

2. Chill, coldness, and shivering, in the afternoon and evening, not relieved by external warmth. Chill alternating with heat. Want of natural animal heat.

3. Heat after the chill, from evening till midnight. Heat descending the back.

4. Sweat generally during the heat, and after the same, till toward morning. Sweat after eating.

LEDUM PALUSTRE. (Ledum.)

1. Pulse full and quick; frequently the pulse can be felt on one arm, but is imperceptible on the other.

2. Long lasting chill, with shivering and thirst, with the sensation as if cold water was poured over single parts. Coldness and want of animal heat. Chill with thirst, predominates in the morning and forenoon. General coldness, with heat and redness of the face.

3. Heat without thirst, predominates toward evening. Burning of the hands and feet, in the evening. Heat alternating with sweat.

4. Sweat the whole night through, with inclination to uncover. Night-sweat of sourish, or offensive odor. Sweat from the slightest exercise, mostly on the forehead. Sweat causing itching.

LEPTANDRA VIRGINICA. (Leptand.)

1. Pulse diminished in frequency, but full.

2. Chilly sensation, at the shoulders and down the back. Tendency to shiver. Sore and lame feeling in the small of the back. The feet and legs, from the knees down, feel cold and numb.

3. Skin hot and dry, with frequent pains in the bowels.

4. Sweat?

LOBELIA INFLATA. (Lobel. inf.)

1. Pulse; more frequent and weaker than usual; in the evening slower pulse; almost imperceptible; weak and small but of the usual frequency.

2. Chilly feeling. Shuddering towards the middle of the day. Thirst before the chill. Shaking chill and coldness, increased after drinking. Chills down the back with heat in the stomach.

3. Heat with thirst and sweat. Sensation of heat and shuddering in the day time. Flushes of heat. Heat and inclined to sweat, particularly in the face.

4. Sweat begins with the heat, or after the heat has continued for some time. Sweat after the heat, with sleep. More disposed to sweat. Copious night-sweat. Cold sweats.

LYCOPODIUM CLAVATUM. (Lycop.)

1. Pulse somewhat accelerated, only in the evening, and after eating. Excitement of the circulation, in the evening, with restlessness and trembling. Sensation as if the blood ceased to circulate.

2. Chill in the afternoon and evening (4 to 8 P. M.), with numbness of the hands and feet. Chill in the evening, in bed, preventing sleep. Chill of one, generally the left, side. Chill immediately followed by sweat, without intervening heat. Chill and heat alternating. Want of animal heat.

3. Flushes of heat, over the whole body, mostly toward evening, attended with frequent drinking, of but small quantities at a time, profuse urination, and constipation. Heat of one (left) foot, with coldness of the other (right.)

4. Profuse sweat, during the day, from the slightest exercise; most profuse on the face. Night and morning sweat often with coldness of the face. Clammy night-sweat. Sweat is frequently cold, sour or offensive smelling; or of a bloody, or onion odor.

MAGNESIA CARBONICA. (Magn. carb.)

1. Pulse somewhat accelerated, only at night.

2. Chill and shivering, with external coldness, in the evening and after lying down, passing off slowly. Chill running down the back, seldom ascending from the feet.

3. Heat mostly in the forenoon, frequently with sweat on the head. Heat in the evening, after the chill. Anxious internal heat at night, with restlessness and aversion to uncovering.

4. Sweat the whole night, most profuse toward morning. The sweat is oily, staining yellow, with a sour and offensive odor.

MAGNESIA MURIATICA. (Magn. mur.)

1. Pulse somewhat accelerated, with orgasm of blood while sitting.

2. Chill in the evening, between 4 and 8 o'clock, even when near the warm stove, passing off slowly, after lying down.

3. Heat after the chill, from evening till midnight. Heat in the evening, with sweat only on the head.

4. Sweat, with thirst, lasting from midnight till morning. Morning sweat.

MANGANUM. (Mangan.)

1. Pulse very unequal and irregular, now rapid, and again slow, but always soft and weak.

2. Chill mostly in the evening, with ice-cold hands and feet. Chill with heat of the head, and frontal headache, which continues long after the chill.

3. Sudden flushes of heat, in the face, on the chest, and over the back.

4. Profuse sweat all over, with short anxious breathing. Itching night-sweat, often only on the throat and on the lower legs.

MARUM VERUM. (Mar. ver.)

1. Pulse somewhat accelerated toward evening.

2. Chill, after eating, which spreads as if from the abdomen Chill with trembling, in the evening, particularly when talking about unpleasant things. Want of animal heat.

3. Heat toward evening, with great exaltation and loquacity.

4. Sweat wanting.

MENYANTHES TRIFOLIATA. (Menyanth.)

1. Pulse slow during the chill; during the heat accelerated.

2. Chill predominating. Chill with shivering over the back, icy coldness of the hands and feet, and cold feeling in the abdomen. General chill, which passes off near a warm stove, remaining only in the back. Shuddering without chill, (like from hearing horrible tales), only on the upper body. Chilly sensation, on the fingers and legs.

3. General heat in the evening, most severe on the head,

attended with cold feet. Sensation of heat, particularly in the back, with intermingling of coldness, particularly in the abdomen.

4. Sweat in the evening in bed, immediately after lying down, frequently lasting the whole night.

MERCURIUS CORROSIVUS. (Merc. corr.)

1. Pulse small, weak, and frequently intermitting; at times trembling.

2. Chill from the least motion, and in the open air, almost always with abdominal pains. Chilliness in the evening, particularly on the head. Chill at night, in bed.

3. External heat with yellowness of the skin. Burning and stinging heat in the skin. Heat when stooping and coldness when rising.

4. Night-sweat. The sweat becomes offensive smelling toward morning. Cold sweat, often only on the forehead. General anxious, cold sweat.

MERCURIUS VIVUS. (Merc. viv.)

1. Pulse irregular, generally full and accelerated, with strong beating in the blood vessels; at times weak, slow, and trembling; seldom intermitting. Imperceptible pulse, with warmth of the body. Orgasm of blood with trembling, from slight exertion.

2. Chill in the morning when rising, but more generally in the evening after lying down, like from cold water being poured over one, not relieved by the warmth of the stove. Chill at night with frequent urination. Chill alternating with heat, frequently only on single parts. Internal chill with heat of the face.

3. Heat in bed and chill when out of bed. Heat after midnight, with violent thirst for cold drinks. Anxious heat with pressing together of the chest, alternating with chill.

4. Sweat toward morning with thirst and palpitation of the heart. Much sweat with the least motion even when eating. Sweat in the evening, in bed, before falling asleep. Profuse night-sweat. Very debilitating sweat. Sweat sour or offensive, also cold, oily, or clammy, and causing burning in the skin. Sweat, or at least a moisture of the skin, with all the pains.

MEZEREUM. (Mezer.)

1. Pulse full and hard, accelerated in the evening; at times intermitting.

2. Chill predominating, even in a warm room. Chill with external coldness and thirst for cold water, without desire for warmth. With the chill continuous thirst, with dryness in the back part and increase of saliva in the front of the mouth, but without desire for drink. Chilliness and shivering with almost all complaints. Great sensitiveness to cold air. Chill running from the upper arm, down the back into the feet.

3. Heat, in bed, principally on the head. Internal heat with external coldness.

4. Sweat with sleep, immediately after the chill, without intermediate heat.

MOSCHUS. (Mosch.)

1. Pulse very full and accelerated, with strong orgasm of the blood. Great want of blood, with weak pulse and fainting.

2. Chill with shivering, spreading from the scalp over the body. Sensation, particularly on uncovered parts, as from cold air blowing thereon. External coldness with internal heat. Shivering alternating with heat. One cheek hot without redness, the other red without heat.

3. Burning heat in the evening in bed, frequently only on the right side, attended with restlessness and inclination to uncover. One hand burning hot (and pale), the other cold (and red.)

4. Clammy sweat in the morning, smelling like musk.

MURIATICUM ACIDUM. (Mur. ac.)

1. Pulse weak and slow, frequently every third beat intermits.

2. Chill predominating. Evening chill with cold sensation in the back, but with external warmth and burning in the face. Shivering over the whole body, with hot cheeks and cold hands. Chill and heat, without thirst.

3. Internal heat with inclination to uncover and restlessness in the whole body. Burning heat particularly in the palms of the hands and soles of the feet. Heat at night always with palpitation of the heart.

4. Sweat particularly of the head and back, during the first sleep, lasting till midnight. Night- and morning-sweat. In the evening in bed, the sweat on the feet, is at first cold.

NATRUM CARBONICUM. (Natr. carb.)

1. Pulse excited, mostly at night, with orgasm of the blood.

2. Chill and internal chilliness with shivering the whole day, worse in the forenoon; hands and feet cold, head hot; or, warm hands and cold cheeks. Slight chilliness, in the evening, with dullness of the head, followed by heat with sleep.

3. Heat with lassitude and sleep, (without headache, which with Natr. mur is very violent.) Flushes of heat from the nape down the back, with very irritable mood. Heat with sweat over the whole body at the same time.

4. Profuse anxious sweat with every slight motion. Burning sweat on the forehead, where the hat presses. Profuse night-sweat. Night-sweat alternating with dryness of the skin. Cold anxious sweat with trembling, during the pains.

NATRUM MURIATICUM. (Natr. mur.)

1. Pulse extremely irregular, often intermitting, particularly when lying on the left side; with beating in the blood vessels and puffing up of the same. Pulse at one time quick and weak, then again, full and slow. The beating of the pulse, shakes, visibly, the whole body.

2. Chill predominating; mostly internal as from want of animal heat; with icy coldness of the hands and feet; principally in the evening. Chill of long duration, from morning till noon. (Nursing children: Attack in the morning, ulcers around the mouth and corners of the mouth, the child begins to drink after it shakes.)

3. Flushes of heat with the most violent headache; frequently with shivering over the back, and sweat of the axillæ and soles of the feet. Heat of long duration, in the afternoon, attended with the most violent headache and unconsciousness, which gradually subside during the subsequent sweat. During the heat, generally violent thirst.

4. Profuse sweat, during which are lost, the sufferings attendant on the heat. During the day, much sweat, and great inclination thereto with every motion. Night- and morning-sweat. Debilitating, somewhat sour smelling sweat.

NATRUM SULPHURICUM. (Natr. sulph.)

1. Pulse accelerated.

2. Internal coldness with stretching and yawning. Chills with icy coldness and goose-flesh, 4 to 8 P. M., during catamenia. Chill mostly toward evening, without thirst. Chill in the evening, 7 o'clock, not followed by heat or sweat. Chill in the evening in bed, could not get warm all night. Violent chill, up the back, with chattering of the teeth and shaking, without external coldness. Chilly when in bed and shaking chills when out of it, thirst increased, pulse accelerated.

3. Increased warmth of the whole body, and restlessness. Sudden flushes of heat toward evening. Hot feeling in the top of the head.

4. Sweat without thirst. Sweat at night. After the sweat, very dry in the mouth. Sweat on the face. Sweat on the scrotum.

NITRI ACIDUM. (Nitr. ac.)

1. Pulse uncommonly unequal: frequently after one natural beat, there will follow two small and quick, the fourth intermitting. Alternating hard, quick and small beats.

2. Chill mostly in the afternoon, evening, and after lying down. Chill with internal heat at the same time. Chill in the morning, in bed, subsequent to the heat. Continuous chilliness.

3. Heat, particularly in the face, and of the hands. Flushes of heat, with sweat of the hands. Nightly internal dry heat, with inclination to uncover. After eating, heat with sweat and great lassitude.

4. Sweat every night, or every other night, most profuse on the side on which he lies. Sweat smelling sour, offensive, or like horse urine.

NITRUM. (Nitrum.)

1. Pulse full, hard, and accelerated; Pulse slow in the morning; quick in the afternoon and evening.

2. Chill and coldness in the afternoon and evening; increased from every motion; passing off when lying. Chill with subsequent sweat, without intervening heat. Evening chill with the pains. Coldness with thirst, in the afternoon.

3. Slight heat in the evening. Heat at night without thirst, and without subsequent sweat.

4. Very debilitating sweat from the least exertion. Night-sweat, most profuse on the legs. Morning-sweat, most profuse on the chest.

NUX MOSCHATA. (Nux mosch.)

1. Pulse somewhat accelerated, like from orgasm of the blood.

2. Chill from uncovering, and chilliness in the open, particularly damp cold air, with great paleness of the face, passing off in the warm room. Sensation of coldness in the feet with heat in the hands. Chilliness in the evening, with great sleepiness. Chill and somnolency predominating.

3. Heat in the face and on the hands, in the forenoon, with hypochondriac mood, and dryness of the mouth and throat, without thirst.

4. Slight sweat, which however at times, is red like blood.

NUX VOMICA. (Nux vom.)

1. Pulse full, hard and accelerated, particularly during the heat. Pulse small and quick, the fourth or fifth beat often omits. Pulse imperceptible.

2. Chill and coldness not relieved by external warmth. Chill with shivering during the evening and at night in bed, till morning; aggravated by every motion, and from drinking. Chill with heat of the face, Chill alternating with heat. Chill and shivering during motion in the cold open air. Between the chill and heat, sleep. (Nursing children: chill in morning; children costive.)

3. General internal burning heat. Heat at night without thirst. Heat continues to increase during the least exertion or motion, also in the open air. Heat, with aversion to uncovering, which causes chilliness immediately. Heat with inclination to uncover from which however, symptoms immediately set in.

Heat before the chill. Heat of single parts, with chill and shivering along the blood-vessels. Heat as if streaming from the throat.

4. Sweat after midnight and in the morning. Sour or offensive smelling sweat. Sweat, one-sided; or, only on the upper body. Cold, clammy sweat in the face. Sweat with amelioration, particularly, of the pains in the limbs.

OLEANDER. (Oleand.)

1. Pulse very changeable and irregular. Pulse, full and accelerated in the evening; weak and slow, in the morning.

2. Chill and shivering over the whole body, in attacks; with heat of the face and cold hands. Chilliness and deficient animal heat. External chilly feeling with internal heat at the same time.

3. Flushes of heat, in attacks, excited particularly by mental or bodily exertion.

4. Sweat entirely wanting.

OPIUM. (Opium.)

1. Pulse extremely varied; full and slow with heavy snoring breathing; quick and hard, during the heat, with quick anxious breathing; toward the last, weak and intermitting.

2. Chill and diminished animal heat with stupor; pulse weak, scarcely perceptible. The whole body is stiff and cold. Coldness only on the limbs.

3. Heat with sweat, predominating; spreading from the head, or from the stomach, over the whole body. Burning heat and sweating of the whole body, with great redness of the face, and subsequent snoring sleep. Heat with inclination to uncover. (Nursing children: Hot sweat, during the hot stage; bed and sheet feels hot to the child.)

4. Profuse sweat over the whole body, which is burning hot, with snoring sleep. Profuse hot sweat, in the morning, with inclination to uncover. Sweat of the upper body, with dry heat of the lower part of the body. Cold sweat on the forehead.

OXALICUM ACIDUM. (Oxal. ac.)

1. Pulse omitting a beat now and then, always when thinking about it. Pulse more rapid in the morning. Pulse more fre-

quent and harder than usual. Small contracted pulse. Small, tremulous, intermittent pulse.

2. Creeping of cold, particularly from the lower part of the spine upwards. Sneezing, with chilliness, in the evening. Chill after diarrhœa (afternoon). Shaking chill in the evening, with small contracted pulse, red face, and a feeling of heat without external warmth; hands ice-cold as if dead.

3. Sensation of internal heat, most in the face, during the forenoon. Heat in the face and on the hands. Heat first in the face, afterwards in the left lower leg. Flushes of heat, attended with sweat, in the morning, with pain in the forehead and temples. Typhoid fever, with delirium and involuntary diarrhœa.

4. Clammy sweat; face, hands and feet cold, and covered with a cold sweat; tongue cool. Night-sweat, clammy and cold.

PARIS QUADRIFOLIA. (Paris.)

1. Pulse full, but slow.

2. Chill principally toward evening, with internal trembling. Coldness of one (right) side, with warmth of the other side. During the chill, contractive sensation in the skin, and in all parts of the body. Chilliness with gooseflesh. Cold feet at night, in bed.

3. Heat descending the back, from the neck. Heat with sweat of the upper body.

4. Sweat in the morning when awaking, attended with pungent itching.

PETROLEUM. (Petrol.)

1. Pulse full and accelerated, increased by exercise, but slower again when at rest.

2. Chill mostly toward evening, now early and again later. Slight chilliness through the whole body, with subsequent severe itching. Internal chill with simultaneous heat, in the evening. Chilliness in the open air. Chill with headache, and with marked coldness of the face and hands.

3. Heat in the evening, after the chill, with cold feet. Heat after midnight, and in the morning in bed. Flushes of heat over the whole body, in frequent (6 to 10) attacks, during the day.

Sensation of heat over the whole body, with violent burning in the skin.

4. Profuse sweat every night. Sweats easily, particularly on the forearms and lower leg. Sweat immediately after the chill, without preceeding heat.

PHOSPHORUS. (Phosphor.)

1. Pulse various: generally accelerated, full and hard; at times however, weak and small; rarely slow, or intermittent. Orgasm of blood with beating of the carotids.

2. Chill generally in the evening, without thirst; with aversion to uncovering and great distention of the blood-vessels, of the hands. Internal chill and shivering, not relieved by the warmth of the stove. Chill alternating with heat, at night. Chilliness from evening till midnight, with great lassitude and sleepiness. Nightly chill with diarrhœa. Chill ascending the back.

3. Flushes of heat over the whole body, but first in the hands. General anxious heat with burning in the hands and face, in the afternoon and evening. Nightly heat disturbing sleep, mostly after midnight. Heat ascending the back. Heat with somnolency.

4. Sweat most profuse on the head, hands, and feet, with frequent urination. Sweat only on the forepart of the body. After midnight and in the morning hours profuse sweat, with subsequent great debility. Clammy sweats. The transpiration frequently smells like sulphur.

PHOSPHORI ACIDUM. (Phosph. ac.)

1. Pulse irregular, occasionally one or two beats intermit; mostly small, weak, but accelerated; frequently however full and strong. Violent orgasm of blood, with great restlessness. Distended blood-vessels.

2. Chill, with shivering and shaking, always in the evening. Chill and heat alternating, in frequent attacks. Cold feeling in one side of the face. With the chill, a peculiar sensitive coldness in the finger-tips and in the abdomen.

3. Internal dry heat, without thirst, and without complaint,

at all times of the day. General heat, with unconsciousness and somnolency. Anxious heat in the evening, with violent orgasm of the blood. Heat of the head with cold feet.

4. Sweat principally on the occiput and in the nape, when sleeping during the day. Profuse night and morning-sweat, with anxiety. Great inclination to sweat, day and night. Clammy sweat.

PLATINA. (Platin.)

1. Pulse small and weak, often trembling.

2. Chill in the evening, with trembling, and tremulous feeling through the whole body. Shaking chill when going from the room into the open, even warm, air. Chill and chilliness predominating with irritability, which latter, passes off with the heat. Alternation between chill, and the symptoms of the mind and disposition.

3. Heat, with sensation as of burning redness, in the face, yet the color is but natural. Flushes of heat, intermingled with shiverings. Gradually increasing, and in like manner decreasing, heat.

4. Sweat only during sleep, passing off immediately on awaking.

PLUMBUM. (Plumbum.)

1. Pulse variable and unequal: generally small, contracted and slow; at times hard and slow; at times small and accelerated; seldom full and feverish, or intermitting.

2. Chill predominating, increasing toward evening, with violent thirst and redness of the face. Internal chill with external heat, in the evening. Chilliness in all the limbs. Coldness in the open air and when moving.

3. Heat with thirst, anxiety, redness of the face and sleepiness. Internal heat, evening and at night, with yellowness of the entire buccal cavity.

4. Sweat, anxious, cold, or viscid and clammy.

PODOPHYLLUM PELTATUM. (Podophyl.)

1. Pulse slow; scarcely perceptible; pulselessness and collapse.

2. Chilliness while moving about during the fever, and in the act of lying down, with sweat immediately afterwards. Chill in the morning at 7 o'clock, with pressing pains in both hypochondria, and dull aching pains in the knees and ankles, elbows and wrists; backache before the chill. The shaking and sensation of coldness, continue for some time after the heat commences. Some thirst during the chill. The patient is conscious during the chill, but cannot talk, because he forgets the words he wishes to employ.

3. Heat with violent headache and excessive thirst. Delirium and loquacity, during the hot stage, with forgetfulness afterwards of all that passed. Constipation. Dryness of the skin.

4. Sweat with sleep. Warm sweat on the legs; feet feel cold. Sweat of the head with coldness of the skin.

PSORINUM. (Psorin.)

1. Pulse: weak and irregular; small irritated. The circulation seems arrested, with pressure in the centre of the chest.

2. Chill and trembling with the pain in the chest, then heat lasting two hours. Coldness, shivering and chill. Feels cold, and after that, stitching pain in the right ear. Coldness from morning till evening, with thirst. Very severe coldness every afternoon, with thirst. Internal shivering in the afternoon. Flitting chills. Cold shiver running downwards from head to feet, with anxiety; loins and knees feel drawn together, as if he would sink down. Blue circles under the eyes, with shivering.

3. Heat in the afternoon. Heat in the evening, with delirium and much thirst. Heat and sweat in the evening, when riding in a carriage. Feels feverish with tearing headache. Hands burn, face hot and red, much thirst. Continual heat with sweat in the face, heat increased at night. Quivering heat through the body.

4. Sweat in the palms of the hands; and in the face. Profuse sweat 3 A. M. Night-sweat. Very copious sweat when walking. Profuse stinking sweat at night. Sour smelling viscous sweat. Sweat at night, relieving the headache. After the sweat all the complaints cease. Free sweating; also entire want of perspiration.

PULSATILLA. (Pulsat.)

1. Pulse weak and small, often scarcely perceptible, but accelerated; seldom slow. Beating in the blood-vessels, in the evening. Blood-vessels distended during the heat, in the evening.

2. Chill, coldness, and shivering, predominates. Continuous internal chilliness, even in the warm room. Chill increased toward evening. Chill with the pains. Chilliness with occasional warm feelings. One-sided coldness with sensation of numbness. Cold feeling through the back, in the evening. Constant flitting chilliness, without shaking, in the evening and before midnight. Thirst before the chill, or before the heat, seldom during the same.

3. Heat after the chill, with anxiety and redness of the face. General internal dry heat, in the evening, or at night, without external heat. Heat of the face, or of one hand, with coldness of the other. Heat of the body with coldness of the extremities. Attacks of anxious heat, as if hot water was poured over one.

4. Profuse sweat at night, or in the morning. Sweat during sleep, passing off soon after waking. Sweats easily during the day. One-sided sweat, at times only in the face and on the scalp. Night-sweat with stupid slumber. Sweetish acid odor to the sweat. Sweat smells musty, or like musk, and is at times cold.

RANUNCULUS BULBOSUS. (Ran. bulb.)

1. Pulse hard, full and accelerated, in the evening; slower in the morning.

2. Chill predominating with heat of the face, principally in the afternoon and evening. After eating (dinner), slight chilliness with heat of the face. In the open air he feels cold, principally on the external (clothed) chest. The fever frequently consists of the chill only.

3. Heat in the evening particularly in the face, frequently of only the right side, with cold hands (and feet.) Heat with internal chill at the same time.

4. Sweat slight and only in the morning on awaking.

RANUNCULUS SCELERATUS. (Ran. scel.)

1. Pulse quick, full, but soft, with the heat at night.

2. Chill and slight chilliness during meals.

3. Heat in the evening, in the room, after walking in the open air. Dry heat at night with violent thirst and orgasm of the blood, mostly after midnight. Heat predominates.

4. Sweat after the heat, toward morning, most profuse on the forehead.

RHEUM PALMATUM. (Rheum.)

1. Pulse only slightly accelerated.

2. Chill alternating with heat. One cheek red the other pale. Internal shivering with external warmth.

3. Heat over the whole body, strongest on the hands and feet, with cold face. Heat predominates.

4. Sweat from slight exertion. Cold sweat around the mouth and nose. Sweat on the forehead and scalp. The sweat stains yellow and smells of rhubarb.

RHODODENDRON CHRYSANTHEMUM. (Rhodod.)

1. Pulse weak and slow.

2. Chill over the whole body, in the morning in bed, and during the day, when a cold air blows on one. Chill alternating with heat. Ice-cold feet during the evening, continuing long after lying down in bed.

3. Heat in the evening with cold feet. Sensation of warmth, particularly on the hands, although they are cold to the touch. Feverish heat in the evening, with burning in the face.

4. Very profuse debilitating sweat, particularly when moving about in the open air. Offensive smelling sweat of the axillæ. Aromatic smelling sweat. With the sweat, itching and crawling in the skin, like from ants.

RHUS TOXICODENDRON. (Rhus tox.)

1. Pulse irregular: generally accelerated, but weak, flagging and soft; at times imperceptible and intermittent.

2. Chill most frequently during the evening, often beginning in and spreading from the feet, or from the scapulæ. Chill as if cold water was poured over him; or, as if the blood ran cold through the blood-vessels. Cold feeling with every motion. Chill, with increased pains particularly in the limbs. Chill with heat and redness of the face. Chill and heat in quick alterna-

tion. One-sided chill; chill of the right with heat of the left side. Coldness of the head and back, with heat of the forepart of the body. Coldness with paleness, alternating with heat and redness of the face. Cough with the chill, not with the heat. (Dunham.)

3. Heat after the chill, frequently with sweat at the same time, with cessation of the pain in the limbs and other concomitants. General heat as if hot water was poured over one; or, as if the blood, flowing through the blood-vessels, was hot. Flushes of heat with sweat, spreading from the navel, frequently alternating with chill. Heat with nettle-rash.

4. General sweat, usually beginning during the heat; frequently however excepting the face. Profuse night and morning-sweat. Musty, putrid, or, sour smelling sweat. Sweat, with the pains, when sitting. During the sweat, violent itching of the eruption.

RUTA GRAVEOLENS. (Ruta.)

1. Pulse accelerated only during the heat.

2. Internal chill with shivering and shaking, even when near the warm stove. Coldness running over one side of the head. Chill principally in the back, running both up and down. Chill with heat of the face and violent thirst.

3. Heat over the whole body, mostly in the afternoon, without thirst, but with anxiety, restlessness and dyspnœa. External and internal heat of the face, with redness of the cheeks, and cold hands and feet. Frequent attacks of quick flushes of heat.

4. Cold sweat on the face, in the morning, in bed. General sweat, after walking in the open air.

SABADILLA. (Sabad.)

1. Pulse small but somewhat spasmodic. Orgasm of the blood and beating in the blood-vessels. Sensation of stagnation of the blood.

2. Chill in the afternoon, or evening, returning at the same hour; frequently without subsequent heat. Chill predominates, particularly on the extremities, with heat of the face. The chills always run from below—upward. Chill relieved by the warmth of the stove.

3. Heat mostly of the head and face, often interrupted by

shivering, always returning at the same hour. Thirst only between the chill and heat. Sweat frequently during the heat. Internal heat at night, and in the morning.

4. Sweat in the morning and sleep therewith. Hot sweat in the face, with coldness of the rest of the body.

SABINA. (Sabin.)

1. Pulse unequal; mostly quick, strong, and tense. Strong beating in the blood-vessels, through the whole body.

2. Chill in the evening, with attacks of shivering. Great chilliness during the day. Shivering with obscuration of sight, followed by sleepiness. Cold sensation in the whole (right) leg.

3. Unbearable burning heat in the whole body, with great restlessness. Flushes of heat in the face, with chilliness of the rest of the body, hands and feet cold.

4. Sweat every night.

SAMBUCUS NIGRA. (Sambuc.)

1. Pulse mostly small and very quick; at times intermittent; often full and slow. Orgasm of blood in the body.

2. Chill running over the whole body, with crawling sensation here and there. Shivering, with very cold hands and feet.

3. Dry heat over the whole body as soon as he falls asleep, after lying down; with aversion to uncovering, and without thirst. Burning heat of the face, with ice-cold feet.

4. Unusually profuse sweat, day and night, but only when awake; breaking out in the face first; continuing even during the apyrexia. Extremely debilitating sweat. General night-sweat, with the exception of the head, increased toward morning. Continuous sweat when awake, changing to dry heat when asleep.

SANGUINARIA CANADENSIS. (Sanguin.)

1. Pulse tense and quick; extremely irregular. Increased force and frequency of the pulse (from small doses.) Suppressed pulse with fainting (from very large doses.)

2. Chill and shivering in the back, in the evening in bed. Shaking chill, with pain under the shoulder blade on motion. Chill with headache. Chill and nausea. Slight chill, then violent fever, headache, and delirium.

3. Burning heat, rapidly alternating with chill and shivering. Heat flying from the head to the stomach. Sensation as if hot water was poured from the breast into the abdomen. Febrile excitement in the afternoon, with circumscribed redness of the cheeks. Flushes of heat. Fever and delirium.

4. Copious sweat. Cold sweat.

SARSAPARILLA. (Sarsap.)

1. Pulse somewhat accelerated, with strong orgasm of the blood, especially toward evening.

2. Chill predominating, day and night. Frequent shiverings, running from below upwards, mostly in the forenoon. Coldness of the whole body, especially of the feet, even when near the warm stove, the face and chest however are not cold. During the chill he feels the worst.

3. Heat in the evening, with orgasm of blood and palpitation of the heart. Sensation of warmth in the evening, with a feeling as of increased good health.

4. Sweat only on the forehead, in the evening, during the heat.

SCILLA MARITIMA. (Scilla.)

1. Pulse small and slow, but somewhat hard.

2. Internal chill with external heat, at night. Chilliness toward evening when walking, not when sitting.

3. Predominating dry, burning, internal heat of the whole body, with cold hands and feet, and intolerance to uncovering. Sensation of great heat in the whole body, generally with cold feet, in the afternoon and evening. Uncovering during the heat, causes immediately chill and shivering.

4. Sweat entirely wanting. Want of all transpiration, even with the most severe burning heat.

SECALE CORNUTUM. (Secal.)

1. Pulse often unchanged, even during the most violent attacks. Pulse generally slow and contracted, at times intermittent, or suppressed; somewhat accelerated during the heat.

2. Violent chill of but short duration, followed soon after by internal burning heat, with great thirst. Disagreeable sensation of coldness in the back, in the abdomen, and in the limbs.

3. Severe and long lasting dry heat, with great restlessness and violent thirst.

4. Sweat especially on the upper part of the body. General cold and clammy sweat.

SELENIUM. (Selen.)

1. Pulse but little accelerated, even with strong orgasm of the blood.

2. Constant alternation of chill with heat.

3. Only external heat, like burning in the skin, and only on single parts, (chest, abdomen, loins &c.)

4. Very profuse sweat, particularly on the chest, in the axillæ, and on the genitals. Sweat from the slightest exercise. Sweat during every sleep, night or day. Sweats exceedingly easy. The sweat makes yellow, or white stiff spots, in the linen.

SENEGA. (Seneg.)

1. Pulse, unequal; mostly hard and accelerated, with strong orgasm of blood; seldom soft.

2. Chill and chilliness almost only in the open air, with weakness in the legs and difficult breathing. Shivering over the back, with heat of the face, chest symptoms, and other complaints.

3. Only quick flushes of heat. Burning in the left chest (Raue.)

4. Sweat entirely wanting, appears only in the after effect of the drug.

SEPIA. (Sepia.)

1. Pulse quick, full and often intermitting, during the night; during the day slow. Pulse becomes accelerated, especially from anger or motion. Orgasm of blood and beating in the blood-vessels.

2. Chill frequently setting in after heat. Chilliness, evenings, in the open air and from every motion. Chill and heat alternating. Thirst greater during the chill than during the heat. Shivering with the pains. Want of animal heat.

3. Flushes of heat in attacks, during the day, particularly in the afternoon and evening, while sitting as well as when walking in the open air, with excited mood, and generally, with thirst and redness of the face. Attacks of heat, as if hot water was poured over one.

4. Profuse sweat, more after than during motion. Protracted debilitating sweat. Continuous night and morning-sweats. Sweat only on the upper part of the body. Sweat anxious, stinking, sour, or smelling like elder flowers.

SILICEA. (Silic.)

1. Pulse small, but hard and quick; frequently irregular, and then at times slow. The circulation is excited very easily.

2. Severe chill in the evening, in bed, increased by uncovering. Great chilliness, particularly from every motion. Continuous internal chilliness and want of animal heat.

3. Heat predominating. During the day, frequent short attacks of flushes of heat, worse in the face. General severe heat with violent thirst, in the afternoon, evening, or during the whole night. During the day typically returning heat, without preceeding chill, and with subsequent slight sweat.

4. Debilitating sweat during the night, or only in the morning. Sweat from slight motion, most profuse on the head and in the face. Profuse sweat, only on the head. Night-sweat sour or offensive smelling. Entire want of sweat.

SPIGELIA ANTHELMINTICA. (Spigel.)

1. Pulse irregular, generally strong but slow. Trembling pulse. Pulse more rapid in the evening, slower in the morning.

2. Chill, often returning at the same hour in the morning. Chill alternating with heat, or with sweat. Chill of single parts, with warmth of others. General flitting chills, with simultaneous heat. Slight chilliness from the least motion. The chill, begins in and spreads from the chest.

3. Heat particularly in the back. Nightly flushes of heat, with thirst for beer. Heat in the face and on the hands, with chill in the back.

4. Offensive smelling night-sweat, with heat at the same time. Clammy sweat on the hands. Cold sweat.

SPONGIA. (Spong.)

1. Pulse very quick, full and hard. Strong orgasm of the blood and distention of the blood-vessels.

2. Chill, with shaking, even near the warm stove, mostly over the back.

3. Severe heat soon after the chill, with dry burning skin over the whole body, with the exception of the thighs, which remain cold, numb, and chilly. Flushes of heat, in attacks. Anxious heat, with red face and tearful, inconsolable mood.

4. Cool sweat of the face, in the evening. Morning-sweat over the whole body. Worse with the sweat, better after the sweat.

STANNUM. (Stann.)

1. Pulse small and quick.

2. Evening chill particularly over the back, preceeded by heat with sweat. Shivering chill every forenoon (10 A. M.) Chill only on the head. With a slight shivering chill, great chattering of the teeth as from a convulsion of the masseter muscles. During the forenoon chill, a marked numb sensation in the tips of the fingers.

3. Heat in the afternoon (4 to 5 P. M.) returning daily, with sweat at the same time. Burning heat in the limbs, strongest in the hands, every evening. Anxious heat, as if sweat would break out, in repeated attacks. Anxious sensation of heat with the least motion. Predominating sensation of internal heat.

4. Very debilitating sweat, during the night and in the morning hours, most profuse on the neck. Very debilitating general sweat, from slight motion. Musty, or mouldy smelling sweat.

STAPHISAGRIA. (Staphis.)

1. Pulse much accelerated but small, and frequently trembling.

2. Chill and coldness predominating. In the evening chill and coldness, frequently without subsequent heat. Violent chill in the evening, attended with shivering and shaking, and heat of the face. Shivering chill in the afternoon (3 P. M.) better from motion in the open air. Chill, ascending from the back, over the head, even when near a warm stove. Chill running down the back.

3. External heat with thirst, after midnight, succeeded toward morning by a chill. Burning heat at night, particularly of the hands and feet, with inclination to uncover.

4. Profuse sweat and great tendency thereto. (Inability to induce sweat, during a headache with paleness of the face.) Night-sweat smelling like rotten eggs. Cold sweat on the forehead and on the feet.

STRAMONIUM. (Stramon.)

1. Pulse extremely irregular; generally full hard and accelerated; then again small and quick; at times slow and scarcely perceptible; also intermittent, and trembling.

2. Chill and general coldness, with redness of the face and twitchings, frequently of long duration. General coldness in the afternoon, succeeding heat of the head and face, and followed by general heat. During the chill, extreme sensitiveness toward uncovering. Chill running down the back.

3. Heat of the whole body, with bright redness of the face, generally accompanied with sweat. Hot redness of the face, with cold hands and feet. Anxious heat with vomiting.

4. Profuse sweat over the whole body, already during the heat, with great thirst. Greasy, oily, putrid smelling sweat General cold sweat.

STRONTIA CARBONICA. (Strontia.)

1. Pulse full and hard, with strong beating in the blood-vessels.

2. Chill in the forenoon, running from the small of the back over the posterior part of the thighs. Shivering over the head and shoulder blades.

3. Dry heat at night with thirst. Heat, which seems to stream out of the nose and mouth.

4. Sweat in the morning hours. Night-sweat mostly on the affected parts, with increased pains from uncovering the same.

SULPHUR. (Sulphur.)

1. Pulse full, hard and accelerated, at times intermittent.

2. Chill and chilliness mostly internal and without thirst, generally in the evening, but also at other times of the day. External chill, with simultaneous internal heat and redness of the face. Severe chill at night in bed. In the forenoon chill; in the afternoon heat with cold feet. Chill with thirst, preceeded

by heat. Chill spreading from the toes. Chill running up the back.

3. Heat in the afternoon and evening, with dryness of the skin and much thirst. Frequent attacks of flushes of heat. Strong heat at night without thirst, preceeded by chill with thirst.

4. Sweat at night and in the morning hours. Profuse sour smelling sweat, the whole night. Sweat in the evening, most profuse on the hands. Profuse sweating from slight exercise. Anxious, debilitating, empyreumatic-sourish, less frequent offensive smelling, at times also, cold sweat. Night-sweat only on the nape of neck and occiput.

SULPHURIS ACIDUM. (Sulph. ac.)

1. Pulse small and weak, but accelerated.

2. Chill during the day, mostly in the room, better from motion in the open air. Frequent shiverings running down the body.

3. Evening heat, also after lying down in bed. Frequent flushes of heat in the evening, particularly after exercise. Attacks of flushes of heat, with sweat at the same time (during the climacteric years.)

4. Excessive sweat, most profuse on the upper body. Profuse morning-sweat. Sweat from every motion, and continuing a long time after sitting down. Sour-sweat. Cold sweat, immediately after eating warm food.

TARAXACUM. (Tarax.)

1. Pulse?

2. Chill and chilliness, particularly after eating and drinking. General chill with headache. Shivering chill in the open air.

3. Heat particularly in the face and on the hands, at night when awaking.

4. Very profuse sweat, the whole night, most profuse before midnight, during the first sleep. Very debilitating sweat, causing biting sensation on the skin.

THERIDION CURASSAVICUM. (Therid.)

1. Pulse accelerated in the morning, after the nocturnal paroxysm. Slow pulse, with vertigo.

2. Violent shaking chill, during which foam appears at the mouth. Shaking chill during headache, with vomiting. Pain in all the bones, as if every part would fall asunder; feels as if broken, from head to foot; thereupon violent coldness, so that nothing would warm her; without thirst. Cold hands, with flickering of the eyes and nausea. After breakfast heaviness in every limb; he must lie down; grows sleepy; he is attacked by a severe internal chill so that he trembles. Internal coldness, but not cold to the touch, accompanying a peculiar drawing in the right thigh, which began in the hip and passed downward; with a cold sensation below the knee; external warmth was agreeable.

3. Heat?

4. Light perspiration, after walking out. More perspiration after walking and driving. Icy sweat covers the body, with faintness and vertigo, and vomiting at night.

THUYA OCCIDENTALIS. (Thuya.)

1. Pulse, in the morning, slow and weak; in the evening, accelerated and full. Strong beating in the blood-vessels, in the evening. Great distention of the blood-vessels.

2. Chill in attacks, at various times of the day, but mostly toward evening. Chill on the left side, which also feels cold to the touch. Chill without thirst, after midnight and in the morning. Internal chill, with external heat and great thirst.

3. Heat in the evening, particularly in the face. Burning in the face, without redness. Dry heat of the covered parts.

4. Sweat at the beginning of sleep. Sweat of the uncovered parts of the body, with dryness of those covered; also vice versa. Anxious, at times cold sweat. Sweat after the chill, without intervening heat. Sweat often greasy, at times fetid, or smelling sweetish like honey.

VALERIANA OFFICINALIS. (Valer.)

1. Pulse very unequal and irregular; generally much accelerated and somewhat tense, yet at times small and weak.

2. Chill which lasts but a short time, soon passing into a continuous heat. The shivering chill, usually commences at the nape of the neck, and runs down the back.

3. Predominating long lasting and general heat, frequently with sweat in the face. Flushes of heat in the face. Increased heat in the evening and when eating. Heat with thirst, predominating.

4. Profuse sweat particularly at night and during exercise, with continuous strong heat. Frequent sudden attacks of sweat, especially in the face and on the forehead, which again passes off as suddenly.

VERATRUM ALBUM. (Veratr.)

1. Pulse irregular; most frequently small, thread-like, weak and slow; often entirely imperceptible; seldom hard and quick. The blood runs like cold water through the veins.

2. Chill and coldness, mostly external, with internal heat and cold clammy sweat. Shaking chill with sweat, which soon passes off into a general coldness. Chill and coldness, running downward, predominating. Chill and heat alternating. Chill increased by drinking. Icy coldness of the whole body. (Chill, of nursing children.)

3. Heat, mostly internal, with thirst, but without desire to drink. Heat in the evening, with sweat. Heat suddenly alternating with chill. Chill and heat alternating, now here and again there, on single parts.

4. Profuse sweat in the morning, evening, or all night; also with every stool. Cold, clammy, sour, offensive, or, at times bitter smelling sweat; or staining yellow; always with deathly paleness of the face. Cold sweat over the whole body, most profuse on the forehead. Sweats readily during the day, with every motion.

VERBASCUM THAPSUS. (Verbas.)

1. Pulse?

2. Chill and one-sided shivering, like from cold water pouring over one. Internal and external cold feeling, of the whole body. Chill and coldness predominating.

3. Heat?

4. Sweat?

VIOLA ODORATA. (Viol. od.)

1. Pulse full and strong.

2. Chill during the day, consisting of shivering only.

3. Heat?
4. Sweat during the night.

VIOLA TRICOLOR. (Viol. tr.)

1. Pulse accelerated.
2. Chill and chilliness in the forenoon, and in the open air.
3. Dry anxious heat, at night in bed, with great redness of the face. Immediately after eating, general anxious heat.
4. Night-sweat. Hot sweat after eating.

ZINCUM. (Zinc.)

1. Pulse small and quick, in the evening; in the morning and during the day slower. Pulse at times intermittent. Violent beating in the blood-vessels, during the heat.
2. Chill generally after eating (dinner), lasting till late in the evening, even in bed. Chill in the open air, and from touching a cold object. Frequent alternations of chill and heat during the day. Shivering chills, running down the back. Shivering chills on the approach of stormy weather. Continuous external chilliness, with increased internal warmth.
3. Internal heat, with cold sensation in the abdomen and on the feet. Anxious sensation of heat without external heat, during the entire night. Heat of the face with cool body, in the forenoon. Flushes of heat, with violent trembling and short hot breath.
4. Profuse sweat during the entire night, with inclination to uncover. Sweats very easily during the day, when exercising. Offensive smelling sweat.

PART II.

REPERTORY.

CIRCULATION.

Anæmia: *Acon.*, Alum., *Ant. tart.*, Arnic., ARSEN., Bellad., BRYON., CALC. CARB., Carb. veg., Chamom., Cina, *Cinchon.*, *Coccul.*, Coffea, Coloc., *Conium*, Cuprum, Cyclam., Digit., FERR., Graphit., Helleb., Hepar, Ignat., Iod., Kali carb., Laches., *Lycop.*, Magn. carb., Magn. mur., Merc. viv., Mezer., MOSCH., Natr. carb., Natr. mur., *Nitr. ac.*, Nux mosch., NUX VOM., *Phosphor.*, Phosph. ac., PLATIN., Plumbum, PULSAT., Rhodod., Rhus tox., Ruta, Sabina., SCILLA, SEPIA, Silic., Spigel., Stann., STAPHIS., SULPHUR, Valer., Veratr., Zinc.

Blood vessels; beating in the: ACON., ANAC., ANT. TART., ARNIC., Arsen., Asar., Aurum, BELLAD., Bovist., Bryon., Calad., CALC. CARB., *Canthar.*, Capsic., *Carb. an.*, Carb. veg., Cinchon., *Clemat.*, *Coloc.*, *Conium*, Cuprum, Ferr., Graphit., Helleb., HEPAR, IGNAT., *Iod.*, KALI CARB., KREOS., MERC. VIV., Natr. carb., *Natr. mur.*, Nitrum, Nitr. ac., *Nux vom.*, *Phosphor.*, Phosph. ac. Plumbum, PULSAT., *Rhus tox.*, SABAD., SABIN., Sarsap., *Selen.*, SEPIA, Silic., Staphis., STRONTIA, Sulphur, THUYA, *Zinc.*

— **burning,** in the: ARSEN., *Bryon.*, Calc. carb., Hyosc., Natr. mur., Opium, *Rhus tox.*, Veratr.

— **coldness,** sensation of, in the: ACON., Ant. tart., ARSEN., Lycop., *Rhus tox.*, VERATR.

Blood vessels, distention of the; in general: Acon., Alum., Ambra., *Amm. carb.*, Ant. tart., ARNIC., Arsen., Aurum, Baryt., BELLAD., Bovist., Bryon., Calc. carb., *Carb. veg.*, Camphor., Caustic., Chelid., Cicut., CINCHON., Clemat., Coccul., Coloc., Conium., *Crocus.*, Cyclam., *Ferr.*, Fluor. ac. *Graphit.*, Hepar, HYOSC., Kreos., Laches., Lauroc., Lycop., Magn. carb., Menyanth., Mosch., Natr. carb., Natr. mur., *Nux vom.*, Oleand., Opium, *Phosphor.*, PHOSPH. AC., PULSAT., Rheum, Rhodod., Rhus tox., Ruta., Sarsap., Selen., Sepia, Silic., Spigel., SPONG., *Staphis.*, Strontia., SULPHUR, Sulph. ac., THUYA, Zinc.

— — **head,** of the: Arsen., *Bellad.*, Calc. carb., Cinchon., FERR., *Spigel.*, Silic., Staphis., THUYA.

— — **face,** of the: Acon., Ambra., Arsen., *Baryt.*, *Bellad.*, Bovist., Calc. carb., Caustic.; Cinchon., Clemat., *Ferr.*, Graphit., Natr. carb., Natr. mur., Opium, Phosphor., Phosph. ac., Spigel., *Stramon.*, Sulphur, *Thuya.*

— — **neck,** of the: Arnic., *Arsen.*, *Bellad.*, Calc. carb., Conium, Graphit., Hepar, *Laches.*, Lycop., Oleand., *Opium*, Rhus tox., Spong., *Thuya.*

— — **hands,** of the: Acon., Alum., Amm. carb., *Arnic.*, *Baryt.*, Bellad., Bryon., Calc. carb., Caustic., Chelid., Cicut., *Cinchon.*, Cyclam., Fluor. ac., Lauroc., Lycop., *Menyanth.*, Mosch., *Natr. mur.*, *Nux vom.*, Oleand., Opium, *Phosphor.*, Phosph. ac., PULSAT., Rheum, Rhodod., *Rhus tox.*, Ruta, Sarsap., Selen., Sepia., Silic., Staphis., Strontia, *Sulphur*, THUYA.

— — **feet,** of the: Ambra., Ant. tart., ARNIC., *Arsen.*, *Aurum*, Baryt., Bellad., Calc. carb., *Carb. veg.*, Caustic., Coloc., *Cyclam.*, *Ferr.*, Graphit., Kreos., Laches., LYCOP., Magn. carb., NATR. MUR., Nux vom., Phosphor., PULSAT., Rhodod., Rhus tox., Sepia, Silic., Spigel., Spong., Strontia, *Sulphur*, Sulph. ac., THUYA, ZINC.

— **inflammation,** of the: ACON., *Ant. tart.*, Arnic., Arsen., Bellad., Carb. veg., *Chamom.*, Kreos., Laches., Lycop., Nux vom., PULSAT., Rhus tox., Sepia., Silic., Spigel., *Sulphur*, Thuya, Zinc.

Blood vessels; netted, (like marbled skin): Ant. tart., *Arsen.*, Bellad., Calc. carb., Carb. an., *Carb. veg.*, CAUSTIC., Clemat., Graphit., Kreos., Laches., LYCOP., Merc. viv., Natr. mur., Nitr. ac., Nux vom., Petrol., Phosphor., PLATIN., Pulsat., Rhus tox., *Sepia*, Silic., Staphis., Sulphur, Sulph. ac., THUYA.

— **varicose:** *Ambra*, Ant. tart., ARNIC., ARSEN., *Calc. carb.*, CARB. VEG., *Caustic.*, Coloc., *Ferr.*, *Graphit.*, Kreos., LACHES., LYCOP., Magn. carb., *Natr. mur.*, Nux vom., PULSAT., Silic., *Spigel.*, *Sulphur*, Sulph. ac., THUYA, ZINC.

Congestion of blood; in general: ACON., Agar., Agn. cast., Alum., Ambra, Amm. carb., Amm. mur., Angust., Ant. crud., Ant. tart., Apis, ARNIC., Arsen., Asaf., AURUM, Baryt., BELLAD., Borax, Bovist., Brom., BRYON., Calad., CALC. CARB., Camphor., Cann. sat., Canthar., *Carb. an.*, CARB. VEG., Caustic., Chamom., Chelid., CINCHON., Clemat., Coccul., Coffea, Coloc., CONIUM, Crocus, Cuprum, Cyclam., Digit., Dulcam., Euphras., FERR., Fluor. ac., GRAPHIT., Guaiac., Helleb., Hepar, HYOSC., Ignat., Iod., Ipecac., Kali carb., LACHES., Lauroc., Ledum, LYCOP., Magn. carb., Magn. mur., Mangan., *Merc. viv.*, Merc. corr., Mezer., Mosch., *Natr. carb.*, NATR. MUR., Nitrum, NITR. AC., *Nux mosch.*, NUX VOM., Opium, Petrol., *Phosphor.*, *Phosph ac.*, Platin., Plumbum, PULSAT., *Ran. bulb.*, Rhodod., RHUS TOX., Sabin., Sambuc., Sarsap., Scilla, Secal., Selen., SENEG., SEPIA, SILIC., Spigel., SPONG., Staphis., STRAMON., SULPHUR, Sulph. ac., Tarax., THUYA, *Valer.*, Veratr., VIOL. OD., Zinc.

— **head,** to the: *Acon.*, Ambra, Amm. mur., Ant. crud., *Apis*, Arnic., Asaf., AURUM, Baryt., BELLAD., Borax, Bovist., Brom., *Bryon.*, *Calc. carb.*, Camphor., *Cann. sat.*, Canthar., Carb. an., *Carb. veg.*, Caustic., Chamom., Chelid., CINCHON., *Coffea*, Coloc., Conium, Digit., Dulcam., FERR., *Graphit.*, Guaiac., Helleb., *Hyosc.*, Ignat., Iod., *Kali carb.*, Laches., Lauroc., *Lycop.*, Magn. carb., Mangan., *Merc. viv.*, Mezer., *Mosch.*, Natr. carb., *Natr. mur.*, Nitrum, *Nitr. ac.*, Nux mosch., NUX VOM., *Opium*, Petrol., PHOSPHOR., *Phosph. ac.*, Plumbum, *Pulsat.*, Ran. bulb., *Rhus tox.*, Sabin., Seneg., *Sepia*, SILIC., *Spong.*, Staphis., *Stramon.*, SULPHUR, Tarax., *Thuya*, Valer., *Veratr.*, *Viol. od.*, Viol. tr., Zinc.

Congestion of blood; eyes, to the: ACON., Alum., Apis, *Arnic.*, Aurum, BELLAD., Brom., Bryon., CALC. CARB., Carb. veg., Chamom., Clemat., Coffea, Conium, Crocus, Euphras., Hepar, Laches., Lauroc., Lycop., Merc. viv., *Nux vom.*, Phosphor., Plumbum, *Pulsat.*, *Rhus tox.*, Ruta, Seneg., *Sepia*, Silic., SPIGEL., Stramon., SULPHUR, Thuya, Veratr.

— **ears,** to the: Acon., Agar., Agn. cast., *Alum.*, Anac., Ant. crud., Arnic., *Aurum*, Bellad., Borax, Bryon., *Calc. carb.*, Camphor., Cann. sat., Canthar., Carb. veg., *Caustic.*, Cinchon., Coccul., Colchic., *Conium*, Droser., Ferr., *Fluor. ac.*, *Graphit.*, Hepar, Ignat., Iod., *Kali carb.*, Kreos., Ledum, *Lycop.*, Magn. carb., Magn. mur., *Merc. viv.*, *Natr. mur.*, Nitrum, *Nitr. ac.*, *Nux vom.*, Opium, Petrol., *Phosphor.*, Platin., PULSAT., Rheum, Rhodod., Rhus tox., Secal., Selen., SEPIA, Silic., SPIGEL., Spong., Staphis., Stramon., *Sulphur*, Sulph. ac., Veratr., Viol. od.

— **nose,** to the: (nose bleed): ACON., Agar., Alum., Ambra, Amm. carb., Anac., Ant. crud., Apis, Argent., *Arnic.*, Arsen., AURUM, Baryt., BELLAD., Borax, BRYON., CALC. CARB., Cann. sat., Canthar., Capsic., Carb. an., Carb. veg., *Caustic.*, Chamom., Cina, *Cinchon.*, Coffea, Colchic., Conium, CROCUS., *Cuprum*, *Droser.*, Dulcam., Euphras., *Ferr.*, *Graphit.*, Hepar, Hyosc., Iod., *Ipecac.*, KALI CARB., Kreos., Laches., *Ledum*, *Lycop.*, Magn. carb., Magn. mur., *Merc. viv.*, MOSCH., *Natr. carb.*, Natr. mur., NITRUM, NITR. AC., *Nux vom.*, Petrol., Phosphor., *Phosph. ac.*, PULSAT., Ran. bulb., RHUS TOX., Ruta, Sabad., Sabin., Sambuc., Sarsap., *Secal.*, Sepia, SILIC., *Spigel*, Spong., Stann., SULPHUR, *Sulph. ac.*, Tarax., *Thuya*, Veratr.

— **face,** to the: ACON., Alum., Angust., *Ant. crud.*, APIS, Argent., *Arnic.*, Arsen., Aurum, Baryt., BELLAD., Bovist., BRYON., Calad., *Calc. carb.*, Camphor., Cann. sat., Canthar., *Capsic.*, Carb. veg., Caustic., CHAMOM., Chelid.,

Cicut., CINCHON., Clemat., *Coccul.*, *Coffea*, Coloc., Conium, Crocus, *Cuprum*, Digit., *Droser.*, Dulcam., Euphras., *Ferr.*, Graphit., *Hepar.*, HYOSC., Ignat., Kali carb., Kreos., *Laches.*, Lauroc., *Lycop.*, Magn. carb., Menyanth., Merc. viv., Merc. corr., Mezer., Mosch., Mur. ac., Natr. carb., Natr. mur., Nitrum, Nux mosch., NUX VOM., OPIUM, *Phosphor.*, *Phosph. ac.*, Platin., *Pulsat.*, Ran. bulb., *Rhus tox.*, Sabad., Sambuc., Scilla, Secal., Sepia, *Silic.*, Spigel., *Spong.*, Stann., STRAMON., Strontia, *Sulphur*, Tarax., Thuya, Valer., Veratr.

Congestion of blood; chest, to the: ACON., Alum., *Amm. carb.*, Amm. mur., Anac., *Apis*, *Arnic.*, Arsen., Asaf., AURUM, Baryt., *Bellad.*, Bovist., Brom., BRYON., Calad., *Calc. carb.*, CAMPHOR., Cann. sat., Canthar., Capsic., *Carb. veg.*, Chamom., *Cinchon.*, *Coccul.*, Coffea, Cuprum, Cyclam., Digit., Dulcam., Ferr., Graphit., Guaiac., *Hyosc.*, Ignat., Iod., Kali carb., Laches., *Lycop.*, Magn. mur., Mangan., Menyanth., Merc. viv., Mur. ac., Natr. carb., Natr. mur., Nitrum, *Nitr. ac.*, *Nux vom.*, Oleand., Paris, PHOSPHOR., Phosph ac., PULSAT., Ran. bulb., *Rhodod.*, Rhus tox., Sabad., *Scilla*, SENEG., *Sepia*, Silic., SPIGEL, *Spong.*, Stramon., SULPHUR, *Thuya*, Veratr., Zinc.

— **abdomen,** to the: *Acon.*, Alum., Amm. carb., Ant. crud., Ant. tart., *Apis*, *Arnic.*, Arsen., Asaf., BELLAD., Brom., BRYON., Calad., *Calc. carb.*, Cann. sat., Canthar., Capsic., Carb. an., Carb. veg., Chamom., Cicut., CINCHON., Coloc., Digit., Dulcam., Euphorb., Ferr., *Fluor. ac.*, Graphit., Hepar, Hyosc., Ignat., Iod., Ipecac., Kali carb., Laches., Lauroc., *Lycop.*, *Merc. viv.*, Merc. corr., Mezer,, Nitrum, NUX VOM., Opium, Petrol., *Phosphor.*, Phosph. ac., Platin., *Plumbum*, PULSAT., RHUS TOX., Sabin., Sarsap., Scilla, Selen., SEPIA, *Silic.*, Spigel., Spong., Stann. Stramon., SULPHUR, Sulph. ac., *Thuya*, Veratr, Zinc.

— **upper limbs,** to the: *Acon.*, Alum., *Amm. carb.*, Amm. mur., *Apis*, ARNIC., Baryt., Bellad., Borax, Bovist., Brom., *Bryon.*, CALC. CARB., Carb. veg., Caustic., Chamom., Chelid., Cicut., CINCHON., Coccul., Cyclam., Digit., Droser., Dulcam., *Ferr.*, Fluor. ac., Helleb., Hepar, Ignat., Iod., Kali carb.,

Laches., Lauroc., *Lycop.*, Magn. carb., Mar. ver., *Menyanth.*, Merc. corr., *Merc. viv.*, Mezer., Mosch., Nitr. ac., NUX VOM., Oleand., Opium, Paris, PHOSPHOR., *Phosph. ac.*, Platin., PULSAT., Rheum, Rhodod., RHUS TOX., Ruta, Sabad., Sarsap., Scilla, Secal., Selen., SEPIA, *Silic.*, Staphis., Strontia, SULPHUR, Sulph. ac., Tarax., *Thuya*, Valer., Veratr., Zinc.

Congestion of blood; lower limbs: to the: *Acon.*, Agn. cast., Alum., Ambra, Amm. carb., Amm. mur., Anac., Ant. tart., *Apis*, Argent., ARNIC., Asaf., AURUM, *Bellad.*, Borax, Brom., BRYON., CALC. CARB., Cann. sat., Carb. an., CARB. VEG., Caustic., *Cinchon.*, Coccul., Colchic., Coloc., Conium, Cuprum, Cyclam., Dulcam., *Ferr.*, *Graphit.*, Helleb., Hepar, Iod., Kali carb., Kreos., *Laches.*, Ledum, LYCOP., Magn. carb., Magn. mur., Mar. ver., Merc. viv., Mur. ac., Natr. carb., *Natr. mur.*, Nitrum, Nitr. ac., *Nux vom.*, Oleand., Opium, Petrol., *Phosphor.*, *Phosph. ac.*, Platin., Plumbum, PULSAT., Ran. bulb., Rhodod., RHUS TOX., Ruta, Sabad., *Sabin.*, Sarsap., Secal., SEPIA, SILIC., Spigel., Spong., Stann., Staphis., Strontia, SULPHUR, Sulph. ac., *Thuya*, *Zinc.*

Orgasm of blood: *Acon.*, Alum., *Ambra*, Amm. carb., Amm. mur., Ant. tart., Argent., *Arnic.*, Arsen., AURUM, Baryt., *Bellad.*, Borax, BOVIST., BRYON., *Calc. carb.*, Cann. sat., Carb. an., Carb. veg., CAUSTIC., Chamom., Cinchon., Conium, Crocus, Digit., Dulcam., FERR., Graphit., Guaiac., HEPAR, Ignat., IOD., *Kali carb.*, KREOS., LYCOP., Magn. carb., *Magn. mur.*, *Merc. viv.*, MOSCH., Natr. carb., Natr. mur., Nitr. ac., *Nux mosch.*, Nux vom., Opium, Petrol., PHOSPHOR., *Phosph. ac.*, Pulsat., Rhus tox., *Sabad.*, *Sabin.*, SAMBUC., SARSAP., *Selen.*, SENEG., SEPIA, *Silic.*, SPONG., Stann., Staphis., *Sulphur.*, Thuya, Veratr.

Plethora: *Acon.*, Alum., Amm. carb., Arnic., Arsen., *Aurum*, Baryt., BELLAD., BRYON., CALC. CARB., Canthar., *Chamom.*, Chelid., *Cinchon.*, Coloc., *Crocus.*, Cuprum, Digit., Dulcam., FERR., Graphit., Guaiac., Hepar, *Hyosc.*, Ignat., *Ipecac.*, *Kali carb.*, Laches., *Lycop.*, Merc. viv., Mosch., Natr. carb., *Natr. mur.*, Nitrum, Nitr. ac., NUX VOM., Opium, PHOSPHOR., Phosph. ac., PULSAT., RHUS TOX., Sabin.,

Selen., Seneg., *Sepia*, Silic., Stramon., SULPHUR, THUYA, Veratr.

Stagnation, sensation of: Acon., Bellad., Bryon., Caustic., Crocus, Digit., Hepar, Ignat., Laches., LYCOP., Natr. mur., Nux vom., Oleand., Pulsat., Rhodod., SABAD., Seneg., Sepia, Sulphur, Zinc.

Circulation seems arrested: *Lycop.*, *Psorin.*

Palpitation of the Heart; in general: ACON., Agar., Alum., *Ambra*, Amm. carb., Anac., *Angust.*, Ant. tart., Apis, Arnic., *Arsen.*, Asaf., Asar., AURUM., Baryt., *Bellad.*, Bismuth., Borax, BOVIST., *Brom.*, BRYON., CALC. CARB., Camphor., Cann. sat., Canthar., Carb. an., *Carb. veg.*, Caustic., CHAMOM., CINCHON., Clemat., *Coccul.*, Coffea, *Colchic.*, Coloc., Conium, CROCUS, Cuprum, *Cyclam.*, *Digit.*, Dulcam., *Ferr.*, Graphit., Helleb., Hepar, Hyosc., Ignat., IOD., Ipecac., Kali carb., Kreos., Laches., Lauroc., Ledum, LYCOP., Magn. carb., Magn. mur., Mangan., Menyanth., MERC. VIV., Merc. corr., Mezer., Mosch., Mur. ac., *Natr. carb.*, NATR. MUR., *Nitrum*, NITR. AC., *Nux mosch.*, NUX VOM., Oleand., Opium, Paris, Petrol., PHOSPHOR., *Phosph. ac.*, Platin., Plumbum, PULSAT., Ran. scel., Rhodod., RHUS TOX., Ruta, Sabad., Sabin., *Sarsap.*, *Secal.*, Selen., *Seneg.*, SEPIA, Silic., SPIGEL., Spong., *Staphis.*, Strontia, SULPHUR, *Sulph. ac.*, THUYA, Valer., *Veratr.*, Verbasc., *Viol. od.*, *Viol. tr.*, Zinc.

— **anxious:** ACON., Alum., Amm. carb., Anac., Angust., Ant. tart., Arnic., ARSEN., Asaf., AURUM, Bellad., Borax, Brom., *Bryon.*, CALC. CARB., Camphor., Cann. sat., Carb. veg., Caustic., CHAMOM., Cinchon., *Coccul.*, Coffea, Colchic., Coloc., CROCUS, Cuprum, *Cyclam.*, DIGIT., *Ferr.*, Graphit., Helleb., Hyosc., Ignat., Kali carb., Laches., Lauroc., Ledum, LYCOP., Magn. carb., Menyanth., Merc. viv., Merc. corr., Mosch., *Natr. carb.*, NATR. MUR., NITR. AC., *Nux vom.*, Oleand., Opium, Petrol., PHOSPHOR., *Platin.*, Plumbum, PULSAT., *Rhus tox.*, Ruta, Sarsap., *Secal.*, Seneg., *Sepia*, Silic., SPIGEL., Spong., Staphis., SULPHUR, *Sulph. ac.*, Thuya, Valer., *Veratr.*, Viol. od., *Viol. tr.*, Zinc.

PULSATIONS OF THE HEART.

— **fluttering:** *Apis*, Natr. mur., *Phosph. ac.*, Spigel.

— **intermittent:** *Acon.*, *Agar.*, Alum., *August.*, *Apis*, ARSEN., Asaf., Aurum, *Bismuth.*, *Bryon.*, *Canthar.*, CAPSIC., CARB. VEG., *Cinchon.*, *Digit.*, *Hepar*, HYOSC., Kali carb., *Laches.*, Lauroc., Menyanth., *Merc. viv.*, MERC. CORR., *Mezer.*, Mur. ac., NATR. MUR., Nitr. ac., Nux vom., *Opium*, *Phosphor.*, *Phosph. ac.*, *Plumbum*, *Rhus tox.*, *Sabin.*, Sambuc., *Secal.*, Sepia, *Stramon.*, *Sulphur*, Thuya, Veratr., *Zinc.*

— **audible:** ANGUST., Arnic., BISMUTH., Cinchon., COCCUL., *Cuprum*, IOD., Merc. corr., Plumbum, SABAD., *Secal.*, Sepia, Zinc.

— **fill the chest,** seems to: *Baptis.*

— **shaking the chest:** Seneg.

— **felt by the patient:** *Baryt.*, Calc. carb., *Cyclam.*, Dulcam., *Lycop.*, Mur. ac., Plumbum, Rhodod., Rhus tox., Sabin., Spigel., Veratr.

— **trembling:** Ambra, Angust., ANT. TART., *Arsen.*, Aurum, Bellad., CALC. CARB., Camphor., CICUT., Cina, *Coccul.*, Colchic., Conium, *Cuprum*, Iod., Kali carb., Kreos., Laches., Merc. viv., Merc. corr., Natr. mur., Nux mosch., Phosphor., PLATIN., *Rhus tox.*, Ruta, Sabin., Sepia, *Spigel.*, STAPHIS., *Stramon.*, Thuya, Veratr.

— **visible:** *Ant. tart.*, Bovist., Conium, Dulcam., Graphit., Iod., Rhus tox., Secal., SPIGEL., *Sulphur*, *Thuya*, Veratr.

PULSE, ACCORDING TO ITS RHYTHM.

— **quick, (accelerated):** ACON., Act. rac., Æsc. hip., *Agar.*, *Alum.*, AMBRA, AMM. CARB., AMM. MUR., ANAC., *Angust.*, Ant., crud., ANT. TART., APIS, *Argent.*, *Arnic.*, ARSEN., *Arum. tr.*, ASAF., ASAR., AURUM, *Baptis.*, BARYT., BELLAD., Bismuth., *Borax*, BOVIST., BROM., BRYON., *Cact. grand.*, CALC. CARB., Camphor., CANTHAR., CARB. AN., *Carb. veg.*, Caustic., CHAMOM., CHELID., Chin. sulph., CINA, CINCHON., *Clemat.*, *Coccul.*,

Coffea, COLCHIC., COLOC, *Conium*, Corn. flor., CROCUS, *Cuprum*, *Diadem.*, Digit., *Eup. purp.*, *Fluor. ac.*, *Gelsem.*, GUAIAC., HEPAR, *Hydr. ac.*, HYOSC., IGNAT., IOD., IPECAC., *Kali bichr.*, *Kali carb.*, Kali hydr., Kreos., LACHES., *Lauroc.*, LEDUM, Lobel. inf., *Lycop.*, *Magn. carb.*, *Magn. mur.*, *Mangan.*, *Mar. ver.*, *Menyanth.*, MERC. VIV., Merc. corr., Mezer., MOSCH., NATR. CARB., NATR, MUR., Natr. sulph., NITRUM, *Nitr. ac.*, *Nux mosch.*, NUX VOM., *Oleand.*, *Opium*, Oxal. ac., Paris, PETROL., PHOSPHOR., PHOSPH. AC., *Plumbum*, PULSAT., *Ran. bulb.*, *Ran. scel.*, *Rheum*, RHUS TOX., *Ruta*, Sabin., Sambuc., Sanguin., *Sarsap.*, *Secal.*, *Selen.*, SENEG., Sepia, Silic., SPONG., STANN., STAPHIS., *Stramon.*, SULPHUR, SULPH. AC., *Therid.*, THUYA, VALER., *Veratr.*, VIOL. TR., *Zinc.*

Pulse quick in the morning, during the day or evening slow: AGAR., Alum., ARSEN., Calc. carb., Canthar., Cinchon., Graphit., Ignat., KALI CARB., Lycop., Mezer., Nux vom., Phosphor.

— — **afternoons**; morning slow: NITRUM, Thuya, Zinc.

— — **evenings**; morning slow: Argent., Arnic., Asar., Carb. an., Caustic., Cinchon., *Kali carb.*, *Lycop.*, Mar. ver., Mezer., NITRUM, OLEAND., Petrol., Phosphor., Pulsat., RAN. BULB., *Sarsap.*, Sepia, SPIGEL., THUYA, ZINC.

— — **night**; during the day slow: Amm. carb., Borax, *Bryon.*, Calc. carb., Carb. an., Dulcam., Hepar, Magn. carb., Merc. viv., Mur. ac., Natr. carb., Natr. mur., Nitrum, Phosphor., Ran. scel., Sabin., SEPIA, *Silic.*, Sulphur.

— **slow**: Agar., AGN. CAST., *Ant. crud.*, *Ant. tart.*, *Arnic.*, Arsen., Baptis., *Bellad.*, CAMPHOR., CANN. SAT., *Canthar.*, Chin. sulph., CICUT., Cinchon., Colchic., Coloc., CONIUM, CUPRUM, DIGIT., Dulcam., Ferr., Gelsem., HELLEB., Hepar., Hydrast., HYOSC., *Ignat.*, *Kali carb.*, Lachnanth., *Lauroc.*, Leptand., Magn. carb., *Mangan.*, *Menyanth.*, *Merc. viv.*, Mosch., MUR. AC., *Natr. mur.*, Nitrum, *Oleand.*, *Opium*, PARIS, *Petrol.*, Phosphor., Plumbum, Podophyl., *Pulsat.*, Ran. bulb., RHODOD., Rhus tox., *Sambuc.*,

SCILLA, *Secal.*, *Sepia*, *Silic.*, SPIGEL., *Stramon.*, Therid. Thuya, VERATR., Zinc.

Pulse intermittent: *Acon.*, *Act. rac.*, *Agar.*, Alum., *Angust.*, *Apis*, ARSEN., Asaf,. Aurum, *Bismuth.*, *Bryon*·, *Cact. grand.*, *Canthar.*, CAPSIC., CARB. VEG., *Cimex*, *Cinchon.*, *Digit.*, *Hepar*, HYOSC., Kali carb., *Laches.*, Lauroc., Menyanth., *Merc. viv.*, MERC. CORR., *Mezer.*, Mur. ac., NATR. MUR., Nitr. ac., Nux vom., *Opium*, Oxal. ac., *Phosphor.*, *Phosph. ac.*, *Plumbum*, *Rhus tox.*, *Sabin.*, !Sambuc., *Secal.*, *Sepia*, *Stramon.*, *Sulphur*, Thuya, Veratr., *Zinc.*

— — Every 1 or 2 beats, *Phosph. ac.*

— — " 3d beat, *Mur. ac.*, Natr. mur.

— — " 4th beat, NITR. AC.

— — " 4th or 5th beat, *Nux vom.*

— — " 10th to 30th beat, Agar., Laches.

— **irregular:** Acon., Act. rac., Alum., ANGUST., ANT. CRUD., ARNIC., *Arsen.*, Bryon., *Canthar.*, CAPSIC., Carb. veg., *Cinchon.*, CONIUM, *Digit.*, Hepar, Hyosc., Ignat., Kali bichr., Kali carb., Laches., Lachnanth., *Lauroc.*, MANGAN., MERC. VIV., Merc. corr., NATR. MUR., *Nitr. ac.*, OLEAND., OPIUM, PHOSPHOR., PHOSPH. AC., PLUMBUM, *Psorin.*, RHUS TOX., Sambuc., Sanguin., Secal., Seneg., Sepia, *Silic.*, SPIGEL., STRAMON., VALER., VERATR., Zinc.

— **unequal:** AGAR., Ant. crud., ASAF., Bellad., CANTHAR., CARB. VEG., CHAMOM., *Conium*, Cuprum, Digit., IGNAT., KALI CARB., LACHES., LAUROC., MANGAN., NITR. AC., OLEAND., OPIUM, PHOSPHOR., PLUMBUM, SABIN., SAMBUC., SENEG., Sepia, Silic., Stramon., VALER., Veratr., Zinc.

PULSE ACCORDING TO ITS CHARACTER.

— **audible:** Ant. tart., *Camphor.*, Conium, *Digit.*, Helleb., Iod., Kali carb., Kreos., Merc. viv., Phosphor., Plumbum, Sepia, SPIGEL., Sulphur, *Thuya.*

— **bounding:** Calad.

Pulse contracted: Acon., Arnic., Asaf., BISMUTH., Borax, Cinchon., Cuprum, Kali bichr., Laches., Lauroc., Oxal. ac., PLUMBUM, *Secal.*

— **full:** ACON., ALUM., ANT. TART., APIS, *Arnic.*, Asaf., ASAR., Aurum, Baptis., *Baryt.*, BELLAD., Bismuth., BRYON., CALC. CARB., Camphor., CANTHAR., *Chelid.*, Chin. sulph., *Cinchon.*, COLCHIC., COLOC., Conium, Cuprum, *Digit.*, Dulcam., Eup. purp., FERR., GRAPHIT., Helleb., HEPAR, HYOSC., IGNAT., Iod., Kali carb., Kreos., *Laches.*, *Lauroc.*, LEDUM, Leptand., MERC. VIV., MEZER., MOSCH., Mur. ac., *Natr. mur.*, NITRUM, NUX VOM., *Oleand.*, *Opium*, PARIS, PETROL., PHOSPHOR., *Phosph. ac.*, *Plumbum*, Pulsat., *Ran. bulb.*, RAN. SCEL., SABIN., *Sambuc.*, Secal., *Sepia*, Silic., SPIGEL., SPONG., STRAMON., STRONTIA, SULPHUR, THUYA, Valer., Veratr., VIOL. OD.

— **hard:** ACON., AMM. CARB., Apis, *Arnic.*, Arsen., *Baryt.*, BELLAD., BRYON., Cact. grand., CALAD., Camphor., CANTHAR., *Chelid.*, CINA, CINCHON., CLEMAT., *Coccul.*, COLCHIC., COLOC., Conium, Corn. flor., *Cuprum*, *Digit.*, DULCAM., FERR., GRAPHIT., HEPAR, HYOSC., IGNAT., IOD., *Kali carb.*, Laches., Lauroc., Merc. viv., Merc. corr., MEZER., NITRUM, NITR. AC., NUX VOM., Opium, Oxal. ac., PHOSPHOR., *Plumbum*, Pulsat., *Ran. bulb.*, Ran. scel., *Scilla*, Secal., SENEG., SILIC., SPONG., STRAMON., STRONTIA, SULPHUR, *Veratr.*, Zinc.

— **imperceptible:** *Acon.*, *Agn. cast.*, *Ant. tart.*, *Apis*, Arnic., ARSEN., *Cact. grand.*, CAMPHOR., CANN. SAT., *Canthar.*, CARB. VEG., *Cicut.*, *Coccul.*, Conium, CUPRUM, Ferr., *Helleb.*, Hyosc., *Ipecac.*, Laches., *Lauroc.*, *Ledum*, Lobel. inf., *Merc. viv.*, Mosch., *Nux vom.*, Opium, *Pulsat.*, RHUS TOX., Secal., Silic., *Stramon.*, VERATR.

— **jerking:** *Arnic.*, Conium, Natr. mur., Nux vom., Plumbum.

— **large:** Acon., *Bellad.*, Cinchon., Colchic., CONIUM, IOD., Mosch., Opium.

— **small:** *Acon.*, Agar., Amm. carb., Ant. crud., *Apis*, Arnic., ARSEN., ASAF., AURUM, *Bellad.*, Bismuth., Bryon.,

Calc. carb., CAMPHOR., Cann. sat., Canthar., Carb. an., Carb. veg., CHAMOM., CHELID., Chin. sulph., CINA, CINCHON., Clemat., COCCUL., Colchic., *Coloc.*, *Conium*, Crocus, CUPRUM, Digit., DULCAM., Ferr., Graphit., GUAIAC., HELLEB., Hyosc., *Ignat.*, Iod., Kali bichr., KREOS., LACHES., *Lauroc.*, Lobel. inf., *Merc. viv.*, MERC. CORR., Mosch., Nitrum, *Nitr. ac.*, *Nux vom.*, Opium, Oxal. ac., *Phosphor.*, PHOSPH. AC., PLATIN., PLUMBUM, *Psorin.*, PULSAT., Ran. bulb., Ran. scel., Rhodod., Rhus tox., SABAD., SAMBUC., SCILLA, Secal., SILIC., Spong., STANN., STAPHIS., *Stramon.*, Sulphur, SULPH. AC., *Valer.*, VERATR., *Zinc.*

Pulse soft: Æsc. hip., Ant. tart., Baptis., *Bellad.*, Carb. veg., *Cinchon.*, *Cuprum*, Dulcam., GUAIAC., Hydr. ac., Iod., Kali carb., Laches., Lauroc., MANGAN., Mur. ac., Nitrum, Plumbum, RAN. SCEL., RHUS TOX., SENEG., Stramon., Veratr.

— **spasmodic:** ANGUST., Arnic., BISMUTH., Cinchon., COCCUL., *Cuprum*, Iod., Merc. corr., Plumbum, SABAD., *Secal.*, Sepia, Zinc.

— **strong:** *Acon.*, ANT. TART., Apis, Arnic., ASAR., *Bellad.*, Bismuth., Canthar., Chelid., *Cinchon:*, *Corn. flor.*, Cuprum, Digit., Helleb, HYOSC., Iod., Kreos., *Laches*, Lauroc., *Merc. viv.*, Opium, Petrol., PHOSPH. AC., Ran. bulb., SABIN., Sanguin., SPIGEL., *Stramon.*, Strontia, Valer., *Veratr.*, VIOL. OD. (Compare: pulse full.)

— **suppressed:** Acon., Ant. tart., ARSEN., *Carb. veg.*, *Conium*, Iod., Kreos., *Merc. viv.*, Merc. corr., Mosch., Opium, Pulsat., Sanguin., *Secal.*, Silic., Stramon., VERATR.

— **tense:** AMM. CARB., BELLAD., BRYON., Cact. grand., Camphor, CHAMOM., DULCAM., Merc. corr., Mezer., SABIN., Sanguin., Scilla, Secal., *Valer.*, Zinc.

— **thread-like:** *Acon.*, *Apis*, Colchic., IOD., Merc. corr., Stramon., VERATR.

— **trembling:** Ambra, Angust., ANT. TART., *Arsen.*, Aurum, Bellad., CALC. CARB., Camphor., CICUT., Cina,

Coccul., Colchic., Conium, *Cuprum*, Iod., Kali carb., Kreos., Laches., *Merc. viv.*, Merc. corr., Natr. mur., Nux mosch., Oxal. ac., Phosphor., PLATIN., *Rhus tox.*, Ruta, Sabin., Sepia, *Spigel.*, STAPHIS., *Stramon.*, Thuya, Veratr.

Pulse unaltered: *Coffea*, CYCLAM., DROSER., EUPHRAS., Fluor. ac., *Rheum*, Ruta, SECAL., Selen.

— **weak:** Acon., Act. rac., Æsc. hip., Agar., AGN. CAST., Ant. crud., Ant. tart., Apis, *Arnic.*, ARSEN., Asaf., BARYT., Bellad., Bismuth., CAMPHOR., CANN. SAT., *Canthar.*, CARB. VEG., *Chamom.*, Chin. sulph., CICUT., Cimex, Cinchon., *Coloc.*, Conium, CUPRUM, Digit., *Guaiac.*, *Hyosc.*, IOD., *Kali carb.*, KREOS., LACHES., Lauroc., Lobel. inf., MANGAN., *Merc. viv.*, MERC. CORR., *Mosch.*, MUR. AC., *Natr. mur.*, Nux vom., *Oleand.*, *Opium*, *Phosphor.*, PHOSPH. AC., PLATIN., Plumbum, *Psorin.*, PULSAT., RHODOD., RHUS TOX., Secal., Spigel., Stramon., SULPH. AC., *Thuya*, *Valer.*, VERATR.

AGGRAVATION ACCORDING TO TIME.

Morning: Agar., Alum., *Arsen.*, Calc. carb., Canthar., Cinchon., Ferr., Graphit., Ignat., Kali carb., *Lycop.*, Mezer., Natr. carb., *Nux vom.*, Phosphor., *Sepia*, Spigel.

Forenoon: Argent., Cann. sat., Guaiac., Kali carb., *Natr. carb.*, Natr. mur., Sabad., *Sepia*, Sulph. ac.

Afternoon: Alum., *Calc. carb.*, Ferr., *Nitrum*, *Phosphor.*, Plumbum, Staphis., Thuya, Zinc.

Evening: Angust., ARGENT., ARNIC., Asar., *Bellad.*, Bovist., *Calc. carb.*, Canthar., CARB. AN., Carb. veg., CAUSTIC., *Chelid.*, Cinchon., Ferr., Graphit., Ignat., *Kali carb.*, Laches., LYCOP., Magn. carb., Mangan., Mar. ver., Merc. viv., MEZER., Natr. carb., Natr. mur., *Nitrum*, *Nitr. ac.*, Oleand., Petrol., Phosphor., PULSAT., Ran. bulb., Rhus tox., Sabin., Sambuc., *Sarsap.*, Sepia, *Spigel.*, Sulphur, THUYA, *Zinc.*

Night: Amm. carb., Ant. tart., Arnic., *Arsen.*, Borax, *Bryon.*, Calc. carb., Carb. an., DULCAM., Graphit., *Hepar*,

Ignat., Lycop., *Magn. carb.*, *Merc. viv.*, Mur. ac., NATR. CARB., Natr. mur., Nitrum, *Nitr. ac.*, *Phosphor.*, *Ran. scel.*, Sabin., Scilla, SEPIA, SILIC., Sulphur.

AGGRAVATION ACCORDING TO CIRCUMSTANCES.

Anger, after: *Acon.*, CHAMOM.,Coloc., Ignat., Natr. mur., *Petrol.*, SEPIA, Staphis.

Ascending stairs, from: Acon., *Arsen.*, *Baryt.*, Bellad., Bryon., Calc. carb., Graphit., Merc. viv., Natr. carb., Nitrum, NITR. AC., Nux vom., PETROL., Rhus tox., Ruta, Seneg., Sepia, Spigel., *Spong.*, Stann., Staphis., Sulphur., THUYA, Zinc.

Attacks, during the: Acon., Alum., *Bellad.*, Carb. an., Carb. veg., Cuprum, Kali carb., Laches., Nux vom., Sepia, Silic., Thuya.

Awaking, on: Alum., Amm. carb., Ambra, Arnic., *Arsen.*, Baryt., Bellad., Borax, CALC. CARB., Camphor., Carb. an., Carb. veg., Cina, Cinchon., Coccul., Ferr., *Graphit.*, Ignat., Ipecac., *Kali carb.*, *Lycop.*, Magn. carb., Mosch., *Natr. carb.*, *Natr. mur.*, Nitr. ac., *Nux vom.*, Petrol., *Phosphor.*, Phosph. ac., Pulsat., Ran. scel., *Rhus tox.*, Sabin., SEPIA, *Silic.*, *Staphis.*, *Sulphur*, Sulph. ac., Thuya, Veratr., Zinc.

Cough, from: *Acon.*, Apis, *Arnic.*, ARSEN., BELLAD., Bryon., CALC. CARB., Carb. veg., Cinchon., *Ipecac.*, Natr. mur., Nitr. ac., *Nux vom.*, PHOSPHOR., Pulsat., Rhus tox., Sabad., Scilla, Secal., SEPIA, Spong., Sulphur.

Drinking, from, in general: Acon., Anac., Ant. tart., *Arnic.*, ARSEN., Brom., Bryon., CALC. CARB., *Cinchon.*, Coccul., Coloc., CONIUM, Crocus, Cuprum, Ferr., Hepar, Mar. ver., *Natr. mur.*, Nitr. ac., *Nux vom.*, Pulsat., *Rhus tox.*, *Silic.*, Sulphur, Thuya, VERATR.

— **Beer:** Acon., Arsen., Bellad., Coloc., *Ferr.*, Lycop., Nux vom., Pulsat., *Rhus tox.*, Secal., *Sepia*, Stramon., SULPHUR, *Thuya*, Veratr.

— **Brandy:** ARNIC., *Arsen.*, Calc. carb., Cinchon.,

Coccul., FLUOR. AC., Hepar, Ignat., *Laches.*, Ledum, *Nux vom.*, *Opium*, Rhus tox., Stramon., Sulphur, Sulph. ac.

Drinking; Coffee: Canthar., Caustic., CHAMOM., Cinchon., Coccul., *Ignat.*, Ipecac., Merc. viv., *Nux vom.*, Phosph. ac., Pulsat., Rhus tox., Sulphur, Thuya.

— **Tea:** Arsen., Cinchon., *Ferr.*, Hepar, Phosph. ac., SELEN., Thuya, Veratr.

— **Wine:** Ant. crud., Arnic, ARSEN., Borax, Calc. carb., *Carb. veg.*, Coffea, Fluor. ac., *Laches.*, LYCOP., Natr. carb., NATR. MUR., Nux mosch., *Nux vom.*, Opium, Ran. bulb., Sabin., Selen., SILIC., THUYA, *Zinc.*

Eating; before: Calc. carb., CINCHON., Conium, Iod., *Kali carb.*, *Natr. carb.*, Phosphor., Sepia.

— **while:** Amm. carb., Carb. an., Carb. veg., Ignat., *Kali carb.*, Nitr. ac., Sepia, *Spigel.*

— **after:** Acon., Alum., Angust., Asaf., *Bryon.*, *Calc. carb.*, Camphor., CARB. AN., *Carb. veg.*, Caustic., Chamom., Chin. sulph., Cinchon., Conium, Hepar, Ignat., Kali carb., LYCOP., Mezer., *Natr. carb.*, Natr. mur., *Nitr. ac.*, *Nux vom.*, Paris, PHOSPHOR., Phosph. ac., *Pulsat.*, Ran. bulb., SELEN., Sepia, Silic., Sulphur, Sulph. ac., Thuya, Viol. tr., Zinc.

Exertion of the body, from: Acon., *Amm. carb.*, Arnic., Arsen., Bryon., Digit., IOD., Lycop., MERC. VIV., Natr. mur., Rhus tox., Silic., Sulphur, Thuya.

Lying down, after: Agn. cast., *Ambra*, Amm. carb., ARGENT., *Arsen.*, Asaf., *Aurum*, Bryon., CALC. CARB., Capsic., Carb. veg., Chamom., Chelid., Clemat., Cyclam., DULCAM., Ferr., Graphit., Helleb., HEPAR, Hyosc., *Kali carb.*, Lycop., Magn. carb., Magn. mur., Merc. viv., Nux vom., *Phosphor.*, *Platin.*, Plumbum, *Pulsat.*, *Rhus tox.*, Sabad., SAMBUC., Scilla, Selen., Seneg., *Sepia*, Spong., Strontia, Sulphur, Sulph. ac.

Lying; while (in bed): Acon., Agn. cast., Alum., Ambra, Angust., Ant. crud., Ant. tart., *Argent.*, Arnic., Asaf., Asar., Aurum, Borax, Bryon., CALC. CARB., Chamom., Chelid., Coloc., Ferr., Graphit., *Helleb.*, Ignat., Iod., *Kali carb.*, Ledum,

LYCOP., Magn. mur., Mangan., Menyanth., Merc. viv., Mosch., *Natr. mur.*, Nitrum, NITR. AC., Nux vom., Phosphor., *Pulsat.*. *Rhus tox.*, SAMBUC., *Selen.*, Seneg., *Sepia*, Spigel., Strontia, *Sulphur*, Valer., Veratr., *Viol. tr.*

Lying; on the back, while: Alum., Amm. carb., Amm. mur., ARSEN., Caustic., Chamom., Cinchon., Coloc., Cuprum, Ignat., Iod., *Nitrum*, *Nux vom.*, *Phosphor.*, Plumbum, *Pulsat.*, Rhus tox., *Sepia*, *Silic.*, Spigel.

— **on the left side:** *Acon.*, Amm. carb., Anac., Angust., *Baryt.*, *Bryon.*, Calc. carb., Canthar., Carb. an., Carb. veg., Cinchon., *Graphit.*, Ipecac., *Kali carb.*, *Lycop.*, Merc. viv., Mezer., NATR. CARB., NATR. MUR., PHOSPHOR., PULSAT., *Sepia*, Silic., *Stann.*, Sulphur, Thuya.

— **on the right side:** Acon., Amm. mur., Anac., Borax, Carb. an., Ipecac., Lycop., Magn. mur., *Merc. viv.*, Nitrum, NUX VOM., Pulsat., Seneg., Spigel., Spong., *Stann.*, Viol. tr.

Mental prostration, during: Acon., Asar., *Bellad.*, Bismuth., Cicut., *Cinchon.*, Digit., Magn. carb., Natr. mur., *Petrol.*, Phosphor., Spong., Stann., Stramon.

Menses; before the: Alum., Amm. carb., Baryt., *Calc. carb.*, Coccul., Coloc., Conium, CUPRUM, Iod., KALI CARB., *Lycop.*, Merc. viv., Natr. mur., Phosph. ac., PULSAT., Secal., Sepia, *Spong.*, Stann., Sulphur, Veratr.

— **during** the: *Arsen.*, Cinchon., IGNAT., Iod., Phosphor., SEPIA, *Sulphur.*

Mood, change of, from: *Acon.*, Apis, *Aurum*, *Bellad.*, Bryon., Calc. carb., CHAMOM., Coffea, Colchic., *Coloc.*, *Conium*, Cuprum, HYOSC., IGNAT., Kali carb., *Laches.*, Lycop., Magn. carb., Mar. ver., Natr. mur., *Nitr. ac.*, *Nux vom.*, Opium, *Petrol.*, *Phosphor.*, *Phosph. ac.*, Platin., PULSAT., *Sepia*, *Staphis.*, Stramon., Thuya, Veratr.

Motion, from: Acon., Amm. mur., Ant. crud., ANT. TART., Arnic., Baryt., *Bellad.*, *Bryon.*, Cann. sat., Cinchon., Colchic., Digit., Ferr., *Fluor. ac.*, *Graphit.*, Gelsem., IOD., Laches., Ledum, Mezer., NATR. MUR., Nitrum, *Nitr. ac.*, Nux vom.,

Oleand., Paris, PETROL., *Phosphor.*, Sambuc., Scilla, SEPIA, Silic., Spigel., *Staphis.*, Stramon., Sulphur, *Thuya*, Valer.

Music, from: Acon., Calc. carb., Digit., *Lycop.*, NATR. CARB., Nux vom., *Phosph. ac.*, SEPIA, *Staphis.*, THUYA, Viol. od.

Rest, during: Apis, Argent., Arnic., Aurum, Bellad., *Calc. carb.*, Capsic., Chamom., Cinchon., Coloc., Conium, Cyclam., DIGIT., *Dulcam.*, *Euphorb.*, Ferr., *Kali carb.*, KREOS., Lycop., MAGN. MUR., Menyanth., Mosch., Natr. carb., *Natr. mur.*, Nitrum, Paris, *Phosphor.*, Phosph. ac., Pulsat., RHUS TOX., Ruta, Sabad., Sambuc., *Seneg.*, *Sepia*, *Spigel.*, Stann., Sulphur, Tarax., Valer.

Rising, from: *Acon.*, Arsen., Bellad., *Bryon.*, Natr. mur., Nux vom., Opium, Phosphor., Rhus tox., Scilla, Sulphur, *Veratr.*

Room, in the (warm): Agn. cast., Ambra, Amm. carb., Amm. mur., Anac., Angust., Ant. crud., *Apis*, Arsen., Asar., Bellad., Bryon., Calc. carb., *Crocus*, Graphit., IOD., *Ipecac.*, Lauroc., *Lycop.*, Natr. mur., Phosphor., Platin., *Pulsat.*, Rhodod., Rhus tox., *Sabin.*, Selen., Seneg., Spigel., Sulphur, Sulph. ac., Thuya, Verbas.

Sensitiveness, with: Ambra, *Bellad.*, Calc. carb., Ferr., *Merc. viv.*, Nitrum, Nitr. ac., Phosphor., Phosph. ac., Sepia.

Sitting, while: Agar, Alum., *Anac.*, ANGUST., Ant. tart., *Asaf.*, Asar., Baryt., Calc. carb., Capsic., Carb. an., CARB. VEG., Cinchon., Cyclam., *Digit.*, Dulcam., Ferr., Graphit., Lycop., MAGN. MUR., Mangan., Menyanth., Mosch., Mur. ac., NATR. CARB., PHOSPHOR., Phosph. ac., Platin., Pulsat., Rhodod., *Rhus tox.*, Sabad., Seneg., *Sepia*, *Silic.*, SPIGEL., Sulphur, *Valer.*, Verbas., Viol. tr.

Sitting stooped, while: Alum., Angust., Argent., Bryon., Cann. sat., Cinchon., *Digit.*, Menyanth., Merc. viv., Oleand., Phosph. ac., Ran. bulb., Rhodod., *Rhus tox.*, Seneg., *Silic.*, *Spigel.*, Spong., Stann., Staphis.

Sleep, before: Agar., Amm. carb., *Arnic.*, Arsen., ASAR., Baryt., Bellad., Bryon., CALC. CARB., Carb. an., Carb. veg.,

Dulcam., Graphit., Ignat., Laches., *Lycop.*, *Magn. carb.*, Magn. mur., Merc. viv., Mur. ac., Natr. carb., *Natr. mur.*, Nux vom., Phosphor., PULSAT., RHUS TOX., SABAD., Sabin., Sambuc., Sarsap., *Sepia.*, *Silic.*, Sulphur, Thuya.

Siesta, during: Anac., Bryon., Calc. carb., Graphit., Ignat., Nux vom., Phosphor., *Pulsat.*, Selen., *Staphis.*, Sulphur.

Sleep, during: Acon., *Arsen.*, Bellad., *Calc. carb.*, Camphor., Chamom., Cinchon., Hepar, Hyosc., Ignat., Ledum, Merc. viv., *Natr. mur.*, *Opium*, *Phosphor.*, *Phosph. ac.*, Pulsat., *Rheum*, *Sabin.*, *Sambuc.*, Sepia, Silic., Stramon., *Sulphur.*, Viol. tr., *Zinc.*

Sleeplessness, with: Amm. carb., Amm. mur., Arnic., *Arsen.*, Asar., Borax, *Bryon.*, CALC. CARB., Camphor., *Conium*, Dulcam., Hepar, Kali carb., Lauroc., *Lycop.*, Magn. carb., Merc. viv., Natr. mur., Nitr. ac., PHOSPHOR., *Platin.*, PULSAT., Ran bulb., RHUS TOX., SABIN., Sambuc., *Sepia*, SILIC., Sulphur.

Standing, while: AGAR., Aurum, *Conium*, Cyclam., Ferr., Natr. mur., PLATIN., Pulsat., Rhus tox., *Valer.*

Stool, after: Ant. tart., *Arsen.*, Caustic., Nitr. ac., *Opium*, Rhus tox.

Stooping, while: Acon. Alum., Amm. carb., August., Argent., *Bryon.*, Cann. sat., Cinchon., *Digit.*, *Graphit.*, Mangan., *Merc. viv.*, Merc. corr., Natr. carb., Oleand., Phosph. ac., Ran. bulb., Scilla, Seneg., *Sepia*, Silic., SPIGEL., SULPH. AC., Valer.

Talking, from: Alum., *Ambra*, Amm. carb., Anac., *Arnic.*, Bellad., Borax, *Bryon.*, *Calc. carb.*, Cann. sat., Canthar., *Carb. veg.*, Chamom., Cinchon., Coccul., Dulcam., Graphit., *Hepar*, Ignat., Iod., *Kali carb.*, *Ledum*, Mangan., Merc. viv., Merc. corr., Mezer., Mur. ac., Natr. carb., Natr mur., *Phosphor.*, Phosph. ac., *Platin.*, PULSAT., Ran. bulb., *Rhus tox.*, Scilla, *Selen.*, Sepia, Spigel., *Stann.*, Stramon., *Sulphur*, Sulph. ac., Veratr.

Tobacco fumes, (and smoking) from: Acon., Ant. crud., Arsen., Cicut., Cyclam., *Ignat.*, Nux vom., PHOSPHOR., *Pulsat.*, Selen., Seneg., Sepia, Spong., Staphis.

Turning over, in bed: *Acon.*, Amm. mur., ARSEN., Bryon., Cann. sat., Capsic., Carb. veg., Conium, Ferr., *Hepar*, Kreos., *Lycop.*, Natr. mur., Nux vom., PULSAT., Rhus tox., Silic., Staphis., *Sulphur*, Thuya.

Vomiting, with the: Arsen., Cuprum, Ipecac., Mosch., Pulsat., Sulphur, Veratr.

Walking; while: Arnic., Aurum, Bellad., *Bryon.*, Colchic., Digit., Graphit., Ledum, Merc. viv., Merc. corr., Natr. mur., *Nitr. ac.*, *Nux vom.*, *Petrol.*, Phosphor., Sambuc., Scilla, Selen., Spigel., *Staphis.*

— **in the open air,** while: *Ambra*, AMM. CARB., Amm. mur., Anac., Ant. crud., Argent., *Bellad.*, Borax, Camphor., Cinchon., *Coccul.*, Conium, Guaiac., *Hepar*, NUX VOM., Petrol., Phosph. ac., Rhus tox., *Selen.*, SEPIA, *Spigel.*, Staphis., Sulphur, Tarax.

— — after: Agar., *Ambra*, Anac., Arsen., Cann. sat., Carb. veg., Ferr., Hyosc., Ledum, *Lycop.*, Menyanth., Nux vom., *Petrol.*, *Pulsat.*, *Rhus tox.*, Sabad., Sabin., *Sepia*, Stann., Valer.

Warm; **room**: see room.

— **weather,** during: Ant. crud., Asar., *Bryon.*, Carb. veg., Coccul., Colchic., *Graphit.*, IOD., Laches., Lycop., NITR. AC., Opium, Phosphor., Phosph. ac., *Pulsat.*, Secal., Selen., Sepia, *Sulphur.*

CHILL.

Chill; in general, (predominating): *Acon.*, AGAR., AGN. CAST., ALUM., Ambra, Amm. carb., *Amm. mur.*, *Anac.*, Angust., ANT. CRUD., ANT. TART., *Apis*, Argent., ARNIC., *Arsen.*, ASAF., ASAR., AURUM, BARYT., *Bellad.*, Bismuth., BORAX, BOVIST., *Brom.*, BRYON., Cact. grand., *Calad.*, *Calc. carb.*, CAMPHOR., CANN. SAT., *Canthar.*, CAPSIC., *Carb. an.*, *Carb. veg.*, CAUSTIC., Chamom., CHELID., *Chin. sulph.*, CICUT., *Cimex*, *Cina*, *Cinchon.*, *Cist.can.*, Clemat., *Coccul.*, Coffea, COLCHIC., COLOC., *Conium*, Corn. flor., *Crocus*, *Cuprum*, *Cyclam.*, DIADEM.,

Digit., DROSER., *Dulcam.*, EUP. PERF., EUP. PURP., EUPHORB., *Euphras.*, *Ferr.*, *Gelsem.*, *Graphit.*, Guaiac., HELLEB., *Hepar*, Hydrast., HYOSC., *Ignat.*, Iod., *Ipecac.*, Kali bichr., *Kali carb.*, Kali hydr., KREOS., Laches., Lachnanth., *Lauroc.*, LEDUM, Lobel. inf., LYCOP., *Magn. carb.*, *Magn. mur.*, *Mangan.*, *Mar. ver.*, MENYANTH., *Merc. viv.*, *Merc. corr.*, *Mezer.*, Mosch., MUR. AC., *Natr. carb.*, NATR. MUR., *Natr. sulph.*, *Nitrum*, *Nitr. ac.*, NUX MOSCH., *Nux vom.*, *Oleand.*, Opium, *Oxal. ac.*, *Paris*, *Petrol.*, *Phosphor.*, *Phosph. ac.*, PLATIN., PLUMBUM, Podophyl., PULSAT., *Psorin.*, RAN. BULB., Ran. scel., Rheum, *Rhodod.*, *Rhus tox.*, *Ruta*, SABAD., *Sabin.*, Sambuc., *Sanguin.*, SARSAP., Scilla, *Secal.*, Selen., Seneg., *Sepia*, *Silic.*, *Spigel.*, *Spong.*, *Stann.*, STAPHIS., *Stramon.*, *Strontia.*, *Sulphur*, Sulph. ac., Tarax., Therid., *Thuya*, Valer., VERATR., VERBAS., Viol. od., Viol. tr., *Zinc.*

Chill; ascending: *Acon.*, Amm. mur., Carb. an., *Cina*, Crocus, *Digit.*, Dulcam., *Hyosc.*, Kali bichr., *Laches.*, Magn. carb., Natr. sulph., Oxal. ac., *Phosphor.*, Pulsat., Ruta, SABAD., *Sarsap.*, *Sepia*, *Staphis.*, Sulphur, Veratr.

— **descending:** *Agar.*, Baryt., Bellad., *Canthar.*, Caustic., CICUT., Coccul., *Coffea*, Colchic., *Crocus*, Kreos., Laches., Magn. carb., *Mezer.*, MOSCH., Phosphor., *Psorin.*, Ruta, Sabad., *Staphis.*, Stramon., Strontia, Sulphur, *Sulph. ac.*, Thuya, *Valer.*, Veratr., Zinc.

— **external:** ACON., AMM. MUR., Arnic., Arsen., Calc. carb., CHAMOM., Cinchon., Euphorb., *Euphras.*, IGNAT., Laches., Magn. carb., Merc. viv., Mosch., NITR. AC., OLEAND., Ran. bulb., Rhus tox., *Sabad.*, Silic., *Sulphur*, *Veratr.*, Verbas., ZINC.

— **flitting,** (überlaufender): Agar., Alum., Ant. tart., Asaf., ASAR., *Baryt.*, Bellad., Chamom., Cinchon., COLCHIC., KALI CARB., Ledum, Menyanth., Mezer., Natr. mur., Nux vom., Phosph. ac., Psorin., PULSAT., Rhus tox., *Ruta*, SAMBUC., Sarsap., SPIGEL., Thuya, Valer., Veratr., Verbas.

— **goose flesh,** with: Æsc. hip., Angust., Ant. tart., Arsen., Asar., Aurum, Baryt., *Bellad.*, Borax, *Bryon.*,

Camphor., *Cann. sat.*, Canthar., Caustic., Chelid., Cinchon., *Crocus*, HELLEB., Ignat., Lauroc., Ledum, Mangan., Mezer., Mur. ac., Natr. carb., Natr. mur., Natr. sulph., *Nux vom.*, PARIS, Phosphor., Ran. bulb., Rhodod., Ruta, *Sabad.*, Sabin., Sarsap., Spigel., Stann., Staphis., Sulph. ac., Thuya, Veratr.

Chill; internal: Acon., *Agn. cast.*, Alum., Ambra, *Anac.*, *Angust.*, Ant. crud., Ant. tart., *Arnic.*, *Arsen.*, Asaf., Asar., Baryt., Bellad., Bovist., *Bryon.*, *Calc. carb.*, Camphor., *Canthar.*, Capsic., Carb. veg., *Caustic.*, Chamom., *Chelid.*, Cicut., CINCHON., COCCUL., *Coffea*, Colchic., *Conium*, Crocus, DIGIT., *Droser.*, *Euphras.*, Graphit., *Guaiac.*, Helleb., Hepar, *Ignat.*, *Ipecac.*, Kali carb., Kreos., Laches., Lauroc., Lycop., Magn. carb., Mangan., Menyanth., MERC. VIV., Mezer., Mosch., *Natr. carb.*, *Natr. mur.*, Nitr ac., Nux vom., Oleand., Paris, *Petrol.*, *Phosphor.*, Phosph. ac., Platin., PLUMBUM, Psorin., PULSAT., Ran. bulb., Rheum, Rhus tox., *Ruta*, Sabad., Sarsap., *Scilla*, Secal., Sepia, *Silic.*, Spigel., Spong., Strontia, *Sulphur*, Sulph. ac., Therid., *Thuya*, Valer., Veratr., *Verbas.*, Zinc.

— **one-sided:** Alum., Ambra, Anac., Ant. tart., Arnic., Baryt., Bellad., BRYON., *Carb. veg.*, Caustic., Chamom., *Chelid.*, Cinchon., Coccul., Crocus, Digit., *Droser.*, Ignat., Kali carb., *Lycop.*, Natr. carb., NUX VOM., Paris, *Phosphor.*, Phosph. ac., Platin., *Pulsat.*, Ran. bulb., Rheum, RHUS TOX., *Ruta*, Sabad., Sabin., Sarsap., Spigel., *Stann.*, Stramon., Sulphur, Sulph. ac., THUYA, *Verbas.*

— **left side:** Baryt., CARB. VEG., Caustic., *Droser.*, *Lycop.*, Paris, Rhus tox., Ruta, Spigel., *Stann.*, Sulphur, THUYA.

— **right side:** BRYON., Caustic., CHELID., Lycop., Nux vom., *Phosphor.*, *Pulsat.*, Ran. bulb., RHUS TOX., Sabin.

— **shivering,** with: *Acon.*, Agar., Amm. carb., Anac., ANT. CRUD., Apis, Arnic., *Arsen.*, Asar., Aurum, Baryt., BELLAD., BROM., *Bryon.*, Calc. carb., CAMPHOR., CANN. SAT., Canthar., Capsic., Carb. veg., Caustic., *Chamom.*, CHELID., Cicut., CINA, *Cinchon.*, Coccul., Cuprum, Cyclam.,

Dulcam., Ferr., HELLEB., Hepar, Ignat., IOD., *Ipecac.*, KREOS., Laches., Lauroc., Ledum, Lycop., Magn. carb., Magn. mur., Mangan., Merc. viv., Merc. corr., Mur. ac., Natr. carb., Natr. mur., Natr. sulph., Nitrum, Nitr. ac., Nux mosch., *Nux vom.*, Opium, Petrol., Phosphor., *Phosph. ac.*, PLATIN., Pulsat., Ran. bulb., *Rhus tox.*, RUTA, *Sabad.*, Sabin., *Sambuc.*, Sarsap., Secal., Sepia, Silic., Spigel., SPONG., STAPHIS., Stramon., Sulphur, Therid., Thuya, Valer., VERATR.

Chill; trembling, with, (trembling chill): *Acon.*, AGN. CAST., ANAC., ANT. TART., Apis, Arnic., Arsen., Asaf., Bellad., Borax, Brom., *Bryon.*, Calc. carb., Cann. sat., Canthar., Capsic., Carb. an., Cicut., *Cina*, Cinchon., Coccul., Conium, CROCUS, Ledum, MAR. VER., Merc. viv., Natr. carb., *Natr. mur.*, Nitrum, Nux vom., Oleand., *Opium*, PARIS, Petrol., Phosphor., Phosph. ac., PLATIN., Psorin., *Pulsat.*, *Rhus tox.*, Sabad., Silic., Stramon., *Sulphur*, Therid., Valer., Zinc.

— **cold water** poured over one, as from: Agar., *Anac.*, *Ant. tart.*, ARNIC., *Baryt.*, Cinchon., *Ledum*, Magn. carb., MERC. VIV., Mezer., Nux vom., Pulsat., RHUS TOX., Sabad., Valer., Veratr., Verbas.

Slight chilliness, in general: Agar., AGN. CAST., Ambra, Anac., APIS, *Arsen.*, ASAR., Bellad., Bismuth., BORAX, Bovist., *Bryon.*, *Camphor.*, Canthar., CARB. VEG., Chamom., Cina, Cinchon., COCCUL., *Coffea*, Conium, Cuprum, Digit., Droser., Dulcam., Euphorb., Guaiac., *Helleb.*, *Hyosc.*, *Ipecac.*, Kreos., Laches., Lycop., Mar. ver., Merc. viv., Merc. corr., Mezer., Mur. ac., NATR. CARB., Natr. mur., Nitrum, NUX MOSCH., Nux vom., *Paris*, PETROL., *Phosphor.*, Phosph. ac., PLATIN., Plumbum, Psorin., PULSAT., RAN. BULB., Ran. scel., Rhus tox., Sabad., Sambuc., Sarsap., *Scilla*, Seneg., SEPIA, Silic., SPIGEL., Spong., *Stann.*, Staphis., *Sulphur*, Tarax., Thuya, Valer., Zinc.

Chilliness, in general: Æsc. hip., Agar., Agn. cast., Alum., Amm. mur., ANAC., Ant. crud., Ant. tart., *Arsen.*, *Asar.*, Baptis., BARYT., Bovist., *Bryon.*, Calad., CALC.

CARB., CAMPHOR., Cann. sat., Carb. an., *Carb. veg.*, CAUSTIC., Chamom., CHELID., CICUT., *Cinchon.*, Cist. can., Coccul., Conium, Crocus, Diadem., Digit., Dulcam., Euphorb., EUPHRAS., FERR., Gelsem., GRAPHIT., HEPAR, Hydrast., *Ignat.*, *Ipecac.*, Kali bichr., Kali carb., Kreos., Laches., Lachnanth., Lauroc., *Ledum*, Leptand., LYCOP., MAR. VER., Menyanth., *Merc. viv.*, *Merc. corr.*, MEZER., Mosch., Mur. ac., Natr. carb., *Natr. mur.*, Natr. sulph., NITR. AC., NUX MOSCH., *Nux vom.*, OLEAND., Opium, Oxal. ac., Paris, PETROL., *Phosphor.*, Phosph. ac., *Platin.*, PLUMBUM, Podophyl., PULSAT., Ran. bulb., Rhodod., Rhus tox., *Sabad.*, SABIN., SCILLA, SEPIA, SILIC., Spigel., Stramon., Strontia, SULPHUR, TARAX., Valer., *Viol. tr.*

PARTIAL CHILL.

Partial chill, in general: *Acon.*, Agar., Agn. cast., Alum., AMBRA, Amm. carb., Amm. mur., Anac., Ant. tart., Apis, Argent., Arnic., Arsen., Asar., Aurum, *Baryt.*, *Bellad.*, Borax, Bovist., Brom., BRYON., *Calc. carb.*, Camphor., Cann. sat., Canthar., Capsic., Carb. an., Carb. veg., *Caustic.*, CHAMOM., *Chelid.*, Cicut., *Cinchon.*, Coccul., Coffea, Colchic., Coloc., Conium, Crocus, Cuprum, Digit., Droser., Dulcam., Euphorb., Euphras., Graphit., Guaiac., Helleb., Hepar, Hyosc., *Ignat.*, Iod., Ipecac., Kali carb., *Kreos.*, Laches., Lauroc., Ledum, Lycop., Magn. carb., Mangan., *Menyanth.*, *Merc. viv.*, Merc. corr., Mezer., Mosch., Mur. ac., Natr. carb., Natr. mur., Nitrum, Nitr. ac., Nux mosch., *Nux vom.*, Oleand., Opium, Paris, Petrol., Phosphor., *Phosph. ac.*, Platin., Plumbum, *Pulsat.*, *Ran. bulb.*, Rhodod., *Rhus tox.*, Ruta, Sabad., Sabin., Sambuc., Sarsap., Scilla, Secal., Seneg., *Sepia*, Silic., SPIGEL., Spong., Stann., Staphis., Stramon., Strontia, *Sulphur*, Thuya, Valer., VERATR., Viol. tr., Zinc.

Chill; body, upper, on the: Agar., Baryt., CINA, *Euphorb.*, Menyanth., Rhus tox.

— — **lower,** on the: Acon., ARNIC., Nux vom., Pulsat., Sarsap.

— — **anterior,** on the: *Chamom.*, Pulsat.

Chill; body, posterior, on the: *Chamom.*, COCCUL., IGNAT., *Rhus tox.*, Strontia.

— **head,** on the: Acon., Agar., *Agn. cast.*, Ambra, Asar., Baryt., *Calc. carb.*, Cann. sat., Carb. veg., Caustic., Chelid., Cinchon., Dulcam., Kali carb., Kreos., Laches., Lauroc., *Merc. viv.*, MERC. CORR., Mosch., *Nux vom.*, Phosph. ac., Rhus tox., RUTA, Sabin., *Sepia*, Spigel., STANN., Staphis., STRONTIA, *Sulphur*, Thuya, *Veratr.*

— — **spreading** from the: Mosch.

— — — **occiput:** *Valer.*

— **eyes,** on the: Amm. carb., Asar., Calc. carb., Conium, Crocus, Kali carb., Lycop., Paris, *Platin.*

— **ears,** on the: *Calc. carb.*, *Ipecac.*, Kali carb., Laches., Menyanth., *Merc. viv.*, Platin., Seneg., Staphis., Veratr.

— **nose,** on the: Ant. crud., Bellad., Ignat., Menyanth., Merc. viv., *Nux vom.*, Plumbum, Veratr.

— **face,** in the: Acon., Arnic., Baryt., *Calc. carb.*, Camphor., Caustic., *Chamom.*, Cina, Cinchon., Droser., Ignat., Lauroc., *Lycop.*, Merc. viv., Merc. corr., Mosch., *Nux vom.*, Phosphor., Phosph. ac., *Platin.*, Pulsat., Ran. bulb., *Rheum*, Rhodod., Ruta, Sabin., Sepia, Spigel., Strontia.

— — **spreading** from the: *Baryt.*

— **lips,** on the: Apis, Platin., Sepia.

— — — **beginning:** Bryon.

— **pit of the stomach,** in the: Ant. tart., Arsen., Baryt., *Bellad.*, Camphor., Caustic., *Colchic.*, Ignat., *Ipecac.*, Lauroc., Natr. mur., Nux vom., Phosphor., Spigel., Spong.

— — **spreading** from the: Baryt.

— **stomach,** commencing in the: Calc. carb.

— **hypochondria,** about the: Nux vom., Pulsat.

— **abdomen,** on the: Acon., Ambra, *Arsen.*, CALAD., Cinchon., Colchic., Kali carb., Magn. carb., Mar. ver., Menyanth., *Merc. viv.*, Mezer., Nitr. ac., Nux vom., Opium, *Paris*, Phosph. ac., *Pulsat.*, Ran. bulb., Secal., *Spigel.*, Sulphur, Zinc.

— — **spreading** from the: *Calad.*, *Mar. ver.*, Paris.

Chill; neck, on the: Calc. carb., Dulcam., Kali carb., Phosphor., Sulphur, Valer.

— **chest,** on the: Calc. carb., *Cicut.*, Coffea, *Digit.*, Merc. viv., Natr. carb., Nux vom., Paris, *Ran. bulb.*, *Spigel.*, Sulphur.

— — **spreading** from the: *Cicut.*, *Spigel.*

— **shoulders,** on the: Psorin.

— **scapulæ,** on the: Alum., Amm. mur., Aurum, *Caustic.*, Kreos., *Rhus tox.*, Silic., Strontia, Viol. od.

— — **spreading** from the: *Rhus tox.*

— **back,** on the: Acon., Act. rac., Agar., Alum., Amm. mur., ANAC., Apis, Argent., Arnic., Arsen., Asaf., Asar., Aurum, Baryt., BELLAD., BORAX, Bovist., Camphor., Calc. carb., CANTHAR., *Capsic.*, Carb. veg., *Caustic.*, *Cinchon.*, COCCUL., *Coffea*, COLCHIC., Conium, Crocus, *Digit.*, *Dulcam.*, Gelsem., Graphit., Guaiac., Helleb., Hepar, Hydrast., HYOSC., Ignat., Kali bichr., Kreos., Laches., Lauroc., Ledum, Leptand., Lobel. inf., Lycop., MAGN. CARB., MENYANTH., Merc. viv., MEZER., Mosch., Mur. ac., Natr. mur., Natr. sulph., Nux mosch., Nux vom., Opium, PHOSPHOR., Phosph. ac., Platin., PULSAT., Ran. bulb., *Rhus tox.*, RUTA, Sabad., Sarsap., Scilla, *Secal.*, Seneg., SEPIA, Silic., SPIGEL., SPONG., STANN., Staphis., *Stramon.*, *Sulphur*, Thuya, Valer., Veratr.

— — **spreading** from the: Argent., CAPSIC., Crocus, Dulcam., *Eup. purp.*, Kali hydr., *Staphis.*

— **small of the back,** on the: *Bryon.*, Canthar., Carb. veg., Helleb., HYOSC., Kreos., Laches., Lauroc., *Lycop.*, Merc. viv., Merc. corr., Phosph. ac., *Pulsat.*, *Rhus tox.*, Sabad., Sabin., Spong., STRONTIA, *Sulphur.*

— — **spreading** from the: *Eup. purp.*, *Hyosc.*, *Strontia.*

— **upper limbs,** on the, in general: *Acon.*, Amm. carb., Anac., Baryt., BELLAD., *Bryon.*, Cann. sat., *Caustic.*, Chelid., Cinchon., CICUT., Coccul., Crocus, Cuprum, Digit., Dulcam., Euphras., Graphit., Helleb., Hepar, *Ignat.*, Kali bichr., Kali carb., Mangan., Merc. viv., Mezer., Mosch., *Nux vom.*, Petrol., Phosph. ac., *Plumbum*, Pulsat., Ran. bulb., *Rhus tox.*, Ruta,

SABAD., Scilla, Secal., Sepia, Silic., *Spigel.*, Staphis., Thuya, *Veratr.*, Zinc.

Chill; upper arm, on the: Coccul., Graphit., *Ignat.*, MEZER., Phosph. ac., Psorin., Pulsat., Ran. bulb.

— — **spreading** from the: *Mezer.*

— **forearm,** on the: Bryon., Caustic., Ignat., Nux vom., *Rhus tox.*

— **hands,** on the: Ambra, Anac., *Baryt.*, *Bellad.*, Chelid., CUPRUM, *Digit.*, Droser., Iod., Laches., Menyanth., Mosch., *Natr. mur.*, Nux vom., Phosphor., *Rhus tox.*, SABAD., Sambuc., Spigel., Veratr., Zinc.

— — **spreading** from the: Digit., Gelsem.

— — — and **leaving at the heart:** Digit.

— **fingers,** on the: Acon., *Cuprum*, Digit., Kali carb., Kreos., Mangan., MENYANTH., *Merc. viv.*, *Phosph. ac.*, Ran. bulb., Spigel., Sulphur, Thuya.

— — **tips** of the: Bryon., Menyanth., Natr. mur.

— **lower limbs,** on the, in general: Acon., Agar., Ambra, Argent., Arnic., BELLAD., Camphor., Capsic., Carb. an., Carb. veg., Caustic., Chelid., CICUT., *Cinchon.*, COCCUL., Coloc., *Crocus*, Cuprum, Droser., Euphorb., Helleb., Hepar, *Ignat.*, Kali bichr., Kreos., Lauroc., Ledum, Lycop., *Merc. viv.*, Merc. corr., MEZER., Mosch., Natr. carb., Nitr. ac., Nux mosch., Nux vom., Oleand., *Paris*, Petrol., Plumbum, *Pulsat.*, Ran. bulb., Rhodod., *Rhus tox.*, SABAD., Sabin., Sambuc., Secal., SEPIA, *Spigel.*, Spong., Sulphur, Valer., Veratr.

— **thighs,** on the: Agar., Arnic., Bellad., *Bryon.*, Capsic., Cicut., *Cinchon.*, Helleb., Hydrast., Ignat., Lycop., Merc. viv., Mosch., Nitr. ac., Oleand., Psorin., *Pulsat.*, Ran. bulb., Rhodod., Sambuc., Sepia, SPONG., STRONTIA.

— **knees,** on the: Caustic., *Cinchon.*, Coloc., Ignat., Laches., *Menyanth.*, Nitr. ac., Phosphor., *Pulsat.*, Sepia.

— **legs,** on the: Ambra, ARSEN., Baryt., Bellad., CHELID., Cinchon., Kreos., *Pulsat.*

—**feet,** on the: Acon., *Amm. carb.*, Anac., Argent., Arsen., *Baryt.*, *Bellad.*, *Brom.*, Chelid., Coloc., Crocus, CUPRUM,

Digit., *Droser.*, Ignat., Kreos., Lauroc., Lycop., *Magn. carb.*, MENYANTH., Merc. viv., Mezer., Natr. mur., Nux mosch., Paris, Pulsat., Ran. bulb., *Rhus tox.*, SABAD., Sambuc., Sepia, *Sulphur*, Valer., Veratr.

Chill; feet, spreading from the: *Baryt.*, Digit., Hyosc., Kali bichr., RHUS TOX., *Sulphur.*

— **toes,** on the: Bryon., Menyanth., Natr. mur.

COLDNESS.

Coldness; in general: Acon., Ambra., Amm. carb., *Amm. mur.*, Anac., *Ant. tart.*, *Arnic.*, *Arsen.*, Asaf., Asar., *Aurum*, Baryt., Bellad., *Bismuth.*, Borax, Bovist., Brom., *Bryon.*, *Calad.*, Calc. carb., CAMPHOR., *Cann. sat.*, *Canthar.*, Capsic., Carb. an., *Carb. veg.*, *Caustic.*, *Chamom.*, *Chelid.*, Cinchon., Coccul., Coffea, Colchic., *Coloc.*, *Conium*, Corn. cir., Crocus, CUPRUM, Cyclam., Digit., Droser., *Dulcam.*, *Euphorb.*, *Euphras.*, *Ferr.*, Graphit., *Helleb.*, *Hydr. ac.*, HYOSC., Ignat., Iod., Ipecac., Kreos., *Laches.*, *Lachnanth.*, *Lauroc.*, *Ledum*, Lobel. inf., *Lycop.*, *Magn. carb.*, Mangan., Menyanth., Merc. viv., Merc. corr., MEZER., *Mosch.*, Mur. ac., *Natr. carb.*, *Natr. mur.*, Natr. sulph., *Nitrum*, Nitr. ac., Nux mosch., *Nux vom.*, Oleand., OPIUM, *Oxal. ac.*, Paris, Petrol., Phosphor., Phosph. ac., Platin., *Plumbum*, *Psorin.*, PULSAT., *Ran bulb.*, *Rhus tox.*, Ruta, Sabad., Sabin., Sambuc., *Sarsap.*, Scilla, Secal., Selen., *Sepia*, Silic., Spigel., Spong., STAPHIS., *Stramon.*, Sulphur, Thuya, Valer., VERATR., Verbas., Zinc.

— **with gooseflesh:** Lachnanth.

PARTIAL COLDNESS.

Coldness; affected parts, of the: *Angust.*, Arsen., Coccul., Dulcam., Laches., *Ledum*, Merc. viv., Petrol., Platin., Plumbum, Rhodod., *Rhus tox.*, Silic., Thuya.

— **one-sided:** Ant. tart., Arnic., Baryt., BRYON., Carb. veg., CAUSTIC., Chelid., Cinchon., Coccul., Digit., DROSER., Ipecac., *Lycop.*, MOSCH., *Nux vom.*, PARIS, Phosphor.,

Phosph. ac., PULSAT., Rheum, *Rhus tox.*, *Ruta*, Sabad., Sulphur, THUYA, Verbas.

Coldness; posterior body, of: *Rhus tox.*

— **left side:** Arnic., *Caustic.*, Cinchon., DROSER., Paris, THUYA.

— **right side:** BRYON., Caustic., *Lycop.*, *Paris*, Phosph. ac., Pulsat., *Rhus tox.*

— **head,** of the: Agar., Alum., Amm. carb., *Apis*, Baryt., CALC. CARB., *Cist. can.*, Graphit., Magn. mur., Mangan., Phosphor., Phosph. ac., Rhodod., RHUS TOX., *Ruta*, Sabad., *Sepia*, *Sulphur*, Veratr.

— **ears,** of the: Dulcam., *Ipecac.*, Kali carb., Laches., Mangan., Merc. viv., *Platin.*, Seneg., Stann., *Veratr.*

— **nose,** of the: Apis, *Arnic.*, Bellad., Cinchon., Cyclam., Droser., Ignat., Natr. mur., *Nux vom.*, Phosph. ac., Plumbum, *Veratr.*

— **face,** of the: Ant. tart., Asar., Bellad., Bismuth., *Camphor.*, Canthar., Carb. veg., Chamom., Cicut., CINA, DROSER., *Hyosc.*, Ignat., *Ipecac.*, LYCOP., *Natr. carb.*, Nitr. ac., PETROL., Platin., Rheum, Rhus tox., VERATR.

— **cheeks,** of the: *Bellad.*, Chamom., Rheum.

— **lips,** of the: Apis.

— **chin,** of the: *Veratr.*

— **mouth,** in the: Acon., *Arsen.*, Camphor., *Carb. veg.*, Caustic., Colchic., Cuprum, Nitrum, Rhus tox., VERATR.

— **tongue,** of the: *Arsen.*, *Carb. veg.*, Colchic., Cuprum, *Oxal. ac.*, VERATR.

— **pit of the stomach,** of the: Ant. tart., Arsen., *Bellad.*, Camphor., Caustic., Ignat., Lauroc., Natr. mur., Nux vom., Phosphor., Spigel., Spong.

— **abdomen,** of the: *Ambra.*, Apis, Calad., Cinchon., Merc. viv., Merc. corr., Opium, *Paris*, Pulsat., *Sepia*, Spigel.

— **genitals,** of the: *Agn. cast.*, Cann. sat., Capsic., Caustic., Merc. viv., *Sulphur.*

— **glans penis,** of the: *Caustic.*, Merc. viv., Sulphur.

Coldness; scrotum, of the: *Agn. cast.*, Capsic.

— **chest,** of the: Cicut., Merc. viv., Merc. corr.

— **back,** of the: *Amm. mur.*, Calc. carb., Camphor., *Caustic.*, Crocus, Dulcam., Menyanth., Natr. mur., *Oxal. ac.*, *Rhus tox.*, *Secal.*, Stann., Thuya.

— **small of the back,** of the: Carb. veg., Phosph. ac., Spong.

— — **spreading,** from the: *Hyosc.*

— **upper limbs,** of the: Amm. carb., Apis, *Arnic.*, BELLAD., Bryon., Camphor., Chamom., Cicut., Cinchon., Digit., Dulcam., Euphorb., *Euphras.*, *Hydr. ac.*, Hyosc., Ipecac., Kali carb., Ledum, Merc. viv., Merc. corr., *Mezer.*, Natr. mur., Nux vom., Oleand., OPIUM, Phosphor., Plumbum, PULSAT., *Rhus tox.*, Ruta, Sabad., Secal., Sepia, Stramon., Sulphur, Thuya, Veratr.

— **hands,** of the: Acon., Agar., Agn. cast., Alum., Ambra, Amm. carb., Ant. tart., Apis, *Arnic.*, Arsen., Asar., AURUM, *Baryt.*, *Bellad.*, Bovist., Bryon., Calad., CALC. CARB., *Camphor.*, Cann. sat., Canthar., Capsic., Carb. an., Carb. veg., *Caustic.*, Chamom., CHELID., Cina, CINCHON., Coccul., Coffea, Colchic., *Coloc.*, Conium, Crocus, Cuprum, CYCLAM., DIGIT., DROSER., Euphras., Ferr., *Helleb.*, Hepar, Ignat., IOD., IPECAC., Kali carb., *Laches.*, Lauroc., Ledum, LYCOP., MANGAN., Mar. ver., MENYANTH., Merc. viv., Merc. corr., *Mezer.*, Mosch., MUR. AC., NATR. CARB., NATR. MUR., Nitrum, *Nitr. ac.*, Nux mosch., *Nux vom.*, OLEAND., *Oxal. ac.*, Paris, PETROL., *Phosphor.*, Phosph. ac., PULSAT., *Ran. bulb.*, *Rhus tox.*, RUTA, SABIN., SAMBUC., Sarsap., *Scilla*, *Selen.*, Sepia, Silic., Spigel., Spong., Stann., STRAMON., *Sulphur*, Sulph. ac., Therid., *Thuya*, *Veratr.*, Verbas., *Zinc.*

— **fingers,** of the: Acon., Amm. carb., Angust., *Ant. tart.*, Apis, Asar., Calad., *Calc. carb.*, Caustic., Chamom., CHELID., Cicut., Coccul., Coloc., Conium, *Digit.*, Helleb., Hepar, Lycop., Merc. viv., Mosch., Mur. ac., Nitr. ac., Paris, Phosphor., *Phosph. ac.*, Ran. bulb., Rhodod., Sarsap., *Sepia*, Spigel., Stann., *Sulphur*, TARAX., THUYA.

Coldness; tips of the fingers, of the: *Ant. tart.*, *Chelid.*, Phosph. ac., Ran. bulb., Sarsap., Spigel., Sulphur, *Tarax.*, *Thuya.*

— **lower limbs,** of the: Apis, *Arsen.*, BELLAD., *Bryon.*, CALAD., Carb. an., *Caustic.*, Chamom., Cicut., Cinchon., Digit., Euphorb., Hydr. ac., Hyosc., Ipecac., *Ledum.*, Lycop., Merc. viv., Merc. corr., *Mezer.*, Natr. carb., Natr. mur., *Nitrum*, NITR. AC., *Nux vom.*, Oleand., OPIUM, Petrol., Phosphor., Plumbum, PULSAT., Rhodod., Sabad., Secal., SEPIA, Stramon., Strontia, *Sulphur*, *Thuya.*

— **thighs,** of the: Agar., *Calad.*, *Calc. carb.*, *Merc. viv.*, Nitr. ac., Nux vom., Oleand., Rhodod., SPONG., *Sulphur*, Thuya.

— **knees,** of the: AGN. CAST., Ambra, Arsen., Aurum, Cann. sat., *Carb. veg.*, Cinchon., Coloc., Mezer., Nitr. ac., Petrol., Phosphor., *Pulsat.*, Sepia, Stann., Sulphur.

— **legs,** of the: Ambra, Arsen., Aurum, *Calad.*, Chelid., Ignat., Ledum, Mangan., Merc. viv., Rhus tox., Sambuc., *Silic.*, Sulphur, Thuya.

— **feet,** of the: *Acon.*, Alum., *Ambra*, AMM. CARB., *Amm. mur.*, Anac., ANT. CRUD., ANT. TART., *Arnic.*, Arsen., Asar., AURUM, Baryt., *Bellad.*, Bovist., BROM., Bryon., *Calad.*, *Calc. carb.*, Camphor., Cann. sat., Canthar., *Capsic.*, Carb. an., Carb. veg., CAUSTIC., Chamom., CHELID., Cicut., CINCHON., Coccul., *Coffea*, Colchic., *Coloc.*, CONIUM, Crocus, Cuprum, Cyclam., DIGIT., DROSER., Euphras., Ferr., GRAPHIT., Helleb., Hepar, Hyosc., Ignat., IOD., IPECAC., *Kali carb.*, KREOS., LACHES., Lauroc., Ledum, LYCOP., Magn. carb., Magn. mur., MANGAN., MENYANTH., Merc. viv., *Merc. corr.*, *Mezer.*, *Mur. ac.*, NATR. CARB., NATR. MUR., NITRUM, NITR. AC., Nux vom., *Oleand.*, PARIS, PETROL., *Phosphor.*, PHOSPH. AC., *Platin.*, Plumbum, PULSAT., Ran. bulb., RHODOD., *Rhus tox.*, RUTA., Sabad., SABIN., SAMBUC., SARSAP., SCILLA, Selen., SEPIA, SILIC., Stann., Staphis., STRAMON., Strontia, SULPHUR, Sulph. ac., THUYA, Valer., *Veratr.*, Verbas., Zinc.

— **toes,** of the: Acon., Brom., *Calad.*, *Digit.*, *Sulphur.*

SENSATION OF COLDNESS.

Sensation of coldness, in general: Acon., Agar., *Arnic.*, Asar., Baryt., Bellad., Bovist., Bryon., *Calc. carb.*, Camphor., Cann. sat., Canthar., *Caustic.*, Chelid., *Cinchon.*, COCCUL., Coffea, Crocus, Digit., Droser., Dulcam., Euphorb., Graphit., Helleb., Ignat., Kali bichr., Kreos., Laches., LAUROC., *Lycop.*, Magn. carb., MENYANTH., *Merc. viv.*, Mezer., MOSCH., *Mur. ac.*, Paris, Phosphor., Phosph. ac., *Platin.*, Plumbum, Phodophyl., *Psorin.*, PULSAT., Rhodod., RHUS TOX., Ruta, *Secal.*, SEPIA., Spigel., Stann., Staphis., SULPHUR, *Veratr.*, VERBAS., Zinc.

(Compare Slight Chilliness and Chilliness.)

PARTIAL SENSATION OF COLDNESS.

Sensation of coldness; head, on the: Agar., *Agn. cast.*, Ambra, Asar., Baryt., *Calc. carb.*, Cann. sat., Carb. veg., Chelid., Dulcam., Kali carb., Laches., Lauroc., Merc. viv., *Merc. corr.*, Nux vom., Phosph. ac., *Sepia*, Spigel., Stann., Staphis., *Sulphur*, *Veratr.*

— — **in** the: *Acon.*, Ambra, Arnic., Arsen., Asar., Baryt., *Bellad.*, CALC. CARB., Cann. sat., *Chelid.*, *Cist. can.*, Crocus., Dulcam., Ignat., Laches., Lauroc., Mangan., Merc. viv., Mosch., Natr. mur., *Phosphor.*, Phosph. ac., Platin., Pulsat., *Sepia*, Spong., Sulphur, Valer., *Veratr.*

— **eyes,** in the: Acon., *Alum.*, Amm. carb., Asaf., *Asar.*, CALC. CARB., Caustic., *Conium*, Crocus, Fluor. ac., Graphit., Kali carb., Lycop., Paris, Phosph. ac., *Platin.*, Seneg., *Thuya.*

— **eyelids,** on the: Asar., Graphit., Kali carb., Phosph. ac.

— **ears,** on the: Calc. carb., *Ipecac.*, Menyanth., Staphis., Veratr.

— **nose,** in the: Anac., ANT. CRUD., Ignat.

— **face,** in the: Acon., Arnic., Baryt., CALC. CARB., Camphor., Caustic., *Cina*, Cinchon., Ignat., *Lycop.*, Merc. viv., Merc. corr., Mosch., Nux vom., Phosphor., PHOSPH. AC., PLATIN., *Ran. bulb.*, Ran. scel., Rheum, Rhodod., Strontia.

Sensation of coldness; face, on one side of the: Phosph. ac.

— **lips,** on the: *Platin.*, Sepia.

— **chin,** on the: *Platin.*

— **teeth,** on the: Alum., Asar., Carb. veg., Droser., Natr. carb., Nitr. ac., Petrol., Phosphor., *Phosph. ac.*, *Rheum*, *Sepia*, SPIGEL.

— **mouth,** in the: Asar., *Veratr.*

— **tongue,** on the: Bellad., Lauroc., Mezer., Veratr.

— **larynx,** in the: *Cist. can.*

— **œsophagus,** in the: *Argent.*, Bismuth., *Carb. veg.*, *Caustic.*, Lauroc., Menyanth., Mezer., Nitrum, Phosphor., Sulphur, *Veratr.*

— **stomach,** in the: Acon., Alum., Amm. carb., Ant. tart., ARSEN., Baryt., Bovist., Camphor., *Capsic.*, Chelid., Cinchon., COLCHIC., *Conium*, Graphit., Ignat., IPECAC., Laches., Lauroc., Magn. carb., Mezer., Natr. mur., *Nitrum*, Nitr. ac., Nux vom., *Phosphor.*, Phosph. ac., *Pulsat.*, Rhus tox., Sabad., Spigel., Spong., *Sulphur*, Sulph. ac., Veratr., Zinc.

— **hypochondria,** in the: Natr. carb.

— **abdomen,** in the: Acon., Alum., *Ambra*, Angust., ARSEN., Asaf., Bovist., *Calc. carb.*, *Camphor.*, Caustic., Cinchon., *Colchic.*, Helleb., KALI CARB., Kreos., Lauroc., Magn. carb., *Mar. ver.*, MENYANTH., *Merc. viv.*, Mezer., Natr. carb., Nux vom., *Oleand.*, Paris, *Petrol.*, *Phosphor.*, *Phosph. ac.*, Plumbum, *Pulsat.*, Ruta, Sabad., Sarsap., SECAL., *Sepia*, Sulphur, ZINC.

— **genitals,** on the (Scrotum): *Brom.*, Merc. viv.

— **trachea,** in the: *Argent.*, Arnic., *Arsen.*, Brom., *Bryon.*, Camphor., *Carb. veg.*, Cinchon., Merc. viv., Mur. ac., Phosphor., *Rhus tox.*, *Sulphur*, *Veratr.*

— **throat and neck,** on the: *Calc. carb.*, Phosphor., Sulphur.

— **chest,** in the: Alum., *Apis*, Arnic., ARSEN., Brom., BRYON., *Calc. carb.*, Camphor., Carb. an., Cicut., Graphit., *Laches.*, NATR. CARB., *Natr. mur.*, Nux vom., *Oleand.*,

Paris, Petrol., Ran. bulb., Rhus tox., Ruta, Spigel., *Sulphur*, *Zinc.*

Sensation of coldness; chest, (external) on the: *Calc. carb.*, Digit., Natr. mur., Paris, Ran. bulb.

— **scapulæ,** on the: Alum., Amm. mur., Aurum, *Caustic.*, Kreos., *Rhus tox.*, Viol. tr.

— — **between** the (like ice): Lachnanth.

— **back,** on the: Acon., Amm. mur., Angust., Apis, Arnic., *Arsen.*, Asar., Bellad., Borax, *Calc. carb.*, Camphor., Canthar., Capsic., Carb. veg., *Caustic.*, Cinchon., COCCUL., Coffea, Colchic., Conium, *Crocus*, Digit., Dulcam., Guaiac., Helleb., Hepar, *Hyosc.*, Ignat., Kreos., Laches., Lauroc., Ledum, Lycop., Menyanth., Mezer., Mosch., MUR. AC., Natr. mur., Nux mosch., Nux vom., Opium, PULSAT., Ran. bulb., *Rhus tox.*, Ruta, Sabad., Scilla, SECAL., *Sepia*, Silic., *Spong.*, *Stann.*, Staphis., Stramon., Sulphur, Veratr.

— **small of the back,** on the: *Bryon.*, Canthar., Helleb., Lauroc., Lycop., Merc. viv., *Merc. corr.*, Pulsat., *Rhus tox.*, Sabad., Sabin., Spong., Strontia.

— **upper limbs,** on the: *Acon.*, Ambra, Anac., Baryt., Bellad., *Bryon.*, Cann. sat., CAUSTIC., Chelid., Cicut., Cinchon., Coccul., Crocus, Digit., Dulcam., Euphras., Graphit., Helleb., Hepar, *Ignat.*, Mangan., Menyanth., Mezer., Mosch., Nux vom., Petrol., Phosphor., Phosph. ac., Plumbum, Pulsat., Ran. bulb., *Rhus tox.*, Ruta, Sambuc., Scilla, SECAL., Sepia, Spigel., Staphis., Thuya, Veratr., Zinc.

— **hands,** on the: Acon., Menyanth., Mosch., Spigel., Zinc.

— **fingers,** on the: Kali carb., Kreos., *Menyanth.*, Merc. viv., *Phosph. ac.*, Ran. bulb., Spigel., Sulphur, Thuya.

— **tips of the fingers,** on the: *Phosph. ac.*

— **lower limbs,** on the: *Acon.*, Agar., Camphor., Carb. veg., Caustic., Cicut., Cinchon., Hepar, *Ignat.*, Kreos., *Merc. viv.*, Mezer., Natr. carb., Nux vom., Paris, Petrol., Plumbum, Pulsat., Rhodod., Rhus tox., SABIN., *Sambuc.*, SECAL., SEPIA, Spigel., Spong.

— — **right,** on the: *Sabin.*

Sensation of coldness; thighs, on the: Arnic., Bellad., CAPSIC., Helleb., *Lycop.*, Mosch., Oleand., Pulsat., Ran. bulb., Rhodod., *Spong.*

— **knees,** on the: Cinchon., Coloc., Digit., Ignat., Menyanth., Phosphor., Veratr.

— **legs,** on the: Ambra, *Arsen.*, Baryt., Bellad., Chelid., Cinchon., Ignat., Kreos., Ledum, Menyanth., Mosch., *Pulsat.*, Rhodod., Rhus tox., Ruta, *Sambuc.*, Strontia, *Therid.*, Valer.

— **feet;** on the: Acon., Argent., Arsen., Bellad., Chelid., *Coloc.*, Droser., Ignat., Kreos., Lauroc., Merc. viv., NITR. AC., NUX MOSCH., Sambuc., Sulphur, Valer., Veratr., ZINC.

— **toes,** on the: Acon., Ran. bulb., Sulphur, Veratr.

SHIVERING.

Shivering; in general: Acon., Agar., Alum., Amm. carb., Anac., Angust., *Apis*, Argent., Arnic., *Arsen.*, Asaf., Asar., *Aurum*, Baryt., Bellad., Borax, Bryon., Calad., Calc. carb., *Camphor.*, *Cann. sat.*, *Capsic.*, *Carb. an.*, Carb. veg., *Caustic.*, *Chamom.*, *Chelid.*, *Cina*, *Cinchon.*, *Clemat.*, *Coccul.*, *Coffea*, COLCHIC., COLOC., Conium, Crocus, *Cyclam.*, Digit.,*Droser.*, Dulcam., *Euphorb.*, *Eup. perf.*, *Eup. purp.*, *Ferr.*, Guaiac., Helleb., Hepar, Hyosc., *Ignat.*, Ipecac., Kali carb., Kreos., *Laches.*, *Lauroc.*, *Ledum*, Leptand., Lobel. inf., Lycop., *Magn. carb.*, Magn mur., Mangan., *Menyanth.*, Merc. viv., Merc. corr., Mezer., *Mosch.*, *Mur. ac.*, *Natr. carb.*, Natr. mur., Nitrum, Nitr. ac., *Nux vom.*, *Oleand.*, Opium, *Oxal. ac.*, Paris, PHOSPHOR., *Phosph. ac.*, *Platin.*, Plumbum, *Podophyl.*, *Psorin.*, PULSAT., Rheum, Rhus tox., *Ruta*, Sabad., Sanguin., Sarsap., SEPIA, Silic., Spigel., Spong., Stann., *Staphis.*, Stramon., Sulphur, Sulph. ac., *Tarax.*, Thuya, Valer., Veratr., VERBAS., Viol. od., *Zinc.*

— **ascending:** *Acon.*, Agar., Carb. an., *Cina*, Colchic., Hyosc., *Laches.*, Pulsat., Sabad., *Sarsap.*, Spigel., Strontia, Sulphur.

Shivering; descending: Agar., *Bellad.*, Caustic., *Chelid.*, Coffea, Colchic., *Crocus*, Mosch., Psorin., *Sabad.*, Staphis., Sulph. ac., *Valer.*, *Zinc.*

— **flitting,** (überlaufender): Acon., ANAC., *Angust.*, ASAF., Aurum., *Colchic.*, *Conium*, KALI CARB., *Menyanth.*, Paris, Secal., Silic., Spigel., Thuya.

— **Goose-flesh,** with: Angust., Aurum, Baryt., *Camphor.*, Cann. sat., *Caustic.*, Cinchon., Ignat., Lauroc., Ledum., Mezer., SABAD., Sabin., Sarsap., Staphis., Sulph. ac., Thuya, Veratr.

— **internal:** *Chelid.*, COFFEA, Droser., Helleb., IGNAT., PHOSPHOR., *Psorin.*, Rheum.

— **one side,** of: Alum., Ambra, Anac., Ant. tart., Arnic., Baryt., *Bellad.*, Bryon., *Caustic.*, Chamom., Cinchon., *Coccul.*, Crocus, Digit., Ignat., Kali carb., Lycop., Natr. carb., NUX VOM., Paris, Phosphor., Phosph. ac., Platin., *Pulsat.*, *Rhus tox.*, Ruta, Sabad., Sarsap., Spigel., Stann., Stramon., Sulphur, Sulph. ac., Thuya, VERBAS.

— **wandering:** Baryt., Chamom., *Colchic.*, Rhus tox.

PARTIAL SHIVERING.

Shivering; head, on the: Argent., Arnic., Baryt., Bellad., Capsic., *Caustic.*, Chamom., Cina, *Coccul.*, *Menyanth.*, Merc. viv., Mosch., Phosph. ac., Platin., Ruta, Seneg., Sepia, *Silic.*, Staphis., STRONTIA, Sulphur, Thuya, Valer., Veratr.

— — **spreading,** from the: *Mosch.*, Valer.

— — — **occiput:** Bellad., Silic., *Valer.*

— **face,** in the: Acon., *Arnic.*, Calc. carb., *Caustic.*, *Chamom.* Ignat., Lauroc., Merc. viv., Phosph. ac., PULSAT., *Rhodod.*, Ruta, Staphis., Stramon.

— spreading from the: *Caustic.*

— **chin,** on the: Stramon.

— **pit of the stomach,** in the: *Bellad.*, Caustic.

— **hypochondriæ,** about the: Pulsat.

— **abdomen,** on the: *Bellad.*, Camphor., Cann. sat.,

Chamom., Coffea, *Coloc.*, Phosph. ac., Pulsat., Sabad., Spigel., Staphis., Zinc.

Shivering; scrotum, on the: August., Zinc.

— **throat and neck,** over the: Amm. carb., Bellad., Caustic., Chamom., Conium, Crocus., *Graphit.*, Staphis., Valer.

— **chest,** over the: Acon., Carb. an., Cina, Cinchon., Coccul., *Digit.*, Guaiac., Hepar, MENYANTH., Nitrum, *Nux vom.*, *Platin.*, Ruta, Spigel., Staphis.

— **scapulæ,** over the: *Bellad.*, Bryon., *Nitr. ac.*, Ran. bulb., STRONTIA.

— **back,** over the: Acon., ANAC., *August.*, ASAF., Aurum, BELLAD., Borax, Bovist., Canthar., Capsic., Carb. an., Carb. veg., *Caustic.*, Chamom., CHELID., *Cinchon.*, *Coccul.*, Coffea, COLCHIC., CROCUS, DIGIT., *Graphit.*, Guaiac., Hepar, Kali carb., LACHES., Ledum, Mangan., MENYANTH., Merc. viv., Mezer., Mosch., NATR. MUR., Nitr. ac., Nux vom., Paris, Phosphor., Phosph. ac., Platin., PULSAT., Rhus tox., Ruta, SABAD., Sabin., Sanguin., SENEG., Sepia, Spigel., Spong., Staphis., Strontia, Sulphur, Thuya, Veratr., ZINC.

— **spreading from the back:** Bovist., CROCUS.

— **small of the back,** over the: Asaf., *Nitr. ac.*, Rhodod., Strontia.

— **upper limbs,** on the: Acon., Arnic., Baryt., *Bellad.*, Camphor., *Chamom.*, Chelid., *Cinchon.*, Helleb., Ignat., Lauroc., MENYANTH., Merc. viv., Mezer., *Platin.*, Pulsat., Ran. bulb., Rhus tox., Spigel., Staphis., Sulphur, Veratr.

— **spreading from the arms:** Helleb.

— **lower limbs,** on the: Arnic., Bryon., Camphor., *Cann. sat.*, *Caustic.*, Cina, *Cinchon.*, *Coccul.*, Coloc., Conium, Graphit., Ignat., *Kali carb.*, Lycop., Magn. mur., Menyanth., Phosphor., *Platin.*, Pulsat., Ran. bulb., Sambuc., Sarsap., Spigel., Strontia.

— **knees,** on the: Cinchon., Sambuc.

— **legs,** on the: *Kali carb.*, Menyanth.

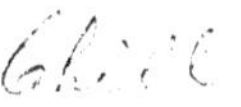

AGGRAVATION.

ACCORDING TO TIME.

Morning: Acon., Agar., Ambra, Anac., ANGUST., Ant. crud., Ant. tart., Apis, *Arnic.*, *Arsen.*, Baryt., Bellad., BOVIST., *Bryon.*, Calad., CALC. CARB., Carb. an., Carb. veg., Caustic., Cina, Cinchon., Coccul., Coffea, Coloc., CONIUM, *Cyclam.*, Droser., EUP. PERF., Euphras., *Gelsem.*, Graphit., Helleb., Hepar, Hydrast., Kali carb., Kreos., LEDUM, Lycop., Magn. carb., Magn. mur., Mangan., *Merc. viv.*, Mezer., *Mur. ac.*, Natr. carb., NATR. MUR., NITR. AC., Nux mosch., *Nux vom.*, *Phosphor.*, Phosph. ac., Plumbum, Pulsat., Rheum, *Rhodod.*, Rhus tox., Sarsap., Sepia, Silic., SPIGEL., *Staphis.*, Sulphur, Sulph. ac., *Therid.*, *Thuya*, *Veratr.*

Forenoon: Agar., Alum., AMBRA, Amm. carb., ANGUST., *Ant. crud.*, Ant. tart., Arnic., ARSEN., *Asar.*, Baryt., Bellad., Bovist., Bryon., CACT. GRAND., CALC. CARB., Cann. sat., Carb. an., *Carb. veg.*, Chamom., *Cinchon.*, CYCLAM., DROSER., *Euphras.*, Graphit., Guaiac., Kali carb., *Ledum*, Lycop., Magn. carb., Magn. mur., Merc. viv., Mur. ac., NATR. CARB., NATR. MUR., Nitrum, Nitr. ac., Opium, Paris, Petrol., Phosphor., *Phosph. ac.*, Platin., Plumbum, Pulsat., Ran. bulb., Rhodod., Rhus tox., *Sabad.*, *Sarsap.*, *Sepia*, Silic., STANN., Staphis., Stramon., STRONTIA, SULPHUR, *Sulph. ac.*, Thuya, VIOL. TR., Zinc.

Noon: Alum., *Ant. crud.*, Argent., Asar., Borax, Bryon., Calc. carb., Kali carb., Laches., Lobel. inf., Magn. carb., Natr. mur., Nux vom., *Phosphor.*, Ran. bulb., Stramon., Sulphur.

Afternoon: Æsc. hip., Alum., Amm. carb., Amm. mur., Anac., ANGUST., Ant. crud., Ant. tart., APIS, ARGENT., Arnic., *Arsen.*, ASAF., Asar., Baryt., Bellad., BORAX, *Bryon.*, Calc. carb., Camphor., *Canthar.*, CARB. AN., Carb. veg., *Caustic.*, Chamom., Cina, CINCHON., COCCUL., Coffea, CONIUM, *Crocus*, Digit., Droser., EUPHRAS., Graphit., GUAIAC., Hyosc., Ignat., Ipecac., Kali carb., Kali hydr., *Laches.*, LAUROC., LYCOP., Magn. carb., Magn. mur., Mar. ver., Merc. viv., Mezer., Natr. carb., Natr. mur., NITRUM, NITR.

AC., *Nux vom.*, Petrol., *Phosphor.*, Phosph. ac., *Psorin.*, *Pulsat.*, RAN. BULB., Rhus tox., SABAD., Sepia, Silic., *Spigel.*, Spong., Stann., Staphis., STRAMON., *Sulphur*, Sulph. ac., *Thuya*, Veratr., ZINC.

Evening: *Acon.*, Act. rac., Agar., *Agn. cast.*, ALUM., Ambra, AMM. CARB., *Amm. mur.*, Ant. crud., Ant. tart., *Apis*, *Argent.*, ARNIC., Arsen., Asar., *Aurum*, Baryt., BELLAD., *Borax.*, BOVIST., BRYON., *Calad.*, *Calc. carb.*, Camphor., *Canthar.*, *Capsic.*, *Carb. an.*, *Carb. veg.*, Caustic., Chamom., *Chelid.*, *Cina*, CINCHON., *Coccul.*, Coloc., Conium, *Crocus*, CYCLAM., *Dulcam.*, *Ferr.*, GRAPHIT., *Guaiac.*, Helleb., *Hepar*, Hydrast., Hyosc., Ignat., *Ipecac.*, KALI CARB., Kali hydr., *Laches.*, Lauroc., Ledum, LYCOP., *Magn. carb.*, *Magn. mur.*, *Mangan.*, Mar. ver., MERC. VIV., *Merc. corr.*, Mezer., *Mur. ac.*, *Natr. carb.*, *Natr. mur.*, Natr. sulph., NITRUM, *Nitr. ac.*, *Nux mosch.*, *Nux vom.*, Opium, Oxal. ac., *Paris*, PETROL., PHOSPHOR., *Phosph. ac.*, *Platin.*, PLUMBUM, *Psorin.*, PULSAT., *Ran. bulb.*, Ran. scel., *Rhodod.*, Rhus tox., *Sabad.*, *Sabin.*, Sambuc., Sanguin., Sarsap., *Scilla*, *Sepia*, *Silic.*, Spigel., Spong., *Stann.*, STAPHIS., Stramon., Strontia, SULPHUR, Sulph. ac., *Thuya*, Veratr., *Zinc.*

Night: Agar., Alum., AMBRA, Amm. carb., AMM. MUR., Angust., Ant. tart., Argent., *Arsen.*, AURUM, *Baryt.*, *Bellad.*, *Borax*, BOVIST., *Bryon.*, *Calad.*, Calc. carb., Canthar., Capsic., Carb. an., Carb. veg., CAUSTIC., Chamom., Cinchon., Conium, DROSER., Euphras., FERR., HEPAR, HYOSC., IOD., Ipecac., Kali carb., Kali hydr., Kreos., Lauroc., Lycop., Magn. carb., Magn. mur., Mangan., MERC. VIV., *Merc. corr.*, Mur. ac., Natr. mur., Natr. sulph., Nitr. ac., NUX VOM., Opium, PARIS, Petrol., PHOSPHOR., Phosph. ac., Pulsat., Ran. scel., Rhus tox., *Sabad.*, Sarsap., Scilla, Sepia, Silic., Spigel., Spong., Staphis., *Stramon.*, SULPHUR., Thuya, Veratr., Zinc.

Midnight; before: *Amm. carb.*, *Argent.*, Aurum, Cact. grand., Calad., Carb. an., Cinchon., Mur. ac., *Phosphor.*, PULSAT., Rhodod., Sabad., Sulphur, Veratr.

— **about:** *Arsen.*, CAUSTIC., Hepar, Silic., Stramon.

Midnight; after: Amm. mur., *Arsen.*, *Borax*, CALAD., Canthar., Caustic., Chamom., Coccul., Droser., Ferr., Kali carb., Lauroc., Nitrum, *Nux vom.*, Petrol., Phosphor., Ran. scel., Rhus tox., Scilla, *Sulphur*, Thuya.

Day, during the: Alum., *Ant. crud.*, Ant. tart., *Asar.*, DROSER., HELLEB., Hepar, *Kali carb.*, Natr. carb., Oxal. ac., Psorin., *Rhodod.*, *Sabin.*, Silic., Spigel., *Sulph. ac.*, Veratr. Viol. od.

Hour, returning at the same: *Ant. crud.*, Apis, BOVIST., CACT. GRAND., CHIN. SULPH., Cina, Conium, DIADEM., Gelsem., Graphit., *Helleb.*, Hepar, *Kali carb.*, *Lycop.*, Magn. mur., Phosphor., SABAD., SPIGEL., Stann., Staphis., *Thuya.*

— 7 A. M.: *Podophyl.*

— 7 to 9 A. M.: *Eup. perf.*

— 10 A. M.: STANN.

— 10 to 11 A. M.: *Arsen.*, NATR. MUR.

— 11 A. M. and 11 P. M.: CACT. GRAND.

— 12 noon: Elaps.

— noon to 2 P. M.: Laches.

— 2 P. M.: Calc. carb.

— 3 P. M., towards: Angust., *Apis*, *Conium.*, Staphis., Thuya.

— 4 and 8 P. M., between: *Bovist.*, Graphit., Helleb., *Hepar*, LYCOP., *Magn. mur.*, Natr. sulph.

— 9 P. M. to 10 A. M.: Magn. sulph.

Different times of the day: Eup. purp.

Every 14 days, returning: Arsen., Calc. carb., Cinchon., Pulsat.

Yearly return: Arsen., Carb. veg., Laches., Sulphur.

ACCORDING TO CIRCUMSTANCE.

Air, in the cold: AGAR., *Arsen.*, Bryon., *Camphor.*, CAPSIC., Caustic., Chamom., COFFEA, *Cyclam.*, Digit., Helleb., Hepar, Kali carb., MEZER., Mosch., Nux mosch.,

NUX VOM., Petrol., Phosphor., *Rhodod.*, *Rhus tox.*, Sabad., Sepia, Silic., Spigel., Veratr.

Air, in the open: AGAR., *Alum.*, *Amm. carb.*, ANAC., *Arsen.*, ASAR., Bellad., Borax, *Bryon.*, Calad., Cann. sat., Carb. an., Carb. veg., Caustic., *Chamom.*, *Chelid.*, *Cinchon.*, Coccul., Coffea, *Conium*, Dulcam., *Euphorb.*, Guaiac., HEPAR, Ignat., Kali carb., Kreos., Lauroc., Magn. mur., Mangan., Merc. viv., *Merc. corr.*, Mosch., Nitrum, *Nitr. ac.*, NUX MOSCH., NUX VOM., PETROL., Phosph. ac., PLATIN., PLUMBUM, Ran. bulb., Rhodod., *Rhus tox.*, Sarsap., Selen., SENEG., SEPIA, Silic., Spigel., Stramon., Strontia, Sulphur, Sulph. ac., *Tarax.*, Thuya, *Viol. tr.* ZINC.

— walking in the open: Anac., Ant. tart., *Arsen.*, Bellad., Borax, Bryon., Carb. an., Carb. veg., CHELID., *Cinchon.*, Coccul., Colchic., Conium, Digit., EUPHORB., Hepar, Mangan., *Merc. viv.*, *Merc. corr.*, Nux mosch., NUX VOM., Phosph. ac., Selen., *Silic.*, *Spigel.*, *Sulphur*, Sulph. ac., Tarax.

— — after: Agar., Amm. carb., Anac., *Arsen.*, Bryon., Cann. sat., Carb. veg., Kali carb., Lauroc., Nitr. ac., Nux vom., *Pulsat.*, *Rhus tox.*, *Sepia*, Spong., Staphis., Zinc.

Alternation of chill, with symptoms of the mind: Crocus, *Platin.*

— with pains: Cinchon., *Helleb.*, Kali carb., Natr. mur.

Anger, after: Acon., Arsen., *Bryon.*, Mar. ver., Nux vom.

Awaking, when: ALUM., *Ambra*, ARNIC., Arsen., *Bryon.*, Calc. carb., Caustic., Hepar, *Lycop.*, Merc. viv., Nitr. ac., Nux vom., Phosphor., Pulsat., Sabad., Sambuc., Sarsap., *Sepia*, Silic., Staphis., Sulphur, Thuya, Veratr.

Bed, in: *Acon.*, Agn. cast., ALUM., *Ambra*, Amm. carb., Amm. mur., *Angust.*, Ant. tart., Argent., Arnic., *Arsen.*, AURUM, Baryt., *Bellad.*, Borax, Bovist., *Bryon.*, Calad., Calc. carb., Canthar., Capsic., CARB. AN., Carb. veg., Caustic., CHELID., CINCHON., Clemat., Coloc., DROSER., FERR., Graphit., Guaiac., Helleb., HEPAR, HYOSC., Iod., Ipecac., *Kali carb.*, Kreos., Lauroc., Ledum, LYCOP., *Magn. carb.*, Magn. mur., Mangan., Menyanth., MERC. VIV., *Merc. corr.*,

Mur. ac., Natr. carb., Natr. mur., Natr. sulph., Nitrum, NITR. AC., *Nux vom.*, *Paris*, Petrol., *Phosphor.*, *Phosph. ac.*, Platin., PULSAT., *Rhodod.*, Rhus tox., *Sabad.*, Sabin., Sambuc., Sanguin., Sarsap., Scilla, *Selen.*, Sepia, SILIC., Spigel., Spong., Stann., Staphis., Strontia, SULPHUR, Sulph. ac., Thuya, Veratr., *Zinc.*

Bed, after getting out of: Acon., *Amm. mur.*, Borax, Bryon., CALC. CARB., Canthar., Carb. veg., *Chamom.*, Coloc., Euphras., Graphit., *Helleb.*, *Laches.*, Lauroc., Mangan., MERC. VIV., Mezer., Natr. carb., Natr. mur., Natr. sulph., *Nux vom.*, *Phosphor.*, Pulsat., Ran. bulb., *Rhus tox.*, *Spigel.*, Staphis., Sulphur, Veratr.

Cold; after taking: Acon., Arsen., Bellad., *Bryon.*, Calc. carb., *Camphor.*, Chamom., Cinchon., Graphit., *Lycop.*, *Merc. viv.*, *Nux vom.*, Phosphor., *Pulsat.*, Rhus tox., *Sepia*, Silic., Spigel., Sulphur, Veratr.

— — from **getting wet through**: Bellad., *Bryon.*, Calc. carb., Colchic., Hepar, Lycop., Nux mosch., Pulsat., *Rhus tox.*, Sarsap., SEPIA.

— **things,** from touching: Natr. mur., Silic., *Zinc.*

Coryza, during the: Anac., *Ant. tart.*, Bryon., Calad., Capsic., Caustic., *Chamom.*, GRAPHIT., Hepar, Natr. carb., *Nux vom.*, PULSAT., Spigel., Spong., Sulphur.

Cough, with the: *Arsen.*, Bryon., Calc. carb., Carb. veg., *Conium*, Cuprum, Hyosc., *Mezer.*, Nux vom., Phosphor., PULSAT., *Rhus tox.*, *Sabad.*, Sepia, Sulphur, *Veratr.*

Denudation: see uncovering.

Draught, in a: Bellad., *Calc. carb.*, Canthar., CAPSIC., Cinchon., Hepar, Kali carb., Selen., Silic., Sulphur.

Drinking, after: Ant. tart., Arnic., ARSEN., ASAR., Bryon., Cann. sat., CAPSIC., CINCHON., Coccul., Crocus, Eup. perf., Hepar, *Lobel. inf.*, Mezer., Natr. mur., Nitr. ac., NUX VOM., Pulsat., *Rhus tox.*, *Silic.*, Sulphur, *Tarax.*, VERATR.

Eating, before: Ambra, Bovist., Calc. carb., *Carb. an.*, Carb.

veg., Cinchon., Euphorb., *Graphit.*, Iod., Lauroc., Lycop., *Natr. carb.*, Phosphor., Pulsat., Rhus tox., Sepia, Sulphur.

Eating, while: Carb. an., Carb. veg., Coccul., Conium., EUPHORB., Kali carb., Nitr. ac., *Ran. scel.*, Sepia, *Staphis.*

— after: Agar., Alum., Amm. carb., Amm. mur., Anac., *Arsen.*, ASAR., Bellad., Borax, *Bryon.*, *Calc. carb.*, CARB. AN., Carb. veg., *Caustic.*, Chamom., Cinchon., *Conium*, Crocus. Cyclam., Graphit., Ignat., *Ipecac.*, KALI CARB., Laches., *Lycop.*, MAR. VER., Natr. carb., Natr. mur., Nitr. ac., *Nux vom.*, Petrol., Phosphor., Phosph. ac., Pulsat., RAN. BULB., *Rhus tox.*, Selen., Sepia. Silic., Staphis. *Sulphur*, TARAX., *Therid.*, (breakfast). *Veratr.*, ZINC.

— **warm things,** from: *Alum.*, *Bellad.*, Bryon., Pulsat.

Epileptic attacks, after: Arsen., *Calc. carb.*, Camphor., Carb. veg., Coccul., CUPRUM, Silic., Sulphur, Veratr.

Fright, after: Acon., Bellad., Ignat., *Merc. viv.*, Nux vom., Opium, Platin., *Pulsat.*, Silic., *Veratr.*

Indisposition, after every attack of: CUPRUM.

Lying down in bed: see in bed.

Lying, on the side on which he is: *Arnic.*, Thuya.

Menses, before the: Acon., Amm. carb., Baryt., CALC. CARB., Carb. veg., Chamom., Coloc., Conium, Kali carb., Kreos., LYCOP., Mangan, Merc. viv., Nux vom., Phosphor., PULSAT., Ruta, *Sepia*, *Sulphur*, *Thuya*, *Veratr.*

— during the: *Amm. carb.*, Amm. mur., Bellad., Calc. carb., Carb. an., *Chamom.*, Coccul., GRAPHIT., Ignat., Kali carb., Kreos., Lycop., Magn. carb., Natr. carb., *Natr. sulph.*, *Nux vom.*, *Phosphor.*, PULSAT., Sepia, Sulphur, *Veratr.*

— after the: Borax, *Graphit.*, Kreos., Lycop., Natr. mur., Nux vom., Phosphor., *Pulsat.*

Motion, during: Acon., Alum., Ant. tart., APIS, Arnic., Asar., Baryt., Bellad., *Bryon.*, Cann. sat., Caustic., Chelid., Cinchon., Coccul., COFFEA, Colchic., Conium, Helleb., Hepar, Kali carb., Lachnanth., Ledum, Merc. viv., *Merc. corr.*, Mezer., Natr. mur., *Nitrum*, Nux vom., *Plumbum*, *Psorin.*, Ran. bulb.,

Rhus tox., SCILLA, Selen., *Sepia*, SILIC., SPIGEL., Staphis., Thuya.

Motion, after: Agar., *Arsen.*, Cann. sat., Kali carb., Nux vom., Phosphor., PULSAT., *Rhus tox.*, Sepia, Stann., Valer., Zinc.

Overheating, after: Acon., *Ant. crud.*, Bellad., *Bryon.*, Camphor., Carb. veg., Digit., Kali carb., Natr. mur., *Nux vom.*, Opium, Phosphor., *Pulsat.*, Rhus tox., Sepia, Silic., Thuya, Zinc.

Pains, with the: Angust., *Arsen.*, Baryt., BOVIST., Bryon., Coccul., COLOC., DULCAM., *Euphorb.*, *Graphit.*, Hepar, *Ignat.*, Kali carb., Laches., Ledum, Lycop., MEZER., Natr. mur., *Nitrum*, Plumbum, PULSAT., Ran. bulb., *Rhus tox.*, *Scilla*, SEPIA, Silic., Sulphur.

— after the: *Kali carb.*

Raising up, from: Acon., Arnic., Arsen., *Bellad.*, *Bryon.*, Chamom., Merc. viv., MERC. CORR., Mur. ac., *Nux vom.*, Phosphor., Pulsat., Rhus tox., Scilla, Sulphur, Veratr.

Sitting, while: Ambra, Capsic., Conium, DROSER., Helleb., Ipecac., KREOS., Lycop., *Phosphor.*, Phosph. ac., Platin., *Pulsat.*, Sepia, Rhus tox.

Sleep, during: Acon., Alum., Ambra, *Amm. carb.*, Arsen., Aurum, Bellad., BORAX, Bryon., Carb. an., Carb. veg., Caustic., Chamom., Cinchon., Hepar., *Lycop.*, Merc. viv., *Mur. ac.*, Natr. mur., Opium, Phosphor., Phosph. ac., *Pulsat.*, Sabad., Sarsap., Sepia, Silic., Staphis., *Sulphur*, Veratr., *Zinc.*

— **after:** see when awaking.

Stool, before: Ant. tart., Baryt., Bryon., *Calad.*, Capsic., Carb. an., Carb. veg., Caustic., Chamom., Digit., Mangan., MERC. VIV., MEZER., Natr. carb., *Pulsat.*, Spigel., Veratr.

— during: Alum., *Arsen.*, Bellad., *Calad.*, Calc. carb., Chamom., Cinchon., *Coloc.*, Conium, Digit., Hyosc., Magn. mur., *Merc. viv.*, Merc. corr., Natr. carb., Nitr. ac., Phosphor., PULSAT., Rheum, Rhus tox., Sepia, Silic., SPIGEL., Stann., *Sulphur*, VERATR.

— after: Ambra, Angust., Arsen., Bovist., Calc. carb., *Canthar.*, Carb. an., Carb. veg., Caustic., *Kali carb.*, Laches.,

Magn. mur., *Merc. viv.*, MEZER., Nitr. ac., Nux vom., Phosphor., PLATIN., PULSAT., Selen., Staphis., Sulphur, Veratr.

Talking of unpleasant things, when: Calc. carb., *Gelsem.*, *Mar. ver.*

Toothache, with the: Euphorb., *Kali carb.*, Mezer., PULSAT., Rhus tox.

Touching a cold object, from: Natr. mur., Silic., *Zinc.*

Touched, from being: ACON., Angust., Apis, Bellad., Chamom., *Cinchon.*, Colchic., Hepar, Hyosc., *Lycop.*, NUX VOM., Phosphor., Pulsat., Ran. bulb., Sabin., Sepia, *Spigel.*, Staphis., Sulphur.

Turning over, in bed: Acon., *Bryon.*, Capsic., Hepar, Lycop., Natr. mur., Nux vom., PULSAT., Silic., Staphis., Sulphur.

Uncovering, (undressing, denudation), from: *Acon.*, AGAR., *Amm. mur.*, *Argent.*, *Arnic.*, Arsen., Asar., Aurum, Bellad., *Borax*, Canthar., Capsic., CHAMOM., Cinchon., CLEMAT., Coccul., Colchic., Conium, *Cyclam.*, Digit., Droser., *Hepar*, Laches., Magn. carb., Mezer., *Mosch.*, *Nux mosch.*, NUX VOM., Phosphor., Platin., *Pulsat.*, Rhodod., *Rhus tox.*, Sambuc., SCILLA, SILIC., Spong., *Stramon.*, Strontia, *Thuya.*

Urination, before: Arnic., Borax, Bryon., Coloc., *Nitr. ac.*, Nux vom., Pulsat., Rhus tox., Sulphur, Thuya.

— during: Lycop., Merc. viv., *Nitr. ac.*, Nux vom., Phosphor., PLATIN., Pulsat., Sulphur, *Thuya*, Veratr.

— after: Arnic., Calc. carb., Hepar, Natr. mur., PLATIN., Pulsat., Rhodod., Sulphur, Thuya.

Vertigo, with the: Chelid., Coccul., Ledum, Merc. viv., Plumbum, *Pulsat.*, Rhus tox., Sepia, Veratr., *Viol. tr.*

Vomiting, after: Ant. tart., Cuprum, *Veratr.*

Warm room, in the: *Alum.*, ANAC., ANT. CRUD., APIS, Arsen., Asar., Baryt., *Bovist.*, BRYON., Canthar., Caustic., *Cina*, Cinchon., *Clemat.*, COCCUL., Colchic., Crocus, *Dulcam.*, Graphit., *Guaiac.*, Helleb., IOD., IPECAC., Kali carb., Laches., *Lauroc.*, Lycop., *Magn. mur.*, Mar. ver.,

Menyanth., *Merc. viv.*, MEZER., Mur. ac., Natr. mur., Nux vom., *Phosphor.*, Phosph. ac., Platin., PULSAT., Ran. bulb., Rhus tox., *Ruta*, Sabin., Sarsap., Sepia, Silic., *Spong.*, *Staphis.*, Sulphur, SULPH. AC., Thuya.

Warm stove, by the: *Alum.*, *Anac.*, Ant. crud., APIS, *Arsen.*, Asar., Baryt., *Bovist.*, Bryon., Canthar., Caustic., *Cina*, Cinchon., COCCUL., Colchic., Crocus, *Dulcam.*, Graphit., *Guaiac.*, Helleb., Iod., IPECAC., Kali carb., Laches., *Lauroc.*, Lycop., *Magn. mur.*, Mar. ver., Menyanth., *Merc. viv.*, MEZER., Mur. ac., Natr. mur., *Nux vom.*, *Phosphor.*, Phosph. ac., Platin., PULSAT., Ran. bulb., Rhus tox., *Ruta*, Sabin., *Sarsap.*, Sepia, Silic., *Spong.*, *Staphis.*, Sulphur, Sulph. ac., Thuya.

Weather, during damp, cold: Amm. carb., Calc. carb., *Diadem.*, Lycop., Mangan., Merc. viv., NUX MOSCH., *Rhus tox.*, Sulphur., Veratr.

— **stormy,** during: *Bryon.*, Chamom., Cinchon., Nux mosch., Nux vom., Phosphor., Pulsat., Rhodod., *Rhus tox.*, ZINC.

Yawning, when: Arnic., Caustic., *Cina*, Cyclam., Graphit., Ignat., Ipecac., Menyanth., Mur. ac., *Nux vom.*, Oleand., Phosphor., Rhus tox., Sabad., *Sarsap.*, Staphis.

AMELIORATION.

Air; open, in the: Acon., Alum., *Angust.*, Ant. crud., Argent., ASAR., Baryt., *Bryon.*, Cicut., Crocus, *Graphit.*, Helleb., Ipecac., Lycop., *Magn. carb.*, Magn. mur., Menyanth., *Mezer.*, Phosphor., PULSAT., Ran. scel., *Sabin.*, Spong., Stann., *Staphis.*, Sulphur, *Sulph. ac.*

— — **walking** in the: *Alum.*, Aurum, Capsic., Lycop., Magn. carb., Magn. mur., PULSAT., Rhus tox., Sabin., Sepia, Spong., STAPHIS., SULPH. AC.

Arising from bed; after: *Ambra*, Amm. carb., Ant. tart., Argent., Arsen., *Aurum*, Bellad., Droser., Euphorb., Ferr., Ignat., IOD., Ledum, Lycop., Magn. carb., Merc. viv., Merc. corr., *Natr. carb.*, Platin., *Pulsat.*, Rhodod., Rhus tox., Selen., *Sepia*, Strontia, Sulphur, Veratr.

Bed, in: Bryon., Canthar., *Caustic.*, Coccul., Conium, KALI CARB., *Kali hydr.*, *Lachnanth.*, Magn. carb., MAGN. MUR., Mezer., Natr. carb., NITRUM, Nitr. ac., *Nux vom.*, Pulsat., *Rhus tox.*, Sarsap., *Scilla*, Stramon., Sulphur.,

Drinking, from: Bryon., Carb. an., CAUSTIC., CUPRUM, Graphit., Ipecac., Mosch., *Nux vom.*, Oleand., *Phosphor.*, Rhus tox., Silic., Spigel., Tarax.

Drink, abstaining from: Cimex.

Eating, after: AMBRA, *Arsen.*, Bovist., Cann. sat., Chelid., Cuprum, Ferr., Ignat., IOD., *Kali carb.*, Lauroc., Mezer., *Natr. carb.*, Petrol., Phosphor., Rhus tox., Sabad., Scilla, Strontia.

Lying, while: Arnic., Asar., Baryt., Bellad., *Bryon.*, Calc. carb., Canthar., Coccul., Colchic., Natr. mur., *Nitrum*, *Nux vom.*, Scilla.

Motion, from: *Kreos.*, PULSAT., Sabin., Staphis., Sulph. ac.

Sitting, while: *Bryon.*, Colchic., Cuprum, *Droser.*, Merc. viv., *Nux vom.*, *Scilla.*

Sleep, after: Arnic., Arsen., Calad., Capsic., Cinchon., Colchic., Cuprum, Ferr., Kreos., *Nux vom.*, PHOSPHOR., Sambuc., *Sepia.*

Sun, in the: *Anac.*, *Conium*, Platin., Strontia.

Warmth, from external: ARSEN., Aurum., BARYT., Camphor., Canthar., *Caustic.*, *Cicut.*, Clemat., CONIUM., *Helleb.*, *Hepar*, IGNAT., KALI CARB., *Laches.*, Lachnanth., Lauroc., MENYANTH., Mosch., *Nux mosch.*, *Nux vom.*, *Platin.*, Rhodod., *Rhus tox.*, *Sabad.*, Sambuc., *Scilla*, Silic., Strontia, Sulphur, *Therid.*

Warm room, in the: Agar., Amm. carb., *Arsen.*, *Baryt.*, Calad., *Camphor.*, Canthar., Carb. an., Carb. veg., *Caustic.*, Chamom., CHELID., Cicut., Cinchon., Coffea, Conium, Guaiac., Helleb., *Hepar*, IGNAT., *Kali bichr.*, KALI CARB., Kreos., Laches., Lauroc., Magn. carb., Mangan., MENYANTH., Merc. viv., Merc. corr., NUX MOSCH., *Nux vom.*, Petrol., *Platin.*, Ran. bulb., Rhodod., *Rhus tox.* SABAD., Selen., Sepia, Silic., Spigel., Sulphur, *Sulph. ac.*, Valer., Zinc.

CONCOMITANTS.

Mood; anxious: ACON., Apis, Arnic., ARSEN., Bovist., Calad., CALC. CARB., *Camphor.*, Capsic., *Chamom.*, Cimex, Cinchon., COCCUL., Coffea, Conium, Hepar, Ignat., Merc. viv., Nux vom., Phosphor., Platin., PULSAT., Rheum, Rhus tox., Sulphur, Thuya, *Veratr.*

— **apathetic:** *Arnic.*, Arsen., Calc. carb., Cinchon., *Conium*, OPIUM, PHOSPHOR., PHOSPH. AC., Pulsat., Selen., *Sepia*, Stramon., Veratr.

— **dejected:** *Apis*, Arsen., Cann., CINCHON., CONIUM, Hepar, Ignat., Laches., Natr. mur., Platin., Pulsat., Rhus tox., Sulphur.

— **depressed:** Apis, Baryt., Calc. carb., Camphor., Cinchon., CONIUM, Hepar, Ignat., Lycop., Merc. viv., Pulsat., Rhus tox., *Sepia*, Spigel., Sulphur.

— **despairing:** *Acon.*, Arsen., *Aurum*, Bryon., *Calc. carb.*, *Chamom.*, Graphit., Hepar, IGNAT., Merc. viv., Nux vom., Rhus tox., *Sepia*, Veratr.

— **discontended:** Alum., Anac., Bryon., *Capsic.*, Conium, Natr. carb., Nux vom., Petrol., *Rhus tox.*, Silic.

— **ecstatic:** *Acon.*, Bellad., Laches., Opium, *Phosphor.*, Stramon.

— **excitable:** ACON., Arsen., Aurum, Bellad., Bryon., Calc. carb., Cann. sat., Capsic., Carb. veg., CHAMOM., Coccul., COFFEA, *Hepar*, Ignat., Lycop., Mar. ver., Natr. mur., *Nux vom.*, Phosphor., Sepia, Spigel., Sulphur, Veratr.

— **frenzied:** Bellad., Cimex, Hyosc., Opium, Platin., Stramon., Sulphur, Veratr.

— **listless:** Apis, *Arnic.*, CINCHON., Conium, Ignat., Laches., Opium, PHOSPHOR., PHOSPH. AC., *Pulsat.*, Selen., SEPIA, Silic., Veratr.

— **melancholy:** Arsen., Calc. carb., *Conium*, Helleb., *Ignat.*, *Lycop.*, Natr. mur., Phosphor., Platin., Selen., Sepia, *Veratr.*

— **oversensitive:** ACON., Aurum, Bryon., *Capsic.*,

CHAMOM., Cinchon., COFFEA, Colchic., Conium, Hepar, Natr. carb., *Nux vom.*, Petrol., Phosphor.,Selen., *Sepia*, Veratr.,

Mood; pensive: *Ant. crud.*

— **rage:** Acon., Arsen., *Cann. sat.*, Canthar., Lycop., Nitr. ac., Nux vom., Stramon., Veratr.

— **restless:** ACON., Amm. carb., Anac., Apis, *Arnic.*, ARSEN., Asaf., BELLAD., Bovist., *Calc. carb.*, Carb. veg., Capsic., CHAMOM., Cinchon., Coffea, Ipecac., Kreos., Laches., *Lycop.*, Merc. viv., Mezer., Natr. carb., Natr. mur., NUX VOM., Petrol., Phosphor., *Phosph. ac.*, Platin., Pulsat., *Rhus tox.*, Ruta, Sabad., SEPIA, *Silic.*, Spigel., *Veratr.*

— **serene:** Cann. sat., *Coffea*, *Crocus*, *Natr. carb.*, *Nux mosch.*, OPIUM, Phosphor., PLATIN., Pulsat., Rhus tox., *Sarsap.*, Veratr.

— **sorrowful:** ACON., Calc. carb., Cann. sat., Chamom., Coccul., Conium, *Cyclam.*, *Graphit.*, IGNAT., NATR. MUR., Nitr. ac., Nux vom., Platin., *Pulsat.*, Rhus tox., Sepia, Spigel., Staphis.

— **tearful:** Acon., Arsen., *Aurum*, BELLAD., CALC. CARB., Cann. sat., Carb. veg., CHAMOM., Conium, Hepar, Ignat., Kali carb., LYCOP., Merc. viv., Natr. mur., *Petrol.*, Platin., PULSAT., Selen., Silic., Sulphur, Veratr., VIOL. OD.

— **vexatious:** Arnic., *Arsen.*, Bryon., CALC. CARB., CAPSIC., *Chamom.*, Cinchon., CONIUM, Hepar, Ignat., Kreos., LYCOP., Merc. viv., Mezer., Nitr. ac., Petrol., Phosphor., PLATIN., *Pulsat.*, *Rheum*, Rhus tox., Sabad., Silic., *Spigel.*, *Sulphur*, Thuya.

Confusion of the mind: Arsen., Bellad., Bryon., Ipecac., Nux vom., Pulsat., Rhus tox.

Delirium: Acon., Arsen., *Bellad.*, Bryon., Calc. carb., Carb. veg., *Chamom.*, Cina, Cinchon., Dulcam., *Hyosc.*, Ignat., Iod., Kali carb., Natr. mur., Nux vom., *Opium*, Phosphor., Phosph. ac., Platin., Sambuc., *Stramon.*, Sulphur, *Veratr.*

Dullness of the head: Angust., Bellad., Borax, Bryon., *Calc. carb.*, *Capsic.*, Cicut., Conium, Droser., *Helleb.*,

Ipecac., *Kali carb.*, Ledum, NATR. CARB., Natr. mur., Nux mosch., *Nux vom.*, Opium, Phosphor., Phosph. ac., Plumbum, *Rhus tox.*, Ruta, Sepia, Valer., *Veratr.*

Illusions: Bellad., Bryon., Kali carb., Opium, Phosphor., Rhus tox., Sulphur.

Intellect; brightened: Bellad., Coffea, Laches., Opium, Phosphor., Phosph. ac., Spigel.

— weakness of: Bellad., Bryon., Laches.

Memory, weakness of: Bellad., Conium, Hyosc., Rhus tox., Podophyl. (forgets words.)

Muddled; (düseligkeit): Arsen., Bellad., *Bryon.*, Calc. carb., *Capsic.*, *Chamom.*, Conium, Hyosc., *Ipecac.*, Kali carb., Lauroc., Natr, mur., Nux vom., Opium, Phosphor., Phosph. ac., Pulsat., *Rhus tox.*, RUTA, Valer., Viol. tr.

Stupefaction: *Arnic.*, Arsen., Bellad., Borax, Bryon., Calc. carb., Chamom., Conium, Helleb., Hyosc., Lauroc., *Natr. mur.*, Nux vom., OPIUM, *Pulsat.*, Phosphor., Phosph. ac., Rhus tox., Veratr.

Thought, vanishing of: Bellad., Bryon., Laches., Rhus tox.

Unconsciousness: Acon., Arnic., *Arsen.*, Bellad., *Camphor.*, Capsic., Chamom., Cicut., Coccul., *Conium*, Helleb., HYOSC., Kali carb., Mur. ac., *Natr. mur.*, Opium, *Phosphor.*, *Phosph. ac.*, Rhus tox., Sepia, *Stramon.*, Veratr.

Vertigo: Alum., Apis, Arsen., Bellad., Bryon., *Calc. carb.*, Chelid., Cinchon., Coccul., *Conium*, Ipecac., Kali bichr., Lauroc., Ledum, Nux vom., Phosphor., Phosph. ac., Plumbum, Pulsat., Rhus tox., Sepia, Sulphur, Veratr., Viol. tr.

Reeling, (as if drunk): Alum., Bellad., *Capsic.*, Cicut., Coccul., Nux vom., Opium, Pulsat., Rhus tox., Stramon.

Head; pains in the, in general: *Acon.*, Alum., Amm. carb., Anac., Angust., Ant. tart., *Apis*, Arnic., *Arsen.*, *Bellad.*, Borax, *Bryon.*, Calc. carb., Capsic., Carb. veg., Chamom., Cimex, Cina., Cinchon., Coffea, *Conium*, *Droser.*, Ferr., Gelsem., *Graphit.*,

Helleb., Hepar, Ignat., Ipecac., Kali bichr., *Kali carb.*, Kreos., Laches., Ledum, Lycop., *Mangan.*, Merc. viv., *Mezer.*, Natr. carb., NATR. MUR., Nitrum, Nitr. ac., Nux vom., PETROL., Phosphor., *Psorin.*, *Pulsat.*, Rhodod., *Rhus tox.*, Ruta, *Sanguin.*, Seneg., *Sepia*, Silic., Spigel., Spong., Sulphur., TARAX., *Therid.*, Thuya, Veratr., Viol. tr.

Head; beating, in the: Acon., Borax, Chamom., Seneg., Sepia.

— **burning,** in the: *Acon.*, ARNIC., Arsen., *Asar.*, Aurum, BELLAD., Borax, BRYON., Calc. carb., Canthar., Cinchon., Helleb., *Ipecac.*, Laches., Mangan., Merc. viv., *Natr. carb.*, Nux vom., Phosphor., Phosph. ac., Rhodod., Rhus tox., Sabad., Sepia, Veratr. (Compare color, and heat, of the face.)

— **bursting pain,** in the: Alum., *Bryon.*, Spigel.

— **congestion** to the: Acon., Arsen., CINCHON., Ferr., Nux vom., Phosphor., Pulsat., Rhus tox., *Sepia*, Sulphur.

— **contractive sensation:** Bellad., Cinchon., *Conium*, Ignat., Kali bichr., Laches., *Nitr. ac.*, Nux vom., *Pulsat.*, Sulphur.

— **dartings;** in the: Calc. carb., Caustic., Merc. viv., Pulsat.

— **Heat;** in the: see burning.

— **stitches** in the: Arsen., *Bryon.*, Graphit., Kreos., Mangan., *Pulsat.*, Sepia.

Headache after drinking: Cimex.

External head, hair stands on end: Arnic., BARYT., Canthar., Hepar, Lauroc., Menyanth., *Pulsat.*, Spong., Veratr., Zinc.

— **heat;** of the: *Acon.*, Ant. crud., ARNIC., Arsen., Asar., *Bellad.*, Borax, Bryon., *Calc. carb.*, Cann. sat., Canthar., CAUSTIC .,Cinchon., Coffea, Dulcam., Ferr., Graphit., Helleb., IPECAC., Mangan., Natr. carb., Nux vom., Rhus tox., Staphis., STRAMON., Veratr.

— **puffed up:** Arsen., Cuprum, *Sulphur.*

— **sensitiveness,** of the: HELLEB., *Hepar*, Nux vom., *Sabad.*, Spigel., Sulphur.

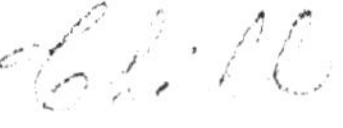

Head; sweat, on the: Arsen., Bryon., *Calc. carb.*, *Chamom.*, Cinchon., Digit., Natr. mur., *Pulsat.*, Rhus tox., *Silic.*

Eyes; pains in general: ACON., Apis, Bellad., *Borax*, Calad., Calc. carb., Canthar., Capsic., Chamom., Coloc., Kreos., Laches., Ledum, Lycop., Mezer., Rhodod., Rhus tox., SENEG., *Sepia.*

— **burning**: Borax, Chamom., Crocus, Seneg., Sepia.

— **glistening**: Bellad., *Laches.*, *Lachnanth.*, Sepia.

— **inflamed**: Acon., Bellad., Kreos., Rhus tox.

— **lachrymation**: *Apis*, Bellad., Kreos., *Mezer.*, Rhus tox.

— **pressing** in the: Kreos., Lycop., *Rhus tox.*, Sepia.

— **pupils; contracted**: ACON., CAPSIC., Chamom., Digit., *Sepia*, Silic., Sulphur, *Veratr.*

— — **dilated**: Apis, BELLAD., Calc. carb., Carb. an., *Cicut.*, Crocus, *Hyosc.*, Ignat., IPECAC., *Mezer.*, *Stramon.*

— **staring**: *Acon.*, Bellad., CICUT., Hyosc., Laches.

— **stitches** in the: Acon., Apis, Borax, *Coloc.*, Rhus tox.

Eyelids; burning: Acon., Apis, Bellad., Kreos., Rhus tox.

— **dryness** of the: Rhus tox.

— **quivering**: Calc. carb., *Rhus tox.*

— **swelling** of the: Apis, Ferr., *Rhus tox.*

Sight; dullness of vision: CHAMOM., KREOS., Lauroc., Lycop., Natr. mur.

— **flames** before the eyes: Bellad., Hyosc.

— **flickering** before the eyes: Chamom., Ledum, Lycop., *Sepia*, Therid.

— **mist** before the eyes: Bellad., Crocus, *Lauroc.*

— **motions** before the eyes: Cicut., Lycop., *Sabad.*

— **obscuration** of: *Bellad.*, Cicut., Cinchon., Digit., Kreos., Laches., Natr. mur., SABIN.

— **photophobia**: Acon., Apis, Arsen., BELLAD., *Borax*, Chamom., Hepar, Kreos., Lycop., *Rhus tox.*, Seneg., Sepia.

8

Sight; trembling before the eyes: Ledum, Lycop., Sabad., Sabin.

— **vanishing** of: *Bellad.*, Hyosc., Laches., Natr. mur.

Ears; pain in general: Acon., Apis, Asar., Calad., Calc. carb., Digit., *Graphit.*, Nux vom., Pulsat., Sulphur.

— **heat** of the: Acon., Alum., Arsen., Bellad., Digit., Merc. viv., *Pulsat.*, Rhus tox.

— — **lobe** of the: Acon., Alum., Kreos., Merc. viv.

— **pressing** in the: Asar.

— **redness** of the: Bellad., Pulsat.

— **stitching** in the: Graphit., Pulsat.

— — **in right**: *Psorin.*

— **swelling of the glands** below the: Cist. cann.

Hearing; dullness of: *Chamom.*, Cinchon., Pulsat., *Rhus tox.*

— **humming** in the ears: *Arsen*, Pulsat.

— **ringing** in the ears: Chin. sulph., Cinchon., Graphit., Rhus tox.

— **sensitve to noise**: Arnic., *Capsic.*

Nose; bleeding of the: Bellad., Bryon., Calc. carb., *Kreos.*, Pulsat., Rhus tox.

— **dryness** of the: Bellad., Calc. carb., *Rhodod.*, Sabad., Silic.

— **heat** of the: Bellad., Rhus tox.

— **itching** of the: *Cina*, Silic., Spigel.

— **pressure** in the: Camphor.

— **redness** of the: Bellad., Rhus tox., Sepia.

Face; color, bluish: Arsen., Camphor., Conium, Cuprum, Hyosc., Laches., *Opium*, Sulphur, Veratr.

Face; color, bluish-red: Bellad., Bryon., Cuprum, Laches., Opium, Sulphur.

— — **earthy:** Arsen., Cinchon., Ferr., Natr. mur., Nux vom., Silic.

— — **pale:** Ant. tart., BRYON., CAMPHOR., Canthar., *Chin. sulph.*, Cicut., CINA, *Cinchon.*, Coccul., Coffea, Crocus, DROSER., Ignat., Ipecac., *Lycop.*, *Merc. viv.*, Mezer., MOSCH., Nux mosch., Nux vom., Phosphor., Phosph. ac., *Pulsat.*, *Rhus tox.*, Silic., *Sulphur*, *Veratr.*

— — **red:** Acon., Agar., Alum., Amm. mur., Anac., Apis, *Arnic.*, Arsen., Bellad., *Bryon.*, Calc. carb., Cann. sat., CHAMOM., *Cinchon.*, Coccul., Coffea, Coloc., Conium, Cyclam., *Digit.*, Droser., FERR., *Hyosc.*, Ignat., Ipecac., *Kreos.*, Laches., *Ledum*, Lycop., Mangan., Merc. viv., *Mur. ac.*, Natr. carb., Nitrum, *Nux vom.*, *Oleand.*, Opium, Oxal. ac., *Plumbum*, Pulsat., Ran. bulb., *Rhus tox.*, Ruta, Seneg., *Sepia*, Silic., Spong., *Staphis.*, STRAMON., *Sulphur*, Thuya, Veratr., Zinc.

— — — **one side** of: Acon., Arnic., CHAMOM., Ipecac., *Mosch.*, Nux vom., *Rheum.*, Rhus tox., Thuya.

— — — — **and cold:** *Mosch.*

— — **alternating** in: Amm. carb., Bellad., Ferr., Ignat., Ipecac., Phosphor., Platin., Rhus tox., Veratr.

— — **yellow:** *Arnic.*, Arsen., Cinchon., Conium, Digit., Ferr., *Helleb.*, Ignat., Laches., Natr. mur., Nitr. ac., Nux vom., Phosphor., Rhus tox., Sepia, Sulphur.

— **coldness** of the: Ant. tart., Asar., Bellad., Bismuth., *Camphor.*, Canthar., Carb. veg., Chamom., Cicut., CINA, DROSER., *Hyosc.*, Ignat., *Ipecac.*, LYCOP., *Natr. carb.*, Nitr. ac., PETROL., Platin., Rheum, Rhus tox., *Veratr.*

— **convulsions** of the: Arsen., Bellad., Calc. carb., Chamom., Cicut., Ignat., Opium, Stann., Stramon.

— **distortion** of the: Bellad., *Cann. sat.*, Cicut., Opium, Stramon.

— **heat** of: Acon., Agar., Alum., Ambra, Anac., *Apis*, *Arnic.*, Arsen., Baryt., Bellad., Bovist., Brom., Bryon., *Calc.*

carb., *Cann. sat.*, Canthar., Carb. veg., CHAMOM., Cinchon., COFFEA, Coloc., Digit., *Euphorb.*, FERR., Graphit., *Helleb.*, Hepar, HYOSC., Ipecac., Kreos., Laches., *Ledum*, Mangan., *Merc. viv.*, Mosch., *Mur. ac.*, Natr. carb., *Nux vom.*, OLEAND., Phosphor., Phosph. ac., Platin., *Pulsat.*, Ran. bulb., *Rhus tox.*, Ruta, *Sabad.*, Sabin., Sambuc., Sarsap., *Seneg.*, Spigel., Stann., Staphis., *Stramon.*, Strontia, Sulphur, Tarax., Thuya, Veratr.

Face; pain (Prosopalgia.): Acon., Cinchon., Laches., Nux vom., Mezer., Rhus tox., *Spigel.*

— **puffed up:** Amm. mur., Arnic., Arsen., Bellad., Chamom., Ferr., Laches., *Lycop.*, Silic.

— **sweat** of the: *Arsen.*, Calc. carb., COFFEA, Euphorb., Laches., Ledum, LYCOP., *Nux vom.*, *Pulsat.*, Sabad., Sulphur, Thuya.

— **tension** of the: Acon., BARYT., Conium, Lycop., Phosphor., Pulsat., Rhus tox.

Lips; color, blue: *Chin. sulph.*, *Eup. purp.*

— **dryness** of the: Acon., Arsen., Bellad., Bryon., Cinchon., Ignat., *Kali bichr.*, *Nux vom.*, Phosphor., Phosph. ac., *Psorin.*, Rhus tox.

— **eruption** on the: *Arsen.*, Bryon., Capsic., Ignat., *Natr. mur.*, *Nux vom.*, Rhus tox.

— **swelling** of the: *Arsen.*, Bryon., Rhus tox.

Teeth; painful: Agar., Apis, Baryt., Calc. carb., Carb. veg., *Graphit.*, Helleb., *Kali carb.*, Ledum, Magn. carb., Merc. viv., Mezer., Natr. mur., Nitr. ac., Pulsat., RHUS TOX., *Sepia*, *Staphis.*

— **chattering** of the: Arsen., Bovist., Bryon., *Camphor.*, CAPSIC., Cinchon., Cuprum, Hepar, Ignat., LACHES., *Natr. mur.*, *Natr. sulph.*, Nux vom., *Phosphor.*, Platin., Ran. bulb., Sabad., STANN., Zinc.

— **grating** of the: Acon., Ant. crud., Apis, Arsen., Bellad., Chamom., Conium, Hyosc., Ignat., Lycop., Phosphor., *Stramon.*

Mouth; burning in the: Arsen., Chamom., Laches., Mezer., *Petrol.*, Veratr.

— **dryness** of the: Acon., Apis, *Arnic.*, Arsen., Baryt., Bellad., Bryon., Chamom., Cinchon., Hyosc., Ignat., Kali bichr., Kali carb., Laches., Lycop., Magn. mur., Merc. viv., *Mezer.*, MUR. AC., Nitr. ac., Nux mosch., *Nux vom.*, Petrol., *Phosphor.*, *Phosph. ac.*, *Psorin.*, Ran. bulb., *Rhus tox.*, Sabad., *Sepia*, Staphis., Stramon., *Sulphur*, *Thuya*, Veratr.

— **foam** at the: *Therid.*

— **odor, offensive:** Anac., *Apis*, ARNIC., Arsen., Aurum, Bellad., Bryon., Carb. veg., Chamom., Dulcam., Graphit., Ipecac., Laches., Lycop., MERC. VIV., Nitr. ac., *Nux. vom.*, Petrol., Pulsat., Rhus tox., Sepia, Silic., *Sulphur*, Sulph. ac.

— **saliva increased:** Acon., *Alum.*, Anac., Arsen., Bellad., Brom., Calc. carb., *Capsic.*, Chamom., Droser., Euphorb., Hepar, Ipecac., Kreos., Laches., Lycop., *Merc. viv.*, MEZER., Natr. mur., Nitr. ac., Nux vom., Phosphor., *Rhus tox.*, Sepia, Silic., Stramon., Sulphur, Veratr.

Tongue; coated: *Ant. crud.*, Arnic., Arsen., Bellad., *Bryon.*, Chamom., Coloc., Graphit., Ignat., Ipecac., Laches., Lycop., Merc. viv., *Nux mosch.*, *Nux vom.*, Opium, *Phosphor.*, Phosph. ac., Pulsat., Rhus tox., Ruta, Sulphur.

— **dryness:** Acon., Arsen., Bellad., Bryon., Hyosc., Lycop., *Natr. mur.*, *Phosphor.*, Phosph. ac., Rhus tox., Sulphur.

Sore throat: Baryt., Bellad., Borax, Bovist., Brom., *Bryon.*, Conium, Droser., Kali carb., Ledum, *Nux vom.*, Phosphor., Phosph. ac., Pulsat., *Rhus tox.*, SEPIA, Spigel., Zinc.

Aversion to food (want of appetite): Alum., Anac., *Ant. crud.*, Ant. tart., Apis, Arnic., *Arsen.*, Bryon., Canthar., Chamom., Cinchon., *Conium*, Hepar, Ignat., *Ipecac.*, Kali carb., Laches., Ledum, Mezer., Natr. mur., Nux mosch., *Nux vom.*, *Phosphor.*, Pulsat., Rheum, Rhus tox., SABAD., Sepia, SILIC., Staphis.

Loathing of food: Amm. carb., *Ant. crud.*, *Apis*, Arnic., *Arsen.*, *Bryon.*, *Chamom.*, Cinchon., Coccul., Helleb., *Ipecac.*,

Kali carb., Laches., Merc. viv., Nux vom., Petrol., Pulsat., *Rheum.*

Desire for; beer: Ant. crud., *Nux vom.*, Pulsat.

— **refreshing things:** *Coccul.*, Phosphor., Phosph ac., Pulsat.

Hunger: Ant. crud., Arsen., Calc. carb., Chamom., *Cina*, *Cinchon.*, Nux vom., Phosphor., Pulsat., Silic., Veratr.

Thirst: *Acon.*, Alum., Amm. mur., Angust., Ant. crud., *Apis*, *Arnic.*, Arsen., Baryt., Bellad., Borax, *Bovist.*, BRYON., Calad., CALC. CARB., Camphor., CANN. SAT., *Capsic.*, *Carb. veg.*, Chamom., *Chelid.*, Cimex, CINA, Cinchon., *Crocus*, Droser., *Dulcam.*, *Eup. perf.*, *Eup. purp.*, Ferr., Hepar, *Ignat.*, *Ipecac.*, Kali bichr., Kali carb., Kali hydr., Kreos., Lauroc., *Ledum*, Magn. mur., Menyanth., MEZER., Mur. ac., Natr. carb., NATR. MUR., Natr. sulph., *Nitrum*, Nux vom., Opium, Phosphor., Podophyl., *Plumbum*, Psorin., Pulsat., Ran. bulb., Rhus tox., *Ruta*, Sabad., Scilla, Secal., SEPIA, Silic., Spong., Stann., Staphis., Sulphur, Thuya, Valer., Veratr.

— **before** the chill: Amm. mur., Angust., *Arnic.*, ARSEN., Bellad., Capsic., Carb. veg., *Cina*, CINCHON., Eup. perf., Ignat., Laches., Lobel. inf., Magn. carb., Natr. mur., *Nux vom.*, PULSAT., Rhus tox., Sepia, *Sulphur.*

— **between** the chill and heat: *Amm. mur.*, Arsen., Bryon., *Canthar.*, CINCHON., Droser., Helleb., Kreos., Natr. carb., Nux vom., Psorin., PULSAT., SABAD., *Sepia.*

Thirstlessness: *Agar.*, Agn. cast., Alum., Amm. carb., Amm. mur., Angust., Ant. crud., *Ant. tart.*, ARSEN., Asar., *Aurum*, Bellad., Borax, Bovist., Bryon., Calc. carb., *Canthar.*, Capsic., Carb. veg., CAUSTIC., Chelid., Cina, *Cinchon.*, Coccul., Coffea, Coloc., *Conïum*, *Cyclam.*, *Droser.*, Dulcam., Euphorb., Guaiac., *Helleb.*, Hepar, *Hyosc.*, Ipecac., Kali bichr., Kali carb., *Kreos.*, Laches., Ledum, *Lycop.*, Mangan., Menyanth., Merc. viv., MOSCH., MUR. AC., Natr. carb., Natr. mur., Natr. sulph., Nitrum, Nitr. ac., *Nux mosch.*, Nux vom., Oleand., Opium, Petrol., PHOSPHOR., *Phosph. ac.*, PULSAT., Rhodod., *Rhus tox.*, SABAD., Sabin., *Sambuc.*, Sarsap., Scilla, SPIGEL., Spong., *Staphis.*, Stramon., *Sulphur*, Tarax., Therid., THUYA, Zinc.

Taste; bitter: Acon., Alum., ANT. CRUD., *Arnic.*, ARSEN., *Bryon.*, *Chamom.*, *Cinchon.*, Coloc., *Hepar*, Ignat., Natr. mur., Nux vom., Phosphor., *Pulsat.*, *Sepia*, Spong.

— **insipid:** Arsen., *Aurum*, Borax, Bryon., Cinchon., Ignat., Pulsat., Staphis.

— **loss** of: Amm. mur., ARSEN., *Droser.*, Pulsat., Silic.,

— **metallic:** Coccul., Cuprum, Ipecac., Nux vom., Rhus tox., Zinc.

— **putrid:** Arnic., Kali carb., Merc. viv., Nux vom., *Pulsat.*, *Rhus tox.*, *Staphis.*

— **salty:** Arsen., Bellad., Cinchon., Merc. viv., Phosphor., Pulsat., Sepia.

— **sour:** Bellad., Calc. carb., Cinchon., Ignat., Natr. mur., Nux vom., Petrol., Phosphor., Pulsat., Sulphur.

— **sweetish:** Acon., Alum., Digit., Phosphor., Plumbum, Pulsat., Sabad., Scilla.

Eructations: *Alum.*, Ant. crud., Arnic., *Bryon.*, Carb. veg., Cina, Cinchon., Ipecac., *Nux vom.*, Phosphor., Ran. bulb., *Rhus tox.*, *Sabad.*, Sarsap., Sepia, Sulph. ac.

Heart-burn: Capsic., Cinchon., Conium, Lycop., Nux vom., Pulsat.

Nausea: Acon., Alum., *Ant. crud.*, *Apis.*, ARSEN., Asar., *Aurum*, *Bellad.*, Bovist., *Bryon.*, Canthar., Carb. veg., *Chamom.*, *Chelid.*, Cina, *Cinchon.*, Coccul., Coffea, Conium, Corn. flor., Droser., Dulcam., Euphorb., *Hepar*, *Ignat.*, *Ipecac.*, Kali bichr., Kali carb., Kreos., Laches., Lauroc., *Lycop.*, Merc. viv., Mezer., Mosch., Natr. carb., Nitr. ac., *Nux vom.*, Opium, *Phosph. ac.*, Platin., *Pulsat.*, RHUS TOX., SABAD., *Sanguin.*, SEPIA, Sulphur, Sulph. ac., Therid., Thuya, Valer., *Veratr.*

Qualmishness: Arsen., Bryon., Cina, Ignat., Lycop., Mezer., Nux vom., Sabad., *Silic.*, Sulphur.

Disposition to vomit: Apis, Arsen., *Aurum*, Bellad., *Chamom.*, Droser., Ipecac., Natr. carb., Pulsat., *Rhus tox.*, Sabad., Sepia, Veratr.

Vomiting: *Ant. crud.*, *Arnic.*, *Arsen.*, Borax, Bryon., *Capsic.*, Carb. veg., *Chamom.*, *Cina*, *Cinchon.*, Conium, Corn. flor., Droser., Eup. perf. (between chill and heat), Ferr., Hepar, *Ignat.*, *Ipecac.*, Kali carb., Laches., Lauroc., *Lycop.*, Natr. mur., Nux vom., Phosphor., *Pulsat.*, Stramon., Sulphur, Therid., Thuya, Valer., Veratr.

— **bitter:** *Ant. crud.*, Arnic., ARSEN., Borax, CHAMOM., Cina, *Cinchon.*, Ignat., Lycop., *Nux vom.*, *Pulsat.*, Veratr.

— **black:** Arsen., Cinchon., Ipecac., Nux vom., Veratr.

— **bloody:** Arnic., *Arsen.*, Cinchon., Ferr., Ipecac., Nux vom., Phosphor., Pulsat.

— **ingesta** of the: Arsen., *Cina*, Ferr., Ignat., Ipecac., Nux vom., Phosphor., Pulsat., Sulphur.

— **mucous:** Ant. crud., Arsen., *Capsic.*, Chamom., Cina, Droser., Ignat., Ipecac., Nux vom., *Pulsat.*, Sulphur.

— **sour:** Arsen., Chamom., Lycop., Nux vom., Phosphor., *Pulsat.*, Sulphur.

— **watery:** Bryon., Droser., Ipecac., Nux vom.

Stomach; pains in the: Ant. crud., Arnic., *Arsen.*, *Bryon.*, *Caustic.*, Chamom., Cina, Cinchon., COCCUL., Euphorb., Ferr., Ignat., Ipecac., Lycop., Merc. viv., *Nux vom.*, Phosphor., PULSAT., *Rhus tox.*, Sabad., Sepia, *Silic.*, Sulphur.

— **heat** in the: Lobel. inf.

Hypochondria; pains in the: Podophyl.

Liver; pains in the: Acon., Ant. crud., *Arsen.*, Borax, Bryon., Capsic., Carb. veg., Chamom., Chin. sulph., CINCHON., Coccul., Ignat., Kali carb., Lycop., Magn. mur., Merc. viv., *Nux vom.*, Pulsat., Ran. bulb., *Sepia*, Sulphur, Thuya.

Spleen; pains in the: Acon., Arsen., Asaf., Borax, *Bryon.*,

Capsic., Carb. veg., Chamom., Cinchon., Kali carb., Natr. mur., Nux vom., Ran. bulb., *Rhus tox.*, Sepia, Sulphur, Sulph. ac., Thuya.

Spleen; enlargement of the: Diadem.

Kidneys; pain in the: Arsen., Canthar., Kali carb., Lycop., Nux vom., Pulsat., Zinc.

Abdomen; pains in the: Ant. crud., Ant. tart., Apis, *Arsen.*, Baryt., *Borax*, *Bovist.*, Bryon., *Calad.*, Calc. carb., Carb. veg., Chamom., Cicut., CINCHON., Coccul., Coffea, COLOC., Corn. flor., Crocus, Ferr., *Ignat.*, Ipecac., Kali carb., Menyanth., *Merc. viv.*, Merc. corr., Mezer., *Nitr. ac.*, Nux mosch., Nux vom., Phosphor., Phosph. ac., *Pulsat.*, Psorin., Ran. bulb., *Rhus tox.*, *Sepia*, Spigel., Strontia, Sulphur.

— **coldness** in the: Arsen., Cist. can., *Menyanth.*, Merc. viv., Mezer., *Phosph. ac.*, Sepia.

— **distention** of the: *Arsen.*, Laches., Mezer., Pulsat., Rhus tox.

Diarrhœa: *Ant. crud.*, Apis, Arnic., Arsen., Bryon., *Calad.*, Chamom., *Cina*, Cinchon., Coffea, Coloc., Conium, Ferr., Hyosc., Ipecac., Lauroc., Merc. viv., Nux mosch., PHOSPHOR., Phosph. ac., *Pulsat.*, *Rhus tox.*, *Spigel.*, Strontia, Sulphur, VERATR.

— **painful:** Bryon., Chamom., Coloc., Merc. viv., Pulsat., Rhus tox., Veratr.

— **painless:** Arsen., Cinchon., Ferr., Hyosc., Phosphor., Phosph. ac.

Constipation: Alum., Ant. crud., Bellad., *Bryon.*, Calc. carb., Cann. sat., COCCUL., Dulcam., *Lycop.*, *Nux vom.*, Opium, Sepia, Silic., Staphis., Sulphur, *Veratr.*

— **through hardness** of the feces: Bryon., Nux vom., Opium, Silic., Sulphur.

— **through inactivity** of the rectum: Alum., Cann. sat., Coccul., Lycop., Nux vom., Opium, Staphis., Veratr.

Urging to stool: Caustic., Hyosc., Mar. ver., Merc. viv., Nux vom., Pulsat., Sulphur.

Tenesmus: Apis, Arsen., Capsic., *Merc. viv.*, *Merc. corr.*, Nux vom., Rheum, Rhus tox., *Sulphur.*

Urination; frequent: *Arsen.*, Bellad., Dulcam., *Lycop.*, MERC. VIV., Phosphor., Phosph. ac., Spigel., Staphis., *Sulphur.*

— **involuntary:** Caustic., Dulcam., Pulsat., Rhus tox., Sulphur.

— **painful:** Canthar., *Chamom.*, Lycop., Merc. viv., Nux vom., Phosph. ac., Pulsat., Sulphur, Thuya.

— **seldom:** Arnic., Canthar., Hyosc., Opium, Stramon.,

Urinate; urging to: *Ant. tart.*, Bryon., Cinchon., Dulcam., Lycop., Nux vom., Phosphor., Phosph. ac., Pulsat., Sulphur.

— — **ineffectual:** Arnic., Arsen., Canthar., Nux vom., Phosphor., Pulsat., Sulphur.

— **retention** of urine: Apis, Arnic., Canthar., Hyosc., Lycop., *Opium*, Pulsat., Stramon.

Sneezing: Bellad., Calc. carb., *Carb. veg.*, Chamom., *Cina*, Laches., Mar. ver., Merc. viv., Pulsat., *Rhus tox.*, SABAD., Staphis., Sulphur.

Coryza; in general: Amm. carb., Ant. tart., Arsen., *Aurum*, Bryon., Calad., Capsic., *Carb. veg.*, Chamom., Kali carb., Laches., Lycop., Merc. viv., Mur. ac., Natr. carb., *Nux vom.*, Pulsat., Rhus tox., Sabad., Spong., Sulphur, Thuya.

— **fluent:** Ant. tart., *Arsen.*, Aurum, *Byron.*, *Carb. veg.*, Chamom., Kali carb., Laches., Merc. viv., Natr. carb., *Pulsat.*, *Rhus tox.*, Sulphur, Thuya.

— **dry:** Bryon., Calad., *Kali carb.*, Lycop., Natr. carb., *Nux vom.*, Rhus tox., Sulphur.

Breathing; affections of, in general: Acon., Anac., Apis, Arnic., ARSEN., Bovist., Bryon., Capsic., Cimex., *Cina*, Cinchon., *Ferr.*, *Ignat.*, *Ipecac.*, KALI CARB., Laches., Lycop., MEZER., Natr. mur., Nux mosch., *Nux vom.*, Phosphor.,

PULSAT., *Rhus tox.*, SENEG., Sepia, Stramon., Sulphur, Veratr., *Zinc.*

Breathing; deep: Bryon., Capsic., Cimex., Ipecac., *Phosph. ac.*

— **loud:** (without mucous rales) *Calad.*, Chamom., Cina., Cinchon., Ignat., Kali carb., Nux vom., Phosphor., Sambuc., Spong., Sulphur, Thuya.

— **quick:** Acon., Arsen., Bellad., Carb. veg., Cuprum, Ignat., Ipecac., Lycop., Nux vom., Phosphor., Pulsat., Rhus tox., Sepia, Sulphur, Zinc.,

— **rattling:** (with mucous rales) Cinchon., Cuprum, Hepar, Lycop., Nux mosch., Stramon.

— **sighing:** Acon., Bryon., Capsic., Coccul., Ignat., *Ipecac.*, Opium, Silic.

— **slow:** Bellad., Capsic., Helleb., Ignat., Opium, Spong.

— **suffocation, attacks** of: *Arsen.*, Hepar, Ignat., Ipecac., Nux vom., Pulsat.

— **unequal:** Angust., Bellad., Cina, Cuprum, Ignat., Mosch., Opium, Pulsat.

Breath; cold: Carb. veg., Cinchon., Veratr.

— **hot:** Acon., Anac., CHAMOM., Rhus tox., Sabad., *Zinc.*

Cough; in general: Acon., *Arsen.*, Borax, *Bryon.*, Calc. carb., Chamom., *Cinchon.*, Conium, Hepar, Hyosc., Ipecac., Kali carb., Kreos., Laches., Lycop., Nux mosch., Nux vom., PHOSPHOR., *Pulsat.*, RHUS TOX., SABAD., Sepia, Spong., Sulphur, Thuya.

— **with** expectoration: *Arsen.*, Bryon., CALC. CARB., Cinchon., Kali carb., Kreos., *Lycop.*, *Phosphor.*, Phosph. ac., *Pulsat.*, *Sepia*, Silic., Sulphur, Thuya.

— **without** expectoration: *Acon.*, Arsen., Bellad., Bryon., Carb. veg., Chamom., Cimex., Cinchon., Hepar, Hyosc., *Ipecac.*, Kali carb., Laches., Nux mosch., Nux vom., *Phosphor.*, Pulsat., Rhus tox., Sabad., Sepia, *Spong.*, Sulphur.

Larynx; affections of the: Borax, Carb. veg., Caustic., Droser., Hepar, Mangan., Phosphor., Spong.

— **cold feeling** in the: Cist. can.

Hoarseness: Acon., Caustic., Droser., Hepar, Nux vom., Phosphor., Sepia.

Neck; stiffness of the: Bellad., *Cicut.*, Lycop., Merc. viv., Silic.

— **glands of the,** swelling of the: Cist. can.

Nape of the neck, pains in the: *Acon.*, *Arsen.*, Calc. carb., Merc. viv., Nux vom., Pulsat., *Staphis.*

Chest; pains in general: *Acon.*, Arnic., *Arsen.*, Bellad., Borax, *Bovist.*, Brom., BRYON., Calad., Calc. carb., Chamom., *Cinchon.*, *Ipecac.*, KALI CARB., Merc. viv., *Mezer.*, Nux mosch., Nux vom., Phosphor., Phosph. ac., Psorin., *Pulsat.*, *Rhus tox.*, Sabad., Seneg., Sepia, Silic., Spigel., Sulphur.

— **burning** in the: Apis.

— **heaviness** in the: Cimex.

— **oppression** of the: Apis, Cimex.

— **stitches** in the: *Acon.*, Amm. carb., BRYON., Cinchon., Kali carb., *Nux vom.*, Phosphor., Pulsat., Sepia, Silic.

— **warmth,** sensation of, in the: Sarsap.

Palpitation of the heart: Acon., Arsen., Brom., Bryon., Calc. carb., CINCHON., Kali carb., Lycop., MERC. VIV., Natr. mur., Phosphor., *Phosph. ac.*, Pulsat., Rhus tox., Sarsap., *Sepia*, Spigel., *Sulphur.*

Scapulæ; pains in the, in general: Bellad., *Cinchon.*, Kreos., Merc. viv., Nux vom., Pulsat., Ran. bulb., *Rhus tox.*, Sanguin., SEPIA, Tarax., Zinc.

— **stitches** in the: Bellad., Cinchon., Merc. viv., Nux vom., Pulsat., *Sepia*, Sulphur, Zinc.

Back; pains in the, in general: Arnic., *Arsen.*, BELLAD., Calc. carb., *Capsic.*, *Caustic.*, Chamom., Chin. sulph.,

Cinchon., Coccul., Hepar, Hyosc., *Ignat.*, Laches., *Lycop.*, *Natr. mur.*, *Nux vom.*, Phosphor., Podophyl., Pulsat., Rhus tox., Sepia, Silic., Sulphur, Veratr.

Small of the back; pains in the, in general: Alum., Arnic., *Arsen.*, Bryon., CALC. CARB., Caustic., Coccul., Hepar, Kali carb., *Laches.*, Lycop., Nux mosch., *Nux vom.*, Phosphor., Phosph. ac., Pulsat., Rhus tox., Sabad., Sepia, Silic., Sulphur, Veratr.

— **lameness,** sensation of, in the: Coccul., Leptand.

— **soreness** in the: Leptand.

Upper limbs; pains in the, in general: Acon., Amm. carb., Apis, Arnic., Bryon., Canthar., Capsic., Caustic., Chelid., Cina, Cinchon., Coccul., Coffea, Droser., Helleb., Ignat., Kali carb., Kreos., Laches., Ledum, Lycop., Menyanth., Merc. viv., Mur. ac., Natr. mur., *Nux vom.*, Petrol., Phosphor., Phosph. ac., *Pulsat.*, Rhus tox., Sabad., Sepia, Spong., Stann., Stramon., Thuya, Veratr.

Elbow; pain at the: Podophyl.

Wrist; pain in the: Podophyl.

Hands; blood-vessels, distention of the: Amm. carb., Phosphor., Thuya.

— **blue:** Amm. carb., Apis, Coccul., *Nux vom.*, Secal., Veratr., Zinc.

— **clenching** of the: Cimex.

— **dead,** as if: Apis, Bryon., Calc. carb., Droser., LYCOP., Mur. ac., Nux vom., Oxal. ac., Petrol., Phosph. ac., Pulsat., Secal., SEPIA, *Stann.*

— **heat** of the: Acon., Agar., Alum., APIS, Asar., Carb. veg., CINCHON., CINA., Droser., Kali carb., Kreos., Lycop., NATR. CARB., *Nux vom.*, Phosphor., Phosph. ac., Pulsat., *Sabad.*, Sepia, Spong., *Stann.*, Thuya.

Fingers; dead, as if: Acon., Amm. carb., Amm. mur., Calc. carb., Chelid., Cuprum, Hepar, Lycop., Mur. ac., Pulsat., Secal., Sepia, *Stann.*, Sulphur, Thuya, Veratr.

Fingers; heat of the: Agar., Magn. carb., Rhus tox., *Sabad.*, Silic., Sulphur, Thuya.

Nails, blue: Arsen., *Aurum*, Chelid., Chin. sulph., Cinchon., *Coccul.*, Digit., Droser., *Eup. purp.*, Natr. mur., *Nux vom.*, Petrol., Silic.

Lower limbs; pains in the, in general: Acon., Amm. carb., Arnic., ARSEN., Baryt., Bellad., Bryon., Calc. carb., Canthar., *Capsic.*, Caustic., Chamom., CINCHON., Coffea, Coloc., Guaiac., Helleb., *Ignat.*, Kreos., Laches., Ledum., Lycop., Mezer., Natr. mur., Nitrum, *Nux vom.*, Phosphor., *Pulsat.*, Rhodod., *Rhus tox.*, Sabad., *Seneg.*, Sepia, Spigel., Spong., *Sulphur*, Tarax., Thuya, Veratr.

— — **hips,** in the: *Arnic.*, Calc. carb., Lycop., Nux vom., Rhus tox., Sepia.

— — **thighs,** in the: *Arsen.*, BORAX, Cinchon., Euphorb., Guaiac., Laches., Natr. mur.

— **right thigh,** drawing in the: Therid.

— **knees, pain** in the: Caustic., Cinchon., Helleb., Nux vom., Podophyl., Pulsat., Rhus tox., Sepia, Sulphur.

— **flexion of the leg,** on the thigh: Cimex.

— **leg, pain** in the: Arsen., Calc. carb., Lycop., Pulsat., Sepia.

— **ankles, pain** in the: Podophyl.

— **toes, pain** in the: Merc. viv., Sulphur, Thuya.

Feet; coldness of the: Agar., Alum., Amm. carb., Cann. sat., *Carb. an.*, Carb. veg., Cina, Cinchon., Cist. can., *Droser.*, Euphorb., Gelsem., Graphit., Hepar, Kreos., Leptand., Lycop., Mangan., Mar. ver., *Menyanth.*, Merc. viv., Mezer., Natr. carb., Natr. mur., Nux vom., *Petrol.*, Phosph. ac., Pulsat., *Sambuc.*, Stann.

— **cold water,** as if in: Gelsem.

— **dead,** as if: Calc. carb., *Lycop.*, Pulsat.

— **heat** of the: Acon., Agar., Arsen., Calc. carb., Lauroc., Lycop., Natr. carb., Nitr. ac., Pulsat., *Spong.*, Sulphur, Sulph. ac.

— **numb feeling:** Leptand.

Feet; swelling of the: Arsen., Cinchon., *Ferr.*, Kali carb., Phosphor., Pulsat., Sepia, Silic., Sulphur.

— **tired feeling:** Cimex.

Limbs; bending and stretching of the: Alum., *Arsen.*, Bellad., Borax, BROM., *Bryon.*, CALC. CARB., Capsic., Carb. veg., *Caustic.*, Chamom., Helleb., Hepar, *Ipecac.*, Kali bichr., Ledum, *Mur. ac.*, Natr. sulph., *Nux vom.*, Pulsat., RHUS TOX., Sepia, Sulphur.

— **go "to-sleep:"** Carb. veg., Coccul., Lycop., Merc. viv., *Nux vom.*, Phosphor., Rhus tox., Silic.

— **heaviness** of the: Bellad., *Cina*, Cinchon., HELLEB., *Kreos.*, Merc. viv., Natr. mur., Nux vom., Phosphor., Pulsat., Rhus tox., Sabad., Sepia, Spigel., Stann., Sulphur, Therid., Veratr.

Beaten; sensation as if: Arnic., Baptis., *Bellad.*, Cinchon., Natr. mur., Nux vom., Rhodod., Sulphur, Veratr.,

Contractions: *Capsic.*, Cimex, Cinchon., Graphit., Lycop., Natr. mur., Nitr. ac., Nux vom., *Paris*, Rhus tox., Sepia.

Crawling sensation: Acon., *Amm. carb.*, Arnic., Caustic., Coloc., Merc. viv., Nux vom., Pulsat., Rhus tox., Sabad., *Sambuc.*, Secal., Sepia, Spigel., Sulphur.

Distention of the blood-vessels: Arsen., *Bellad.*, Calc. carb., CHELID., *Cinchon.*, Ferr., Hyosc., Lycop., Menyanth., Nux vom., PHOSPHOR., Pulsat., Sepia, Sulphur, *Thuya.*

Excitability, nervous: Bellad., Calc. carb., Cinchon., Coffea, *Conium*, Mar. ver., Nux vom., Phosphor., Rhus tox., Sepia.

Exhaustion: Diadem.

Fainting: ACON., Arsen., Bryon., Chamom., Cinchon., *Coffea*, NUX VOM., Opium, Phosphor., PULSAT., Sepia, Stramon., *Valer.*, Veratr.

Floccilation: Arnic., ARSEN., Chamom., HEPAR, HYOSC., IOD., *Opium*, *Phosphor.*, Phosph. ac., Rhus tox., Stramon., *Sulphur.*

Insensibility, to touch: Coccul., Hyosc., Lycop., Mosch., *Opium*, Phosphor., Phosph. ac., *Pulsat.*, Rhus tox., Spong., *Stann.*, Stramon.

Lameness: Arsen., Bellad., Brom., Capsic., Cina, Cinchon., Coccul., *Ignat.*, *Nux vom.*, Phosph. ac., Pulsat., *Rhus tox.*, Sabad., Veratr.

Lassitude: Ambra, Anac., Apis, Arnic., ARSEN., Asar., Bellad., Borax, Bryon., *Calc. carb.*, Capsic., *Carb. veg.*, *Caustic.*, Chamom., CINCHON., Ferr., Helleb., Hepar, Hyosc., Ignat., Ipecac.,Kali carb., Kreos., *Lycop.*, Menyanth., Natr. mur., Nux mosch., *Nux vom.*, PHOSPHOR., Phosph. ac., Pulsat., Rheum, Rhodod., Rhus tox., Sabad., Seneg., *Sepia*, Spong., Stann., Stramon., Sulphur, *Veratr.*

Prostration, bodily: Ant. crud., Calc. carb., Carb. veg., Caustic., Cinchon., Coloc., *Lycop.*, Opium, *Petrol.*, Phosphor., Phosph. ac., Rhodod., Stann.

Restlessness, bodily: Acon., Amm. carb., Arnic., ARSEN., Asaf., BELLAD., Bovist., Bryon., Calc. carb., Capsic., Carb. veg., Chamom., Cimex., Cinchon., Coffea, Ferr., Hyosc., Ignat., *Kreos.*, LYCOP., *Merc. viv.*, Nux vom., Opium, Phosph. ac., RHUS TOX., *Sabad.*, Sepia, Silic., Staphis., Stramon.

Sinking sensation: Psorin.

Joints; stiffness in the: *Acon.*, Bellad., Brom., Bryon., Calc. carb., Capsic., CAUSTIC., Cicut., Coccul., *Coffea*, COLOC., Graphit., HELLEB., Hyosc., Ledum, Lycop., Nux vom., OPIUM, Petrol., Platin., RHUS TOX., *Sepia*, Staphis., Sulphur, Thuya.

— **stitches** in the: Calc. carb., Helleb., Mangan., Merc. viv., Rhus tox., Silic.

Spasms; clonic: Acon., Agar., *Arsen.*, Bellad., Bryon., *Calc. carb.*, *Camphor.*, Caustic., Chamom., Cicut., Cina, HYOSC., Ignat., Laches., Lycop., Merc. viv., *Opium*, Sepia, Stramon., Sulphur.

— **tonic:** Bellad., Caustic., Cicut., Coccul., Coloc., Ignat.,

Lycop., Merc. viv., Mosch., Petrol., Phosphor., Sepia, Sulphur, Veratr.

Tearing; (drawing); bones, in the: Baryt., Bellad., Caustic., Cinchon., Eup. perf., Eup. purp., Kali carb., Lycop., Merc. viv., Phosphor., Rhodod., Staphis., Therid., Veratr.

— **periosteum,** as if in the: *Arnic.*

— **joints,** in the: Bellad., Bryon., Calc. carb., Caustic., *Cimex.*, Cinchon., Kali carb., Ledum, Lycop., Merc. viv., Nux vom., Phosph. ac., RHUS TOX., Sepia, Strontia, Sulphur, Zinc.

— **muscles,** in the: ARSEN., BELLAD., Borax, Calc. carb., Carb. veg., Caustic., Cinchon., Ipecac., Kali carb., Laches., *Ledum*, LYCOP., Merc. viv., Mosch., *Nitrum*, Nitr. ac., *Nux vom.*, Phosphor., Phosph. ac., Pulsat., Rhodod., RHUS TOX., Sepia, Silic., Stann., Staphis., Strontia, Sulphur, Veratr., Zinc.

Tendons were too short; sensation as if: Cimex.

Trembling: Cist. can., Kali bichr.

Trembling sensation; internal: *Calc. carb.*, Iod., Lycop., PLATIN., Rhus tox., Staphis.

Twitchings: Arsen., Caustic., Coloc., Hyosc., Ignat., Laches., *Merc. viv.*, Natr. mur., *Opium*, Phosphor., Staphis., STRAMON., Sulphur.

Twitching of the muscles: Bellad., Iod., Kali carb., Mezer.

Uncover; desire to: Act. rac.

Bending and stretching of the limbs: See page 127.

Yawning: Acon., Ant. tart., Apis, Arnic., ARSEN., BROM., *Bryon.*, Calad., Capsic., *Caustic.*, *Cina*, Cinchon., *Crocus*, Cyclam., Digit., Ipecac., Kali bichr., Kali carb., *Lauroc.*, Lycop., Mar. ver., Menyanth., Mezer., *Mur. ac.*, Natr. mur., Natr. sulph., *Nux vom.*, *Oleand.*, *Paris*, Phosphor., Platin., Psorin., Pulsat., Rhus tox., Ruta, Sepia, Silic., THUYA.

Sleepiness: Acon., *Ambra*, ANT. TART., Apis, Arsen., Bellad., Borax, *Calad.*, Camphor., Capsic., Chamom., Cimex,

Cina, Cyclam., Helleb., Hyosc., Ignat., Kali bichr., Kali hydr., Ledum, Merc. viv., Mezer, *Natr. mur.*, NUX MOSCH., Nux vom., *Opium*, PHOSPHOR., Phosph. ac., Platin., Pulsat., *Rhus tox.*, *Sabad.*, *Sabin.*, Sepia, Staphis., Therid., *Veratr.*

Sleeplessness: Acon., Ambra, Amm. carb., Anac., Arsen., Bellad., Borax., Calc. carb., *Chamom.*, Cinchon., Coffea, Euphras., *Hepar*, Kreos., LYCOP., Mangan., Merc. viv., Natr. mur., Nitr. ac., Nux vom., Phosphor., Platin., *Pulsat.*, Rhodod., Rhus tox., Sepia, Silic., Sulphur.

Frequent waking at night: Act. rac.

Sleep, during; groaning and lamenting: Chamom., Laches., Nux vom.

— **murmuring:** Apis, Phosphor., Phosph. ac., Rhus tox.,

— **talking:** Arsen., Calc. carb., *Chamom.*, Nux vom., Pulsat., Sulphur.

— **bed; sliding down** in: Arsen., *Mur. ac.*

— **snoring:** Bellad., Camphor., *Opium*, Stann.

— **starting:** Arsen., *Lycop.*, Nux vom., Pulsat.

Skin; blueness of the: *Apis*, Coccul., *Laches.*, Merc. viv., *Nux vom.*, Veratr.

— **burning** in the: Petrol.

— — **ulcers** in the: Arsen., Merc. viv.

— **cold, clammy:** Corn. flor.

— **contraction** of the: Paris.

— **itching** in the: *Amm. carb.*, Arsen., Bryon., *Ledum*, *Mangan.*, Merc. viv., Nux vom., *Petrol.*, Rhus tox., Sulphur.

— **stitches** in the: Bryon., Rhus tox., *Sambuc.*

— **yellowness** of the: Ambra, Ant. crud., *Apis*, Arsen., Bellad., Bryon., Calc. carb. *Chamom.*, *Cinchon.*, Conium, Digit., Ferr., Helleb., Ignat., Natr. mur., *Nux vom.*, Opium, *Pulsat.*, *Rhus tox.*, Sepia.

HEAT.

Heat; in general: ACON., Act. rac., Æsc. hip., Agar., Agn. cast., Alum., *Ambra*, Amm. carb., Amm. mur., Anac., August., *Ant. crud.*, ANT. TART., Apis, Argent., *Arnic.*, ARSEN., *Arum tr.*, Asaf., Asar., (Aurum,) *Baptis.*, Baryt., BELLAD., Bismuth., Borax, Bovist., Brom., *Bryon.*, Cact. grand., (Calad.,) CALC. CARB., Camphor., Cann. sat., Canthar., Capsic., Carb. an., Carb. veg., Caustic., CHAMOM., Chelid., Chin. sulph., Cicut., Cimex, Cina, *Cinchon.*, Cist. can., Clemat., Coccul., *Coffea*, Colchic., Coloc., *Conium*, Corn. flor., Crocus, Cuprum, CYCLAM., Diadem., Digit., Droser., Dulcam., Eup. perf., Eup. purp., Euphorb., Euphras., FERR., FLUOR. AC., Gelsem. Graphit., Guaiac., Helleb., Hepar, Hydrast., Hydr. ac., HYOSC., Ignat., Iod., *Ipecac.*, Kali bichr., Kali carb., Kali hydr., Laches., Lauroc., Ledum., Leptand., Lobel. inf., Lycop., *Magn. carb.*, Magn. mur., Mangan., Mar. ver., Menyanth., *Merc. viv.*, Merc. corr., Mezer., Mosch., Mur. ac., *Natr. carb.*, NATR. MUR., Natr. sulph., Nitrum., Nitr. ac., Nux mosch., *Nux vom.*, Oleand., *Opium*, Oxal. ac., Paris, Petrol., Phosphor., Phosph. ac., Platin., Plumbum, Podophyl., Psorin., Pulsat., Ran. bulb., RAN. SCEL., RHEUM, Rhodod., Rhus tox., Ruta, Sabad., Sabin., Sambuc., Sanguin., Sarsap., SCILLA, SECAL., Selen., Seneg., *Sepia*, SILIC., SPIGEL., SPONG., *Stann.*, Staphis. STRAMON., Strontia, *Sulphur*, SULPH. AC., Tarax., Thuya, VALER., Veratr. (Verbas.,) (Viol. od.,) VIOL. TR., Zinc.

— **anxious:** ACON., Alum., AMBRA, Amm. carb., Anac., Apis, Argent., Arnic., ARSEN., *Asaf.*, *Baryt.*, BELLAD., *Bovist.*, Bryon., *Calc. carb.*, *Canthar.*, Capsic., Carb. veg., CHAMOM., Cina, Cinchon., *Coccul.*, Coffea., Colchic., *Conium*, Cyclam., Droser., Euphorb., Ferr., Graphit., Hepar, Hyosc., Ignat., IPECAC., Laches., Lauroc., Lycop., *Magn. carb.*, Magn. mur., MERC. VIV., Mur. ac., Natr. carb., Natr. mur., Nitr. ac., NUX VOM., Opium, Paris, Petrol., PHOSPHOR., *Phosph. ac.*, Platin., *Plumbum*, PULSAT., *Rheum*, Rhodod., Rhus tox., *Ruta*, Sabin., *Secal.*, Sepia, Spigel., SPONG., STANN., Staphis., *Stramon.*, Sulphur, Thuya, Valer., *Veratr.*, *Viol. tr.* *Zinc.*

Heat; ascending: see direction.

— **burning:** ACON., *Agn. cast.*, Apis, Arnic., ARSEN., *Asar.*, BELLAD., *Bismuth.*, Brom., *Bryon.*, *Cann. sat.*, *Canthar.*, Capsic., Carb. an., CARB. VEG., *Chamom.*, Cinchon., Coccul., *Coloc.*, Conium, *Dulcam.*, Euphorb., *Helleb.*, *Hepar*, HYOSC., Ignat., Ipecac., Laches., Lauroc., Ledum, Leptand., Lycop., Magn. carb., Merc. viv., *Merc. corr.*, *Mosch.*, *Mur. ac.*, *Nux vom.*, OPIUM, Petrol., Platin., Psorin., Pulsat., Rhodod., Rhus tox., Sabad., *Sabin.*, SAMBUC., Sanguin., *Scilla*, SECAL., Selen., Silic., Spigel., SPONG., *Stann.*, *Staphis.*, Stramon., *Thuya*, Veratr.

— — **between the skin and flesh,** like: Brom.

— — **sparks,** like from: *Alum.*, Amm. carb., Ant. crud., Baryt., Calad., Cina, *Clemat.*, Graphit., Kali carb., Ledum, Lycop., Magn. mur., Mezer., Nitr. ac., Rheum., Secal., *Selen.*, *Sulphur*, Viol. od.

— **direction; ascending:** *Acon.*, Agar., Amm. mur., Argent., Calad., Canthar., Carb. an., *Cina*, Colchic., Digit., *Hyosc.*, Kali carb., LACHES., *Ledum*, Magn. carb., *Mangan.*, PHOSPHOR., Plumbum, Pulsat., SABAD., *Sarsap.*, Sepia, Spigel., Staphis., Strontia, SULPHUR.

— — **descending:** Acon., Agar., *Alum.*, Baryt., Bellad., Canthar., Caustic., Chelid., CICUT., *Coffea*, Colchic., CROCUS, Euphras., *Lauroc.*, Magn. carb., Mezer., *Mosch.*, *Natr. carb.*, *Opium*, *Paris*, Ruta, Sabad., *Staphis.*, Strontia, *Sulph. ac.*, Thuya, *Valer.*, Veratr., Zinc.

— **dry:** ACON., Æsc. hip., Alum., Ambra, Amm. mur., Anac., Ant. crud., Ant. tart., *Apis*, Argent., *Arnic.*, ARSEN., *Arum tr.*, Baryt., BELLAD., *Bismuth.*, *Bryon.*, Calc. carb., Camphor., Cann. sat., Canthar., Capsic., Carb. veg., Caustic., Chamom., *Chelid.*, Cinchon., *Clemat.*, *Coccul.*, *Coffea*, *Colchic.*, *Coloc.*, Conium, Crocus, Cuprum, Cyclam., *Dulcam.*, FERR., *Graphit.*, Helleb., *Hepar*, Hyosc., *Ignat.*, IOD., IPECAC., Kali carb., Kreos., *Laches.*, Lachnanth., Lauroc., Ledum, Leptand., *Lycop.*, Mangan., *Merc. viv.*, Mosch., Mur. ac., Natr. carb., Natr. mur., Nitrum, *Nitr. ac.*, Nux mosch., *Nux vom.*, Opium, Paris, PHOSPHOR., *Phosph. ac.*, Plumbum, Podoyhyl.,

Pulsat., Ran bulb., *Ran. scel.*, Rheum, Rhodod., Rhus tox., Ruta, Sabad., Sabin., *Sambuc.*, SCILLA, SECAL., Selen., Sepia, Silic., Spigel., *Spong.*, Stann., Staphis., Stramon., *Strontia*, SULPHUR, Sulph. ac., Tarax., *Thuya*, Valer., Veratr., *Viol. tr.*, Zinc.

Heat; external: ACON., AGN. CAST., Alum., *Anac.*, Ant. crud., *Arsen.*, Asar., Baryt., BELLAD., *Bismuth.*, *Bryon.*, *Calc. carb.*, Camphor., CANTHAR., Carb. veg., *Chamom.*, *Chelid.*, Cinchon., *Coccul.*, COFFEA, *Colchic.*, *Coloc.*, CONIUM, *Digit.*, Dulcam., Guaiac., *Helleb.*, Hepar, *Hyosc.*, IGNAT., Iod., Ipecac., Kali carb., Laches., Lauroc., Lycop., Menyanth., *Merc. viv.*, *Merc. corr.*, Mur. ac., Nitrum, Nitr. ac., Nux vom., Opium, Phosphor., Phosph. ac., *Plumbum*, Pulsat., *Rheum*, *Rhus tox.*, Ruta, SCILLA, SELEN., Sepia, *Silic.*, Spigel., Spong., Staphis., Stramon., Sulphur, *Thuya*, Valer.

— **flushes:** Acon., Agn. cast., Alum., Ambra, Amm. carb., *Amm. mur.*, Ant. tart., Apis, *Arnic.*, Arsen., Asaf., Asar., *Baryt.*, Bellad., BISMUTH., *Borax*, *Bovist.*, Bryon., CALC. CARB., Cann. sat., Canthar., Carb. an., CARB. VEG., *Caustic.*, Chamom., Cinchon., Clemat., *Coccul.*, Coffea, *Coloc.*, Corn. cir., *Crocus*, *Cuprum*, *Digit.*, Droser., *Eup. perf.*, Graphit., *Hepar*, Hydrast., IGNAT., IOD., Ipecac., Kali bichr., Kali carb., Kali hydr., *Kreos.*, Lachnanth., Lauroc., Lobel. inf., *Lycop.*, Magn. carb., Magn. mur., *Mangan.*, Mar. ver., Menyanth., Merc. viv., *Natr. carb.*, NATR. MUR., Natr. sulph., *Nitr. ac.*, Nux vom., *Oleand.*, Opium, Oxal. ac., *Petrol.*, PHOSPHOR., Phosph. ac., *Platin.*, Plumbum, Psorin., Pulsat., Ran. bulb., *Rhus tox.*, *Ruta*, Sabad., *Sabin.*, Sambuc., Sanguin., *Seneg.*, SEPIA, SILIC., *Spigel.*, *Spong.*, Stann., Staphis., *Sulphur*, SULPH. AC., *Thuya*, *Valer.*, Viol. tr., *Zinc.*

— **hot water was poured over one,** as if: ARSEN., Bryon., Phosphor., Phosph. ac., *Pulsat.*, *Rhus tox.*, Sanguin., *Sepia.*

— — **breast to abdomen,** from: Sanguin.

— **internal:** ACON., Alum., Ambra, Amm. carb., Amm. mur., Anac., Angust., Ant. crud., Ant. tart., Apis., Argent.,

Arnic., ARSEN., Asaf., Asar., Baryt., BELLAD., Bismuth., Borax, Bovist., *Brom.*, *Bryon.*, CALAD., Calc. carb., Camphor., Cann. sat., Canthar., *Capsic.*, Carb. an., Carb. veg., Caustic., *Chamom.*, *Chelid.*, *Cicut.*, Cina, Cinchon., *Clemat.*, Coccul., COFFEA, Colchic., *Coloc.*, CONIUM, *Crocus*, *Cuprum*, CYCLAM., Digit., Droser., Dulcam., *Euphorb.*, Graphit., Guaiac., *Helleb.*, Hepar, Hyosc., IGNAT., IOD., Ipecac., KALI CARB., Kreos., *Laches.*, Lauroc., *Ledum*, Lycop., *Magn. carb.*, Magn. mur., Mangan., Mar. ver., *Menyanth.*, Merc. viv., Merc. corr., *Mezer.*, *Mosch.*, *Mur. ac.*, Natr. carb., Natr. mur., Nitrum, *Nitr. ac.*, Nux mosch., *Nux vom.*, Oleand., Opium, Oxal. ac., Paris, *Petrol.*, Phosphor., *Phosph. ac.*, Platin., *Plumbum*, *Pulsat.*, Ran. bulb., Ran. scel., *Rhodod.*, *Rhus tox.*, Ruta, *Sabad.*, Sabin., Sambuc., Sarsap., *Scilla*, Secal., Seneg., Sepia, SILIC., Spigel., Spong., STANN., *Staphis.*, Stramon., Strontia, *Sulphur*, Sulph. ac., Tarax., Thuya, Valer., VERATR., Viol. tr., ZINC.

Heat; quivering, through the body: Psorin.

PARTIAL HEAT.

Heat; one side, of: Acon., Agar., *Agn. cast.*, ALUM., Amm. mur., Anac., Ant. crud., Ant. tart., *Arnic.*, Arsen., *Asaf.*, Asar., Baryt., *Bellad.*, Borax, Bovist.. Brom., *Bryon.*, Calc. carb., Cann. sat., Capsic., Carb. an., *Carb. veg.*, *Caustic.*, CHAMOM., *Chelid.*, Cina, Clemat., Coccul., Coffea, Colchic., Coloc., Cyclam., DIGIT., Droser., Dulcam., Euphorb., *Graphit.*, Helleb., Hyosc., Ignat., *Kali carb.*, Lauroc., LYCOP., Magn. carb., Magn. mur., *Mangan.*, Mar. ver., Menyanth., Merc. viv. Mezer., MOSCH., *Mur. ac.*, *Natr. carb.*, Natr. mur., Nitr. ac., NUX VOM., Oleand., PARIS, Phosphor., Phosph. ac., *Platin.*, Plumbum, PULSAT., Ran. bulb., Rheum, RHUS TOX., Ruta, Sabad., Sarsap., Scilla, Seneg., Sepia, *Spigel.*, Stann., *Staphis.*, *Strontia*, *Sulphur*, Sulph. ac., *Tarax.*, Thuya, Veratr., Verbas., Viol. od., Zinc.

— **left side:** Acon., Agar., Anac., Bellad., Calc. carb., Capsic., Chelid., Cina, Coccul., Coffea, Cyclam., Euphorb.,

Graphit., Helleb., Hyosc., Ignat., *Lycop.*, Mar. ver., Menyanth., Merc. viv., Mezer., Natr. mur., Nitr. ac., Nux vom., Paris, Phosph. ac., Platin., *Ran. bulb.* Rheum, *Rhus tox.*, Ruta, Sarsap., Seneg., Sepia, Spigel., Sulphur, Sulph. ac., Tarax., Thuya, Viol. od., Zinc.

Heat; right side: ALUM., Amm. mur., Ant. crud., Ant. tart., Arsen., Asaf., Asar., Baryt., Borax, Bovist., Brom., Bryon., Cann. sat., Carb. veg., Chamom., Clemat., Colchic., Coloc., Droser., Dulcam., Ignat., Kali carb., Lauroc., Lycop., Magn. carb., Magn. mur., Mosch., Mur. ac., Natr. carb., Oleand., Phosphor., Plumbum, Pulsat., *Ran. bulb.*, Rhus tox., Scilla, Sepia, Staphis., Strontia, Thuya.

— **anterior body,** of: Amm. mur., Canthar., Capsic., *Chamom.*, Cicut., Cina, *Crocus*, IGNAT., Iod., Ledum, Mezer., Mosch., Ran. bulb., RHUS TOX., Secal., Selen.

— **posterior body,** of: Amm. carb., Calc. carb., Carb. an., Carb. veg., Caustic., CHAMOM., Lycop., Menyanth., Mur. ac., Natr. carb., Natr. mur., Rhus tox., Sepia, Silic., Stann., Sulphur, Thuya.

— **upper body,** of the: Acon., AGAR., *Anac.*, Arnic., Bismuth., Bryon., Cina, Crocus, *Droser.*, Euphorb., Kali bichr., Menyanth., Nux vom., *Paris*, Rhus tox., Sabad., Selen.

— **lower body,** of the: Caustic., Hepar, Kali carb., Lycop., Natr. carb., Natr. mur., *Opium*, Pulsat., Stann.

— **covered parts,** of the: *Thuya.*

— **head,** on the: ACON., Amm. carb., Ant. crud., *Arnic.*, Arsen., Asaf., *Asar.*, *Aurum*, *Bellad.*, BISMUTH., Borax, Bryon., *Calc. carb.*, Cann. sat., Canthar., Carb. veg. *Caustic.*, Chamom., *Cina*, Cinchon., Coffea, Coloc., *Crocus*, Cuprum, *Droser.*, Dulcam., *Euphorb.*, Ferr., Gelsem., Graphit., Helleb., Hepar, Hydr. ac., *Ipecac.*, Lycop., *Mangan.*, *Menyanth.*, Merc. viv., *Mezer.*, Mosch., Mur. ac., *Natr. carb.*, Natr. sulph., Nitr. ac., Nux vom., Oleand., OPIUM, Petrol., *Phosphor.*, PHOSPH.

AC., *Rhus tox.*, Ruta, SABAD., Sanguin., Selen., Sepia, Silic., Spigel., Spong., Stann., Staphis., *Stramon.*, Sulphur, Veratr., Viol. tr.

Heat; head, spreading from the: *Acon.*, *Opium.*

— **head,** in the: ACON., Alum., Ambra, Amm. mur., Anac., Ant. tart., Apis, *Arnic.*, ARSEN., Aurum, Baryt., BELLAD., Brom., *Bryon.*, *Calad.*, Calc. carb., Canthar., Capsic., Carb. an., Carb. veg., Caustic., Chamom., Chelid., Cicut., Cinchon., Clemat., Coccul., *Coffea*, Coloc., Conium, Crocus, Cuprum, *Cyclam.*, Digit., Dulcam., Euphorb., Euphras., *Helleb.*, Hepar, Hyosc., *Ignat.*, Iod., Ipecac., KALI CARB., *Laches.*, Lauroc., Ledum, Lycop., Magn. carb., MAGN. MUR., Menyanth., Merc. viv., Mezer., Mosch., Mur. ac., Natr. carb., Natr. mur., *Nitr. ac.*, Nux mosch., *Nux vom.*, *Petrol.*, PHOSPHOR., *Phosph. ac.*, Platin., Plumbum, Psorin., *Pulsat.*, Ran. scel., Rhodod., *Rhus tox.*, Ruta, Sabad., Sabin., Scilla., Secal., SEPIA, *Silic.*, Spigel., Spong., *Stann.*, Staphis., Stramon., Strontia, *Sulphur*, VERATR., Viol. od., *Zinc.*

— **top of the head,** on the: *Carb. veg.*, Caustic., Graphit., *Hyper.*, Lauroc., *Magn. sulph.*, *Phosphor.*, Stann.

— **eyes,** of the: *Acon.*, Alum., Ambra, Amm. carb., Amm. mur., Angust., Apis, Arnic., Arsen., *Asaf.*, Asar., BELLAD., Bovist., *Bryon.*, *Calc. carb.*, Canthar., Capsic., Carb. an., *Carb. veg.*, CAUSTIC., CHAMOM., Cicut., Clemat., Coloc., Crocus, *Euphras.*, Ferr., GRAPHIT., *Hepar*, Ignat., *Kali carb.*, Laches., Lauroc., *Lycop.*, Magn. carb., Mangan., *Merc. viv.*, Natr. carb., Natr. mur., Nux mosch., Nux vom., Opium, Paris, Petrol., PHOSPHOR., Phosph. ac., Plumbum, Pulsat., Rhodod., Rhus tox., Ruta, *Sepia*, Silic., *Spigel.*, Spong., Staphis., SULPHUR, Sulph. ac., Tarax., Thuya, Valer., VERATR., Verbas., Viol. od., Zinc.

— **eyebrows,** on the: Apis, Bellad., Coloc., Digit., Droser., Kali carb., Merc. viv., Spigel., Sulphur, Thuya.

— **eyelids,** on the: Acon., *Apis*, *Arsen.*, *Bellad.*, *Bryon.*, *Calc. carb.*, Caustic., Clemat., Conium, Graphit., Lycop., Merc. viv., Nux vom., Oleand., Phosphor., Phosph. ac., Rhus tox., Seneg., Sepia, Spigel., *Sulphur*, Viol. od.

Heat; canthi, in the: Agar., Amm. mur., Aurum, Baryt., *Calc. carb.*, Carb. veg., Clemat., Natr. mur., Nux vom., Paris, *Phosphor.*, *Phosph. ac.*, Pulsat., Sepia, Silic., Staphis., Strontia, *Sulphur*, Thuya.

— **ears,** on the: Acon., Agar., *Alum.*, Angust., Ant. crud., Apis, Arnic., *Arsen.*, Asar., Brom., Bryon., Calc. carb., Camphor., Canthar., *Carb. veg.*, Cinchon., Clemat., Hepar, Ignat., Kali carb., Kreos., Magn. carb., *Merc. viv.*, Natr. mur., Nitrum, Oleand., PULSAT., Rhodod., Sabad., Sabin., *Sepia*, Spigel., Spong., Zinc.

— **ears,** in the: Acon., Alum., Arnic., *Arsen.*, Asar., *Bellad.*, Bryon., CALC. CARB., Canthar., Caustic., Hepar, Ignat., *Kali carb.*, Kreos., *Merc. viv.*, Natr. mur., Nux vom., Paris, *Pulsat.*, Rhodod., Sabin., *Sepia*, Silic., Spong., Sulph. ac., Zinc.

— — **spreading** from the: Oleand., *Sepia.*

— **lobe of the ear,** on the: Acon., *Alum.*, Angust., Arnic., Bryon., Camphor., Carb. an., Caustic., Cinchon., Kali carb., Kreos., Merc. viv., Nitrum, *Sabad.*, Silic.

— **face,** in the: ACON., Act. rac., Agar., *Agn. cast.*, Alum., Ambra, Amm. carb., Amm. mur., *Anac.*, *Angust.*, Ant. crud., Ant. tart., *Apis*, Argent., *Arnic.*, Arsen., *Asaf.*, *Asar.*, *Aurum*, Baryt., BELLAD., *Bismuth.*, Bovist., *Bryon.*, Calc. carb., Camphor., *Cann. sat.*, Canthar., CHAMOM., *Cina*, Cinchon., Cist. can., Clemat., COCCUL., *Coffea*, *Coloc.*, Conium, *Crocus*, *Cyclam*, *Digit.*, *Droser.*, *Dulcam.*, *Euphorb.*, Euphras., *Ferr.*, Gelsem., *Graphit.*, *Guaiac.*, *Helleb.*, Hepar, *Hyosc.*, IGNAT., Ipecac., Kali bichr., Kali carb., Kreos., Laches., Lauroc., *Ledum*, *Lycop.*, *Mangan.*, Menyanth., *Merc. viv.*, Merc. corr., Mosch., *Mur. ac.*, Natr. carb., Natr. mur., Nitrum, *Nitr. ac.*, *Nux mosch.*, *Nux vom.*, *Oleand.*, Opium, Oxal. ac., Petrol., *Phosphor.*, *Phosph. ac.*, *Platin.*, Plumbum, Psorin., *Pulsat.*, *Ran. bulb.*, Ran. scel., RHODOD., *Rhus tox.*, RUTA, SABAD., *Sabin.*, *Sambuc.*, Scilla, Seneg., Sepia, SILIC., Spigel., Spong., Stann., *Staphis.*, STRAMON., Strontia, *Sulphur*, *Tarax.*, THUYA, *Valer.*, Veratr., Viol. od., Viol. tr., *Zinc.*

— — **spreading** from the: *Acon.*, Alum.

Heat; forehead, on the: BELLAD., Chamom., Euphras., *Hepar*, Ledum, Phosphor., *Phosph. ac.*, *Rhus tox.*, SEPIA, Sulphur.

— **cheeks,** on the: ACON., Agar., Alum., *Angust.*, *Ant. crud.*, Arnic., Arsen., Asar., AURUM, BELLAD., *Bovist.*, BRYON., *Calc. carb.*, Cann. sat., Canthar., *Capsic.*, Carb. an., Carb. veg., Caustic., CHAMOM., Cina, CINCHON., Clemat., COCCUL., Coffea, Coloc., Crocus., Droser., *Dulcam.*, *Euphorb.*, *Ferr.*, Helleb., HEPAR, *Hyosc.*, IGNAT., Iod., Ipecac., KALI CARB., Kreos., Laches., *Ledum*, *Lycop.*, Mangan., MERC. VIV., *Merc. corr.*, Mosch., Mur. ac., Nitrum, *Nitr. ac.*, *Nux vom.*, Oleand., *Opium*, *Phosphor.*, Phosph. ac., PLATIN., Plumbum, Pulsat., Ran. bulb., Rhodod., RHUS TOX., *Ruta*, *Sabad.*, *Sambuc.*, SEPIA, *Silic.*, Spigel., STANN., *Staphis.*, STRAMON., Sulphur., *Thuya*, *Valer.*, *Viol. tr.*, Zinc.

— **one cheek,** of: *Acon.*, *Arnic.*, Baryt., *Bellad.*, Borax, *Cann. sat.*, Canthar., CHAMOM., Cinchon., Coloc., *Droser.*, IGNAT., Ipecac., *Mosch.*, Nux vom., *Phosphor.*, Phosph. ac., Plumbum, Pulsat., *Ran. bulb.*, Rheum, Stramon., Sulph. ac., Thuya, Veratr., *Viol. tr.*

— **pale cheek,** of the: Mosch.

— — **uncovered,** of the: *Thuya*, Viol. tr.

— **nose,** on the: Agar., Alum., Ant. crud., Arnic., *Arsen.*, Aurum, Baryt., BELLAD., Bovist., Calad., *Cann. sat.*, CANTHAR., Capsic., *Carb. an.*, Caustic., *Cina*, Cinchon., Coffea, Graphit., Helleb., Hepar, Hyosc., Iod., *Kali carb.*, *Ledum*, Magn. mur., Merc. viv., Mezer., Mosch., Natr. carb., Natr. mur., *Nitrum*, Nitr. ac., Nux vom., Petrol., Phosph. ac., PULSAT., Rhus tox., Ruta, Sarsap., Spigel., Stann., Strontia, Sulphur, *Thuya*, Veratr.

— — **in the:** Amm. mur., Arnic., ARSEN., Asar., Aurum, *Bellad.*, Calad., Cann. sat., Canthar., Caustic., Chamom., *Cina*, Cinchon., Hyosc., *Merc. viv.*, *Mezer.*, Mosch., Nux vom., PULSAT., Rhus tox., Silic., Sulphur.

— — **as if streaming out** of the: Strontia.

— **lips,** on the: Ambra, Amm. carb., Amm. mur., Apis,

Arnic., ARSEN., Asaf., Bellad., Borax, Brom., *Bryon.*, Canthar., Capsic., Carb. an., Caustic., Cicut., Cina, Cinchon., Clemat., Hyosc., Kreos., *Merc. viv.*, MEZER., Mur. ac., Natr. mur., *Nux vom.*, Phosphor., Phosph, ac., Pulsat., Rhodod., *Rhus tox.*, Sabad., Sepia, Spigel., *Staphis.*, Sulphur, Thuya, Veratr.

Heat; lip, upper, on the: Ant. crud., Arsen., Baryt., Bellad., Brom., Cicut., Graphit., Kali carb., Kreos., Merc. viv., Mezer., Natr. carb., Rhus tox., Sepia, *Spigel.*, Staphis., *Sulphur*, Thuya, Veratr.

— — **lower,** on the: Asaf., Bellad., Borax, *Bryon.*, Caustic., Clemat., Hepar, *Ignat.*, *Mezer.*, Oleand., Phosph. ac., *Pulsat.*, Sabad., *Sepia*, *Thuya.*

— **jaw, lower,** on the: Acon., Bovist., Canthar., *Caustic.*, Chamom., Natr. carb., Paris, Phosphor., Pulsat., Rhus tox., *Staphis.*, Zinc.

— **chin,** on the: Agar., Anac., Ant. crud., Apis, *Arsen.*, Bellad., Bovist., *Caustic.*, Clemat., Euphras., Kreos., Mangan., Merc. viv., Mezer., Platin., *Rhus tox.*, Sepia, *Silic.*, Spong., Sulphur, Thuya, Veratr., Zinc.

— **mouth,** in the: Acon., Amm. carb., *Apis*, ARSEN., Asaf., Asar., Bellad., BORAX, Bovist., *Calc. carb.*, Camphor., Canthar., Carb. an., *Carb. veg.*, *Chamom.*, Colchic., Cuprum, Kreos., Lauroc., Magn. mur., *Merc. viv.*, Merc. corr., MEZER., Natr. carb., Natr. mur., Nitr. ac., Petrol., PHOSPHOR., Platin., Plumbum, Pulsat., Sabad., Sepia, Silic., *Spigel.*, Spong., Stramon., Strontia, *Sulphur*, *Veratr.*, Zinc.

— — **as if streaming out** of the: Strontia.

— **tongue,** on the: *Acon.*, *Apis*, Arnic., ARSEN., Asar., Baryt., BELLAD., Bryon., Canthar., Carb. an., Carb. veg., *Caustic.*, Coffea, *Colchic.*, Conium, Hepar, Hyosc., Laches., Magn. mur., Mangan., MERC. VIV., Merc. corr., Natr. carb., PHOSPHOR., *Phosph. ac.*, Platin., PLUMBUM, *Pulsat.*, Ran. scel., Rhodod., Rhus tox., *Sabad.*, *Seneg.*, Stramon., SULPHUR, Thuya, Veratr.

— **teeth,** in the: *Arnic.*, BARYT., Caustic., Cinchon., Graphit., *Kali carb.*, *Magn. carb.*, *Merc. viv.*, Merc. corr.,

Mezer., Natr. mur., *Nux vom.*, PHOSPH. AC., Silic., Spong., Sulphur, Zinc.

Heat; gums, of the: Arsen., BELLAD., CHAMOM., *Lycop.*, Magn. carb., MERC. VIV., Merc. corr., Mur. ac., *Nux vom.*, Petrol., Phosph. ac., Pulsat., Rhus tox., Sepia, Strontia.

— **palate,** on the: Apis, Bellad., Calc. carb., *Camphor.*, Canthar., Capsic., *Carb. veg.*, Chamom., Coccul., DULCAM., Euphorb., Ignat., Laches., Magn. carb., *Merc. viv.*, Merc. corr., Mezer., *Nux mosch.*, Nux vom., Paris, *Petrol.*, Phosphor., Phosph. ac., Ran. bulb., *Scilla*, Seneg., Spigel., Staphis., Thuya.

— **throat, as if streaming out** of the: *Nux vom.*

— **œsophagus,** in the: *Acon.*, Alum., Amm. carb., *Apis*, Argent., Arnic., *Arsen.*, *Asaf.*, Aurum., Baryt., BELLAD., Bismuth., Borax, Bovist., Brom., Calc. carb., *Camphor.*, Cann. sat., *Canthar.*, Capsic., Carb. an., *Carb. veg.*, Caustic., *Chamom.*, Chelid., Cinchon., Coccul., Colchic., Conium, Cuprum, Droser., *Dulcam.*, *Euphorb.*, Graphit., Guaiac., Hepar, Hyosc., Ignat., Iod., Kreos., *Laches.*, Lauroc., Lycop., Mangan., MERC. VIV., *Merc. corr.*, *Mezer.*, Natr. carb., NITR. AC., Nux mosch., NUX VOM., Oleand., Paris, Petrol., *Phosphor.*, Phosph. ac., Platin., *Pulsat.*, Ran bulb., Ran. scel., *Rhodod.*, *Rhus tox.*, SABAD., Scilla, *Secal.*, Seneg., Sepia, Spong., Stramon., *Strontia*, Sulphur, Thuya, VERATR.

— **stomach,** in the: *Acon.*, Amm. mur., APIS, ARSEN., Asaf., Bellad., Bismuth., *Bryon.*, *Calad.*, Calc. carb., *Camphor.*, Cann. sat., *Canthar.*, Capsic., *Carb. an.*, Carb. veg., Caustic., Chamom., Chelid., CICUT., *Colchic.*, Crocus, Digit., Dulcam., EUPHORB., Fluor. ac., *Graphit.*, Helleb., Hyosc., *Ignat.*, Iod., Laches., Lauroc., Lycop., *Mangan.*, Menyanth., Merc. viv., *Mezer.*, Mosch., Nitrum, Nux mosch., *Nux vom.*, Opium, Paris, *Phosphor.*, Phosph. ac., Platin., *Plumbum*, Pulsat., Ran. bulb., Ruta, SABAD., Sabin., Sanguin., *Sarsap.*, SECAL., Seneg., *Sepia*, *Silic.*, *Sulphur*, Sulph. ac., Veratr.

— — **spreading** from the: *Opium.*

— **pit of the stomach** (external), on the: Acon., Ambra, Amm. mur., Ant. crud., *Apis*, Argent., ARSEN., Bellad., *Bryon.*,

Calc. carb., *Capsic.*, *Carb. veg.*, Chamom., Coccul., Euphorb., Ferr., Laches., *Merc. viv.*, Mezer, Mosch., *Natr. mur.*, *Nux vom.*, PHOSPHOR., Platin., Ran. bulb., Ran. scel., SECAL., Sepia, *Silic.*, Sulphur, Thuya, *Veratr.*

Heat; liver, in the region of the: *Acon.*, Amm.carb., Amm. mur., Apis, Arnic., *Arsen.*, Bellad., *Bryon.*, Ignat., *Kali carb.*, Laches., Lauroc., Magn. mur., *Merc. viv.*, Phosphor., Phosph. ac., *Sabad.*, *Secal.*, Sepia, *Stann.*, Sulphur, Thuya.

— **spleen, in the region** of the: Acon., Apis, Arnic., *Arsen.*, *Asaf.*, Bellad., Borax, *Bryon.*, Cann. sat., Carb. veg., Chelid., *Cinchon.*, Graphit., *Ignat.*, Merc. viv., Nux vom., Platin., Pulsat., *Ran. bulb.*, *Rhus tox.*, Secal., Seneg., Spigel., *Sulphur*, Sulph. ac., Thuya.

— **kidneys, in the region** of the: Alum., *Bellad.*, Cann. sat., CANTHAR., *Hepar*, Kali carb., *Lycop.*, *Nux vom.*, Pulsat., Sepia, Thuya.

— **abdomen,** in the: *Acon.*, Alum., Amm. carb., APIS, ARSEN., *Asaf.*, Bellad., Bovist., BRYON., *Camphor.*, *Canthar.*, *Carb. an.*, *Carb. veg.*, Caustic., Chamom., *Cicut.*, Cina, *Coccul.*, *Colchic.*, *Coloc.*, Cuprum, Euphorb., Euphras., IPECAC., Laches., Lauroc., LYCOP., Menyanth., Merc. viv., Merc. corr., *Mezer.*, *Nux vom.*, Paris, PHOSPHOR., *Phosph. ac.*, *Platin.*, Plumbum, Pulsat., Ran. bulb., *Rhus tox.*, Ruta, *Sabad.*, Sabin., Sarsap., SECAL., *Sepia*, SILIC., Spong., Stann., *Sulphur*, Thuya, *Veratr.*

— — **upper part** of the: Amm. mur., *Apis*, *Calad.*, *Camphor.*, CANTHAR., Caustic., Chamom., Nux vom., *Phosphor.*, Thuya.

— — **lower part** of the: *Apis*, ARSEN., Bellad., BRYON., *Calc. carb.*, *Camphor.*, Capsic., Coffea, LYCOP., Nitrum, Phosphor., *Phosph. ac.*, Ran. bulb., Sabin., *Sepia*, *Stann.*, Sulphur, Sulph. ac., Tarax.

— — **external,** on the: Arsen., Bellad., BRYON., Canthar., Carb. veg., Laches., Lycop., Magn. mur., *Merc. viv.*, Natr. carb., *Nux vom.*, Pulsat., RHUS TOX., *Sabad.*, *Selen.*, Sepia, Silic., *Sulphur*, Sulph. ac., Viol. tr.

Heat; umbilicus, spreading from the: *Rhus tox.*

— **groins,** in the: Alum., *Amm. mur.*, ARSEN., Aurum, Canthar., Graphit., *Ignat.*, Kali carb., LYCOP., *Merc. viv.*, Mur. ac., NUX VOM., Rhus tox., Sepia, Silic., Spigel., *Strontia*, SULPHUR, Thuya, Zinc.

— **perinæum,** at the: Ant. crud., Ant. tart., Asaf., CARB. AN., CARB. VEG., *Cyclam.*, Lycop., Mur. ac., *Nux vom.*, Plumbum, Rhodod., Sepia, Silic., Spigel., SULPHUR, Tarax.

— **anus,** at the: Acon., Alum., Amm. mur., Ant. crud., *Apis*, ARSEN., Baryt., Bovist., *Bryon.*, *Calc. carb.*, Canthar., *Capsic.*, Carb. an., CARB. VEG., *Caustic.*, Cinchon., Coccul., Colchic., Coloc., Conium, Euphras., *Graphit.*, Ignat., Iod., Ipecac., *Kali carb.*, Laches., Lauroc., Lycop., Magn. mur., Merc. viv., Mur. ac., Natr. carb., Natr. mur., Nitr. ac., NUX VOM., Oleand., Petrol., PHOSPHOR., Phosph. ac., Pulsat., *Rhus tox.*, *Sepia*, Spigel., Stann., Staphis., Strontia, SULPHUR, Sulph. ac., Thuya, Veratr., Zinc.

— **rectum,** in the: Acon., Alum., Ambra, Ant. tart., *Apis*, ARSEN., *Bellad.*, *Bryon.*, *Calc. carb.*, CANTHAR., Capsic., Carb. an., Carb. veg., Caustic., Cinchon., Conium, Euphorb., Ferr., Ignat., Kali carb., Lauroc., *Lycop.*, Magn. mur., MERC. VIV., Merc. corr., Mezer., Mur. ac., Natr. carb., Natr. mur., Nitr. ac., NUX VOM., PHOSPHOR., Phosph. ac., Pulsat., Rhus tox., SABAD., SEPIA, Strontia, SULPHUR, Thuya, Veratr.

— **bladder,** in the: *Acon.*, Ant. crud., *Apis*, Arnic., *Arsen.*, Bellad., Calc. carb., Cann. sat., CANTHAR., Caustic., Chamom., Cinchon., Coloc., Dulcam., Graphit., Hyosc., Ignat., Laches., *Lycop.*, Merc. viv., Mezer., NUX VOM., Paris., Petrol., Phosphor., Phosph. ac., Pulsat., Rheum, Ruta, Sabin., Sarsap., Scilla, *Sepia*, Staphis., *Sulphur.*

— **urethra,** in the: Acon., Alum., Ambra, Ant. crud., Ant. tart., Apis, Arnic., Arsen., Baryt., Bellad., *Bryon.*, *Calc. carb.*, *Cann. sat.*, CANTHAR., Capsic., *Caustic.*, *Chamom.*, Chelid., *Cinchon.*, Clemat., COLCHIC., Coloc., Conium, Cuprum., Dulcam., Hepar, Ignat., *Ipecac.*, Kali carb., Laches., Lauroc., *Lycop.*, Mar. ver., MERC. VIV., Merc. corr., *Mezer.*,

Mur. ac., Natr. carb., Natr. mur., Nitr. ac., NUX VOM., Paris, Petrol., PHOSPHOR., *Phosph. ac.*, *Pulsat.*, Rheum, Rhus tox., Sabad., Sabin., Sarsap., Seneg., *Sepia*, Silic., Spigel., STAPHIS., SULPHUR, Sulph. ac., THUYA, Veratr., Zinc.

Heat; male genitals, on the, in general: Ambra, Ant. tart., *Arnic.*, *Arsen.*, Calc. carb., Cann. sat., Canthar., Capsic., Carb. veg., Caustic., Conium, Dulcam., Graphit., Ignat., KALI CARB., *Lycop.*, MERC. VIV., Mezer., Natr. carb., Natr. mur., Nitr. ac., NUX VOM., Petrol., Phosphor., *Phosph. ac.*, Platin., Plumbum, PULSAT., *Rhus tox.*, Sabin., Sepia, Spong., Staphis., SULPHUR, Sulph. ac., Thuya.

— **prepuce,** on the: Calad., Calc. carb., *Cann. sat.*, Ignat., MERC. VIV., Merc. corr., Mezer., Natr. carb., *Nitr. ac.*, *Nux vom.*, Phosph. ac., *Rhus tox.*, Sepia, SULPHUR, THUYA.

— **glans,** on the: Ant. tart., Arnic., *Arsen.*, Calc. carb., *Cann. sat.*, Cinchon., Cuprum, Ledum, *Lycop.*, Mangan., MERC. VIV., Merc. corr., *Mezer.*, NITR. AC., *Nux vom.*, *Phosph. ac.*, *Rhus tox.*, Sabin., Sarsap., *Sepia*, Stann., Staphis., Sulphur, THUYA, Viol. tr.

— **penis,** on the: Ant. tart., ARNIC., *Arsen.*, Calc. carb., *Cann. sat.*, CANTHAR., Capsic., CAUSTIC., *Clemat.*, Hepar, *Lycop.*, MERC. VIV., *Mezer.*, Mosch., Mur. ac., Nitr. ac., *Nux vom.*, *Phosphor.*, Phosph. ac., Platin., Plumbum, Pulsat., Sabin., *Sepia*, Spigel., Spong., Staphis., SULPHUR, *Thuya.*

— **scrotum,** on the: ARNIC., ARSEN., CAPSIC., Cinchon., Clemat., Coccul., Dulcam., Euphorb., Graphit., Hepar, *Petrol.*, Phosph. ac., Platin., Plumbum, *Pulsat.*, Rhodod., RHUS TOX., Sepia, Silic., Spong., *Staphis.*, SULPHUR, *Thuya*, Viol. tr.

— **testicles,** in the: ARNIC., Baryt., Capsic., Cinchon., Clemat., Iod., Merc. viv., Nitr. ac., *Nux vom.*, Phosph. ac., *Platin.*, PULSAT., Sepia, Spigel., Spong., *Staphis.*, *Sulphur*, Sulph. ac., Tarax., Thuya, Zinc.

— **spermatic cords,** in the: Ambra, Ant. crud., Apis, *Arnic.*, Clemat., *Mangan.*, Nitr. ac., Nux vom., PULSAT., Spong., STAPHIS., Sulphur, *Thuya.*

Heat; female genitals, on the: Acon., Ambra, Amm. carb., *Apis*, Arsen., Asaf., Bellad., Bryon., CALC. CARB., Canthar., Carb. an., *Carb. veg.*, Caustic., Chamom., Conium, Ferr., Hyosc., *Kali carb.*, Kreos., LYCOP., *Merc. viv.*, Nitr. ac., NUX VOM., PULSAT., Rhus tox., *Sabin.*, SEPIA, Staphis., SULPHUR, *Thuya.*

— — **pubes,** on the: Ambra, Amm. carb., Apis, Arsen., *Bellad.*, CALC. CARB., CANTHAR., Carb. an., Carb. veg., Chamom., Cinchon., Conium, Fluor. ac., Hyosc., Kali carb., Kreos., *Lycop.*, *Merc. viv.*, Mezer., Nitr. ac., *Nux vom.*, Platin., PULSAT., Rhus tox., *Sabin.*, Secal., SEPIA, Staphis., SULPHUR, Sulph. ac., *Thuya*, Zinc.

— **larynx and trachea,** in the: ACON., Amm. mur., Ant. crud., *Apis*, Arsen., Bellad., Brom., Bryon., *Canthar.*, *Carb. veg.*, Caustic., *Chamom.*, Euphorb., Hepar, Iod., Laches., Lauroc., Mangan., Merc. viv., Merc. corr., Mezer., Nitrum, Nitr. ac., NUX VOM., Paris, PHOSPHOR., Phosph. ac., Pulsat., *Rhus tox.*, *Sabad.*, *Seneg.*, *Sepia*, *Spong.*, Stann., *Sulphur*, Veratr., Zinc.

— **neck,** on the: Arnic., *Arsen.*, Baryt., BELLAD., *Bryon.*, Calc. carb., CAUSTIC., Chamom., *Cyclam.*, Ferr., Graphit., Ignat., *Laches.*, LYCOP., Mangan., Merc. viv., Mezer., PHOSPHOR., Phosph. ac., *Pulsat.*, *Rhus tox.*, Scilla, *Sepia*, Staphis., Strontia, *Sulphur*, Tarax., Thuya, Veratr., Zinc.

— **nape of the neck,** on the: Amm. carb., *Apis*, Arnic., *Arsen.*, Asar., BARYT., Bellad., Bryon., *Calc. carb.*, CARB. VEG., Caustic., Cinchon., Colchic., Cyclam., Graphit., IGNAT., Kali carb., Laches., *Lycop.*, *Merc. viv.*, Mezer., NATR. CARB., NUX VOM., PARIS, *Phosphor.*, *Phosph. ac.*, Platin., *Pulsat.*, Rhodod., *Rhus tox.*, *Sepia*, Silic., STAPHIS., SULPHUR, Tarax., Thuya, Zinc.

— **chest,** in the: ACON., Alum., Amm. carb., Ant. tart., APIS, *Arnic.*, ARSEN., Asaf., Aurum, BELLAD., Bismuth., BRYON., *Calc. carb.*, Camphor., CANTHAR., Carb. an., *Carb. veg.*, Caustic., *Chamom.*, *Cicut.*, *Cinchon.*, *Coccul.*, *Coffea*, Colchic., Cuprum, Digit., Dulcam., Euphorb., Graphit., Iod., Kali carb., Kreos., Laches., Lauroc., *Ledum.*, LYCOP., Magn.

mur., *Mangan.*, *Merc. viv.*, Merc. corr., Natr. mur., Nitr. ac., NUX VOM., Opium, PHOSPHOR., *Phosph. ac.*, Platin., *Pulsát.*, *Ran. bulb.*, *Rhus tox.*, *Ruta*, Sabad., *Sarsap.*, *Seneg.*, *Sepia*, Silic., Spigel., Spong., *Stann.*, SULPHUR, Sulph. ac., Thuya, *Zinc.*

Heat; cardiac region, in the: ACON., Argent., Arnic., Arsen., Bellad., Brom., Bryon., *Calc. carb.*, Cann. sat., Canthar., *Carb. veg.*, Caustic., Coccul., Kali carb., Laches., Lycop., Merc. viv., Nitr. ac., Nux vom., *Opium*, PHOSPHOR., PULSAT., Rhus tox., *Sepia*, *Spigel.*, SULPHUR, Veratr.

— **chest,** on the (external): Ambra, *Apis*, ARNIC., ARSEN., Baryt., *Bellad.*, BISMUTH., *Bryon.*, *Calc. carb.*, Canthar., Carb. veg., *Caustic.*, Cicut., Cinchon., Dulcam., Euphorb., Iod., Lauroc., Ledum, LYCOP., MANGAN., Merc. viv., Merc. corr., Mezer., Mur. ac., Natr. carb., *Nux vom.*, Oleand., PHOSPHOR., Phosph. ac., Platin., *Pulsat.*, *Rhus tox.*, *Selen.*, Seneg., Sepia, SPIGEL., Stann., *Staphis.*, Strontia, SULPHUR, Tarax., Veratr.

— **mammæ:** *Acon.*, *Apis*, Arnic., ARSEN., Baryt. BELLAD., BRYON., Calc. carb., *Cann. sat.*, *Carb. an.*, Carb. veg., Chamom., Clemat., Coccul., Conium, Graphit., Hepar., Lauroc., Lycop., *Merc. viv.*, Nitr. ac., PHOSPHOR., *Pulsat.*, Rhus tox., Sepia, *Silic.*, SULPHUR.

— **axillæ,** in the: *Carb. an.*, *Carb. veg.*, Caustic., Clemat., KALI CARB., Lauroc., Lycop., *Natr. mur.*, Nitr. ac., Phosphor., *Rhus tox.*, Sepia, Silic., *Spigel.*, Sulphur, Sulph. ac., Zinc.

— **scapulæ,** on the: ACON., Alum., *Arsen.*, Asaf., *Baryt.*, Bellad., *Calc. carb.*, Carb. veg., *Caustic.*, *Chelid.*, Cinchon., Kali carb., Lycop., *Merc. viv.*, Mezer., Mur. ac., *Natr. carb.*, *Natr. mur.*, NUX VOM., *Plumbum*, PULSAT., RHUS TOX., Sabin., SEPIA, Silic., Spigel., Stann., Staphis., *Sulphur*, Tarax., *Thuya*, Veratr.

— **back,** in the: Acon., Alum., Angust., Ant. tart., *Apis*, ARNIC., ARSEN., Asaf., *Baryt.*, *Bellad.*, Bismuth., *Bryon.*, Calc. carb., CANN. SAT., *Canthar.*, *Carb. an.*, CARB. VEG., CAUSTIC., Chelid., Cinchon., Coccul., Coffea, Conium,

10

DULCAM., *Ignat.*, *Kali carb.*, Laches., LYCOP., Magn. mur., MANGAN., MENYANTH., Merc. viv., Mezer., Mur. ac., NATR. CARB., Natr. mur., Nitr. ac., NUX VOM., PARIS, PHOSPHOR., *Phosph. ac.*, Platin., PULSAT., *Rhus tox.*, Ruta, Selen., Seneg., SEPIA, *Silic.*, SPIGEL., STANN., Staphis., SULPHUR, *Thuya*, *Veratr.*, Zinc.

Heat; small of the back, in the: *Acon.*, *Apis*, Argent., Arnic., ARSEN., Asar., Baryt., *Borax*, *Bryon.*, Calc. carb., *Carb. an.*, Carb. veg., CAUSTIC., Chamom., Cinchon., Coccul., *Ignat.*, *Kali carb.*, Kreos., *Lycop.*, Magn. mur., *Merc. viv.*, Mur. ac., Natr. mur., NUX VOM., PHOSPHOR., *Phosph. ac.*, *Pulsat.*, RHUS TOX., Ruta, Sabin., SEPIA, *Silic.*, Stann., Staphis., SULPHUR, Tarax., *Thuya*, Veratr.

— **os coccygis,** at the: Agar., Alum., Arnic., ARSEN., Borax, Calc. carb., Carb. an., CARB. VEG., CAUSTIC., Cinchon., Colchic., Graphit., Hepar, Ignat., Lauroc., Ledum, *Merc. viv.*, Mur. ac., PHOSPHOR., *Phosph. ac.*, Platin., RHUS TOX., Spigel., Staphis., *Sulphur*, Zinc.

— **upper limbs,** in general: Acon., Agar., Alum., Amm. carb., Ant. crud., Apis, Bovist., BRYON., Calc. carb., Carb. an., CARB. VEG., *Caustic.*, Coccul., Cuprum, Cyclam., Digit., *Graphit.*, KALI CARB., Laches., Ledum, Lycop., Magn. mur., Merc. viv., Mezer., MUR. AC., Natr. carb., Nitr. ac., Petrol., PHOSPHOR., *Phosph. ac.*, Platin., PULSAT., Ran. bulb., Rhodod., RHUS TOX., Ruta, *Sepia*, Silic., Spigel., Spong., STANN., *Staphis.*, SULPHUR, Tarax., *Zinc.*

— **shoulders,** on the: ACON., Amm. mur., Bellad., *Bryon.*, *Carb. veg.*, *Kali carb.*, Lycop., Magn. carb., Menyanth., Merc. viv., Nux vom., Paris, *Phosphor.*, Phosph. ac. Plumbum, *Pulsat.*, RHUS TOX., *Sepia*, Spong., Strontia, Sulphur.

— **shoulder joint,** in the: Bryon., Calc. carb., Carb. veg., Ferr., Graphit., *Ignat.*, Kali carb., Natr. carb., Pulsat., *Rhus tox.*, Sepia, *Staphis.*, Strontia, SULPHUR, Thuya, Zinc.

— **arm,** on the: Acon., *Agar.*, Alum., Amm. carb., Argent., *Arsen.*, ASAF., Bellad., *Borax*, *Bryon.*, Carb. veg., COCCUL., Colchic., Coloc., Digit., Dulcam., *Ferr.*, Graphit., *Ignat.*, Kali carb., Mangan., Mezer., Mur. ac., Natr. mur., Nux vom., Oleand., Phosphor., Phosph. ac., *Sepia*, Valer., Zinc.

Heat; elbow, on the: Alum., Argent., Asaf., Carb. an., Carb. veg., *Caustic.*, Graphit., KALI CARB., Merc. viv., Natr. carb., Nitrum, Phosphor., Phosph. ac., *Platin.*, RHUS TOX., *Sepia*, *Stann.*, Strontia, SULPHUR, Thuya.

— **forearm,** on the: Agar., Amm. carb., Amm. mur., Arnic., Asaf., *Bryon.*, *Calc. carb.*, CAUSTIC., Euphorb., *Graphit.*, LEDUM, *Lycop.*, MERC. VIV., Mur. ac., Oleand., Phosph. ac., Ran. scel., RHUS TOX., *Staphis.*, *Sulphur*, Tarax., Thuya, Zinc.

— **wrist,** at the: Apis, Argent., Bovist., BRYON., Calc. carb., Carb. veg., *Caustic.*, Graphit., *Kali carb.*, Ledum, Natr. carb., RHUS TOX., Ruta, *Sabin.*, *Sepia*, Silic., *Strontia*, SULPHUR, Thuya.

— **hands,** on the: ACON., Æsc. hip., Agar., Alum., *Amm. carb.*, *Anac.*, Ant. tart., *Apis*, Arsen., Asar., Bellad., Borax, BRYON., CALC. CARB., Camphor., Cann. sat., Canthar., Capsic., Carb. an., CARB. VEG., Chamom., Cina, Coccul., Crocus, CYCLAM., Dulcam., *Ferr.*, Graphit., Guaiac., HELLEB., Hepar, *Ignat.*, Kali bichr., Kali carb., Kreos., LACHES., *Lauroc.*, LEDUM, LYCOP., Magn. carb., Merc. viv., Mosch., Mur. ac., NATR. CARB., Natr. mur., NITR. AC., NUX MOSCH., *Nux vom.*, OPIUM, Oxal. ac., *Petrol.*, PHOSPHOR., *Phosph. ac.*, Platin., *Psorin.*, PULSAT., *Rheum*, RHODOD., *Rhus tox.*, *Sabad.*, Sabin., Sarsap., SCILLA, SECAL., SEPIA, Silic., SPIGEL., Spong., *Stann.*, STAPHIS., *Strontia*, SULPHUR, TARAX., Veratr., Zinc.

— **one hand,** on: DIGIT., Mosch., PULSAT.

— **spreading from the hands:** Laches., Ledum, Phosphor.

— **dorsum of the hands,** on the: Angust., Apis, Calc. carb., Cyclam., Kreos., NATR. CARB., Nux vom., RHUS TOX., Sambuc., *Sepia*, *Sulphur*, Thuya.

— **palms of the hands,** on the: *Acon.*, Amm. mur., *Anac.*, *Apis*, ASAR., Borax, BRYON., Canthar., Chelid., Cinchon.,

Coffea, Dulcam., Graphit., IPECAC., Kreos., LACHES., Lauroc., LYCOP., Magn. carb., Merc. viv., Mezer., MUR. AC., Natr. carb., Natr. mur., NUX VOM., *Petrol.*, PHOSPHOR., Pulsat., *Ran. bulb.*, Ran. scel., Rheum, Rhus tox., SAMBUC., *Selen.*, SEPIA, SPIGEL., STANN., *Sulphur.*

Heat; fingers, on the: *Agar.*, Alum., Amm. carb., *Amm. mur.*, Apis, Asaf., Asar., Borax, Calc. carb., *Caustic.*, Cina, Coloc., Conium, Crocus, Digit., Graphit., *Kali carb.*, Laches., Lauroc., LYCOP., *Magn. carb.*, *Mar. ver.*, Merc. viv., Mezer., *Mosch.*, Mur. ac. Natr. carb., Nitr. ac., *Oleand.*, Paris, Petrol., Phosphor., Phosph. ac., Platin., *Pulsat.*, Ran. bulb., Ran. scel., RHUS TOX., Sabad., Secal., Sepia, SILIC., *Spigel.*, Staphis., SULPHUR, Sulph. ac., Tarax., *Thuya*, Veratr.

— — **tips** of the, on the: *Amm. mur.*, Ant. tart., Apis, Canthar., *Crocus*, Lauroc., MAR. VER., Nitr. ac., *Oleand.*, Phosphor., SABAD., Secal., SILIC., Spigel., Staphis., Sulphur, THUYA.

— **lower limbs,** in general: Alum., *Arsen.*, Baryt., *Borax*, *Bryon.*, CALC. CARB., Carb. an., Carb. veg., Caustic., Cina, Cinchon., Coloc., *Kali carb.*, *Laches.*, Lauroc., LEDUM, LYCOP., Magn. carb., Magn. mur., Mangan., Merc. viv., Mezer., Natr. carb., Nitr. ac., Nux vom., Oleand., Phosphor., *Phosph. ac.*, Platin., Pulsat., Rhus tox., Ruta, Sepia, *Silic.*, Spigel., Stann., STAPHIS., Sulphur, Thuya, Zinc.

— **hips,** on the: Arnic., Bellad., *Carb. veg.*, *Caustic.*, Chelid., Cicut., Euphorb., Helleb., Kali carb., *Lycop.*, Mezer., Pulsat., *Rhus tox.*, Ruta, *Sepia*, *Sulphur*, Thuya, *Valer.*, Zinc.

— **hip joints,** in the: Angust., Ant. crud., Argent., Arnic., BELLAD., BRYON., *Calc. carb.*, CAUSTIC., CHELID., Cinchon., Coccul., Coloc., Dulcam., Euphorb., Ferr., Helleb., Ignat., *Kali carb.*, Kreos., Ledum, *Lycop.*, *Merc. viv.*, *Natr. carb.*, Natr. mur., Nitr. ac., *Nux vom.*, *Phosphor.*, Phosph. ac., Pulsat., RHUS TOX., *Sepia*, Silic., *Stann.*, *Strontia*, SULPHUR, Thuya, Veratr.

— **nates,** on the: Caustic., *Graphit.*, Kali carb., LYCOP., Merc. viv., Mezer., *Phosphor.*, *Phosph. ac.*, *Rhus tox.*, Sepia, STAPHIS., *Sulphur*, Thuya, Zinc.

Heat; thighs, on the: Arnic., Asaf., Borax, Bovist., Carb. an., *Carb. veg.*, *Caustic.*, CINCHON., Coccul., Colchic., Droser., Dulcam., Euphorb., Graphit., Guaiac., Lauroc., Lycop., Menyanth., MERC. VIV., Merc. corr., *Mezer.*, Mur. ac., *Nux vom.*, Oleand., Phosphor., Phosph. ac., Plumbum, Rhodod., RHUS TOX., Ruta, Sabin., *Sepia*, *Spigel.*, Staphis., Sulphur, Sulph. ac., *Thuya*, Viol. tr., Zinc.

— **knees,** in the: Anac., Ant. tart., Apis, Argent., *Arsen.*, *Asaf.*, *Baryt.*, Brom., BRYON., Calc. carb., Cann. sat., *Carb. veg.*, *Caustic.*, Cina, *Cinchon.*, Droser., *Ignat.*, Iod., Kali carb., Ledum, *Lycop.*, Menyanth., *Merc. viv.*, Mur. ac., Natr. carb., Natr. mur., Nitrum, Nitr. ac., NUX VOM., Oleand., *Petrol.*, PHOSPHOR., Phosph. ac., Platin., *Pulsat.*, RHUS TOX., Sabad., *Sepia*, Spigel., STANN., *Staphis.*, *Strontia*, SULPHUR, Sulph. ac., TARAX., Thuya, Veratr., Zinc.

— **leg,** on the: *Acon.*, Agar., Anac., Angust., Ant. crud., Argent., Arsen., ASAF., Borax, *Bryon.*, Calc. carb., Cann. sat., Caustic., Chelid., Cinchon., Coffea, Cyclam., Digit., Graphit., Guaiac., Hyosc., Ignat., *Kali carb.*, Laches., LYCOP., *Magn. carb.*, Menyanth., Merc. viv., Mezer., Natr. carb., Nitr. ac., Nux vom., Oxal. ac., Phosphor., *Phosph. ac.*, *Pulsat.*, Ran. scel., RHUS TOX., Sabad., SEPIA, Silic., Spigel., Stann., STAPHIS., Strontia, *Sulphur*, TARAX., Veratr., Zinc.

— **tibia,** on the: Agar., Angust., Asaf., Arsen., Bellad., Calc. carb., *Cyclam.*, Kali carb., Laches., MERC. VIV., *Mezer.*, Nux vom., PHOSPHOR., *Pulsat.*, *Rhus tox.*, Sepia, Tarax., Thuya, Zinc.

— **calves,** on the: Alum., ARSEN., Asaf., *Bryon.*, Calc. carb., Graphit., Ignat., *Lycop.*, Natr. carb., Nitr. ac., *Nux vom.*, Pulsat., RHUS TOX., *Sepia*, Silic., Spigel., STANN., *Staphis.*, SULPHUR, Tarax., Thuya, Veratr., Zinc.

— **ankles,** in the: *Angust.*, Apis, Bryon., Calc. carb., CAUSTIC., *Euphorb.*, *Kali carb.*, Kreos., LYCOP., *Merc. viv.*, Mezer., Natr. carb., Natr. mur., Petrol., Phosphor., RHUS TOX., Ruta, *Sepia*, Silic., Spigel., Strontia, SULPHUR, Tarax., Veratr.

— **feet,** on the: ACON., Agar., Alum., Amm. carb., Anac.,

Apis, Argent., ARNIC., *Arsen.*, BELLAD., Bovist., BRYON., *Calc. carb.*, Camphor., Carb. an., Carb. veg., *Caustic.*, Chamom., Cina, COCCUL., Dulcam., *Graphit.*, Hepar, Ignat., Kali bichr., *Kali carb.*, LACHES., Lachnanth., Lauroc., LEDUM, LYCOP., Magn. mur., Merc. viv., Mezer., Mur. ac., Natr. carb., *Natr. mur.*, Nitr. ac., NUX VOM., Petrol., PHOSPHOR., *Phosph. ac.*, PULSAT., RHEUM., Rhus tox., *Ruta*, Sarsap., SCILLA, SECAL., SEPIA, *Silic.*, *Spigel.*, Spong., STANN., STAPHIS., Stramon., Strontia, SULPHUR, Tarax., Zinc.

Heat; feet, spreading from the: *Laches.*, Ledum.

— **of one foot,** the other cold: *Lycop.*

— **heels,** on the: Arnic., CAUSTIC., Cyclam., Graphit., Helleb., IGNAT., Ledum, *Natr. carb.*, Nitrum, *Pulsat.*, Rheum, *Rhus tox.*, Sabin., *Sepia*, Silic., Spong., STANN., Strontia, *Sulphur*, Sulph. ac., *Thuya*, Veratr., Viol. tr., Zinc.

— **dorsum of the feet,** on the: Ant. tart., Asaf., *Bryon.*, Calc. carb., Camphor., Canthar., CAUSTIC., *Cinchon.*, Hepar, *Ignat.*, Lycop., Mur. ac., Natr. carb., Nux vom., PULSAT., *Rhus tox.*, Spigel., Stramon., Sulphur, *Tarax.*, Thuya.

— **soles of the feet,** on the: Alum., AMBRA, *Amm. mur.*, *Anac.*, *Arsen.*, Asar., Bellad., Bryon., *Calc. carb.*, *Canthar.*, Carb. veg., *Caustic.*, Chamom., Chelid., *Cuprum*, Graphit., Hepar, Kreos., LACHES., *Ledum*, LYCOP., Magn. mur., Mangan., Merc. viv., MUR. AC., Natr. carb., NUX VOM., Oleand., *Petrol.*, *Phosphor.*, PHOSPH. AC., PULSAT., Rhus tox., Ruta, Sabad., Sambuc., Scilla, Sepia, *Silic.*, *Stann.*, Staphis., Strontia, *Sulphur*, *Tarax.*, Verbas., Viol. tr., Zinc.

— **toes,** on the: *Agar.*, *Alum.*, Amm. carb., *Ant. crud.*, Apis, ARNIC., *Asaf.*, *Borax*, Calad., Calc. carb., Carb. an., *Carb. veg.*, CAUSTIC., Conium, *Cyclam.*, Dulcam., Graphit., *Kali carb.*, Kreos., Laches., Lycop., Magn. mur., Merc. viv., Mezer., Mosch., Mur. ac., Natr. carb., Nitr. ac., NUX VOM., Oleand., Paris, Phosphor., *Phosph. ac.*, Platin., *Pulsat.*, *Ran. scel.*, Rhus tox., Ruta, Sabin, Sepia, Silic., STAPHIS., SULPHUR, TARAX., *Thuya*, Viol. tr., *Zinc.*

Heat; tips of the toes, on the: Amm. mur., Ant. tart.,

Arnic., Cinchon., KALI CARB., *Mur. ac.*, Oleand., Pulsat., *Sepia*, Silic., *Thuya*, Zinc.

AGGRAVATION.

ACCORDING TO TIME.

Morning: Amm. mur., Apis, Arnic., BISMUTH., BORAX, Bryon., Calc. carb., Chamom., Cinchon., Coffea, Cyclam., Euphorb., Hepar, Ignat., Ipecac., KALI CARB., Lauroc., Lycop., Magn. carb., Mezer., *Nux vom.*, PETROL., Phosphor., Pulsat., Rhus tox., SABAD., *Sepia*, Staphis., *Sulphur*, Thuya.

Forenoon: Amm. carb., Amm. mur., Ant. crud., ARGENT., Bryon., Calc. carb., Cann. sat., Chamom., Eup. perf., Ignat., *Kali carb.*, MAGN. CARB., Natr. carb., NUX MOSCH., Oxal. ac., Phosphor., Rhus tox., Sabad., Sarsap., Sepia, *Silic.*, Stramon., Valer., *Veratr.*, ZINC.

Noon: ARGENT., Bellad., Kali carb., Merc. viv., Natr. mur., STRAMON., Sulphur.

Afternoon: Agar., Alum., Ambra, Amm. mur., Anac., ANGUST., Ant. tart., ASAF., Asar., Bellad., Bovist., *Bryon.*, Calad., Calc. carb., *Canthar.*, *Cinchon.*, Coffea, Colchic., Conium, Droser., Eup. perf., Ferr., Hepar, Ignat., Iod., Ipecac., *Kali carb.*, Lauroc., Magn. carb., Magn. mur., NATR. MUR., Nitr. ac., Nux vom., Paris, PHOSPHOR., Phosph. ac., Plumbum, Psorin., Pulsat., Rhus tox., RUTA, Sabin., Sambuc., Sanguin., SCILLA, SEPIA, SILIC., STANN., Staphis., SULPHUR, Sulph. ac., Zinc.

Evening: ACON., Agar., AGN. CAST., ALUM., AMBRA, AMM. CARB., ANAC., ANGUST., Ant. crud., *Ant. tart.*, APIS, ARNIC., ARSEN., ASAR., BELLAD., BORAX, Bryon., Calad., CALC. CARB., Carb. an., CARB. VEG. CAUSTIC., *Chamom.*, CHELID., Cina, Cinchon., COFFEA, Cyclam., *Diadem.*, Droser., FERR., GRAPHIT., GUAIAC., HELLEB., *Hepar*, HYOSC., (Ignat.), Iod., IPECAC., Kali carb., LACHES., *Lachnanth.*, LAUROC., LEDUM, LYCOP., MAGN. CARB., MAGN. MUR., MAR. VER., MENYANTH.,

Merc. viv., MOSCH., Natr. carb., Natr. mur., Natr. sulph., NITRUM, Nitr. ac., Nux vom., Paris, PETROL., PHOSPHOR., PHOSPH. AC., Platin., PLUMBUM, PULSAT., Ran. bulb., RAN. SCEL., RHODOD., *Rhus tox.*, Ruta, Sambuc., SARSAP., SCILLA, Selen., SEPIA, SILIC., Spigel., Spong., STANN., Staphis., Stramon., Strontia, SULPHUR, SULPH. AC., THUYA, VALER., VERATR., Zinc.

Nights: Acon., Agar., Alum., Amm. carb., Amm. mur., Anac., August., ANT. CRUD., Apis, Arnic., ARSEN., Baptis., *Baryt.*, *Bellad.*, *Bryon.*, Calc. carb., Camphor., CANN. SAT., CANTHAR., CARB. AN., CARB. VEG., *Caustic.*, *Chamom.*, CINA, Cinchon., CLEMAT., COCCUL., COFFEA, COLCHIC., Conium, DROSER., Dulcam., Eup. perf., GRAPHIT., HEPAR, Ignat., Kali carb., LACHES., Lauroc., Ledum, Lycop., MAGN. CARB., Magn. mur., MERC. VIV., Natr. mur., NITRUM, NITR. AC., Nux mosch., NUX VOM., *Petrol.*, PHOSPHOR., Phosph. ac., PLUMBUM, Psorin., PULSAT., Ran. bulb., RAN SCEL., Rheum, Rhodod., *Rhus tox.*, SABAD., Sabin., *Scilla*, Secal., Sepia, SILIC., SPIGEL., Spong., STAPHIS., STRONTIA, SULPHUR, TARAX., Thuya, Veratr., VIOL. TR., ZINC.

Midnight; before: Alum., Amm. mur., Ant. crud., *Bryon.*, CALAD., Chamom., Ferr., Lachnanth., LAUROC., Lycop., MAGN. MUR., *Pulsat.*, Sabad., Sepia, Veratr.

— **after:** August., Arsen., Bryon., Calc. carb., Cinchon., Coffea, Ignat., Kali carb., Kreos., MERC. VIV., PETROL., PHOSPHOR., Phosph. ac., Pulsat., RAN SCEL., *Rhodod.*, Rhus tox., SABAD., *Sambuc.*, Spong., STAPHIS., Sulphur, Thuya.

3 A. M.: *Psorin.*

From 4 P. M.: *Anac.*, Lycop., *Stann.*

From 6 to 8 P. M.: Caustic.

Hour; returning at the same: SABAD., *Silic.*, *Stann.*

Day; only during the: *Ant. tart.*, *Sepia.*

In repeated short attacks: Agn. cast., AMBRA, Amm. carb., *Amm. mur.*, Ant. tart., ARNIC., Asar., Aurum, *Baryt.*,

Bellad., Borax, CALC. CARB., Carb veg., Chamom., Cinchon., COCCUL., *Cuprum*, Digit., *Euphras.*, HELLEB., HEPAR., Hyosc., *Ignat.*, Iod., Ipecac., Kali carb., Kreos., Laches., Lauroc., Ledum, LYCOP., *Mar. ver.*, NUX VOM., Oleand., Petrol., PHOSPHOR., Phosph. ac., *Rhus tox.*, Ruta, SEPIA, *Silic.*, *Stann.*, SULPHUR, Sulph. ac., THUYA, *Veratr.*, Zinc.

Slowly increasing and slowly decreasing: Cinchon., *Platin.*, Stann., Strontia.

— — **and quickly going off:** Bellad., Sulph. ac.

Quickly coming and going: Thuya.

ACCORDING TO CIRCUMSTANCE.

Anger; after: Acon., *Chamom.*, Nux vom., Petrol., SEPIA, Staphis.

Awaking; when: See Sleep, when awaking from.

Bed; in: ACON., *Agn. cast.*, Amm. mur., Ant. crud., Apis, Arnic., ASAR., Borax, Bryon., CALC. CARB., *Carb. an.*, CARB. VEG., Caustic., Chamom., CHELID., *Coffea*, Graphit., HELLEB., *Hepar*, KALI CARB., Ledum, Lycop., *Magn. mur.*, MERC. VIV., MEZER., *Mosch.*, Nux vom., PETROL., Phosphor., Phosph. ac., *Pulsat.*, *Rhus tox.*, *Sambuc.*, Scilla, Spong., *Sulphur*, SULPH. AC., Thuya, *Viol tr.*

— **after rising** from: *Bismuth.*

Breakfast; after: Chamom., Lauroc., Magn. mur., Phosphor., Plumbum, Sarsap.

Climacteric years; during the: Calc. carb., Laches., Sulphur, *Sulph. ac.*

Coition; after: Calc. carb., Kali carb., Laches., Nux vom., Sepia.

Coryza; during: Acon., Anac., Arsen., Bellad., Bryon., Calc. carb., Camphor., Chamom., Cina, Hepar, *Laches.*, *Lycop.*, Merc. viv., Merc. corr., Mosch., Nux vom., Pulsat., Rhus tox., Sabad., Seneg., *Spigel.*

Coughing; from: Ambra, Amm. carb., Ant. tart., *Arnic.*, *Arsen.*, Bellad., Carb. veg., Hepar, Hyosc., Iod., Ipecac., Ledum,

Lycop., Magn. mur., Natr. carb., Nitrum, Nux vom., Phosphor., Pulsat., Sabad., Scilla, Sulphur.

Covering; from: Acon., Calc. carb., *Chamom.*, Cinchon., Ferr., Ignat., Ledum, Lycop., Mur. ac., Nux vom., Platin., Pulsat., Rhus tox., Staphis., Veratr.

Drinking; beer, after: *Bellad.*, *Ferr.*, Rhus tox., Sulphur.

— **coffee,** from: Canthar., Chamom., Rhus tox.

— **water,** after: Canthar., Ignat., Rhus tox., Sepia.

— **wine,** after: Arsen., *Carb. veg.*, Fluor. ac., Natr. mur., Nux vom., Silic.

Eating; before: Fluor. ac., Phosphor., Sabin.

— **while:** Amm. carb., Chamom., Magn. mur., Nux vom., Psorin., Silic., Spigel., Sulph. ac., *Valer.*

— **after:** Acon., Alum., ANGUST., ASAF., Bryon., CALC. CARB., Caustic., Chamom., Conium, CYCLAM., Digit., Graphit., Laches., Lycop., Magn. carb., Magn. mur., Natr. mur., NITR. AC., Nux vom., Paris, Petrol., *Phosphor.*, Sepia, Silic., Sulphur, Sulph. ac., VIOL. TR., Zinc.

— — **meat:** Magn. carb., Merc. viv.

Exertion; from: Oxal. ac.

Lying: see in bed.

Manual work; from: Merc. viv., Natr. mur., *Oleand.*

Menses; before the: Apis, Calc. carb., Chamom., Conium, Cuprum, Kali carb., Lycop., *Merc. viv.*, Pulsat.

— **during** the: Amm. carb., Bellad., Calc. carb., Chamom., Ferr., *Hyosc.*, Ignat., Lycop., Magn. mur., *Nux vom.*, Phosphor., Pulsat., Sepia, Sulphur.

— **suppression** of the: *Acon.*, Conium, Helleb., Lycop., *Pulsat.*, Silic., Sulphur.

Mental exertion; Ambra, Bellad., NUX VOM., OLEAND., *Sepia*, Silic.

Motion; during: Amm. mur., ANT. CRUD., ANT. TART., *Arsen.*, *Bellad.*, Bryon., CAMPHOR., Cinchon., Eup. perf., *Fluor. ac.*, Ledum, Merc. viv., NUX VOM., Oleand.,

Phosphor., Sambuc., Scilla, Sepia, Spigel., STANN., Staphis., Stramon., Valer.

Motion; after: Amm. carb., AMM. MUR., Arsen., Canthar., Caustic., Nitr. ac., Petrol., Phosphor., Rhus tox., Sepia, Spigel., *Spong.*, *Stann.*, SULPH. AC.

Noise; from: Bryon., Caustic., Coffea, Sepia.

Pains; with the, in general: ACON., Arnic., Arsen., Bellad., Bryon., Carb. veg., Helleb., Ignat., Pulsat., *Rhus tox.*, Silic., Staphis., Sulphur.

Reading: see mental exertion.

Riding in a wagon: *Graphit.*, Psorin., Selen., Sepia.

Room; in the: AMM. MUR., ANGUST., Apis, Caustic., Crocus, Fluor. ac., *Ipecac.*, *Lycop.*, Magn. mur., Nitrum, Nitr. ac., Phosphor., *Pulsat.*, RAN. SCEL., Rhodod., Rhus tox., Valer.

Sitting; when: Alum., Anac., Calc. carb., *Graphit.*, Lycop., Mangan., *Phosphor.*, Rhus tox., SEPIA, Valer.

Sleep; during: Acon., Anac., Arsen., Bellad., Bryon., CALAD., Chamom., Conium, *Dulcam.*, Ignat., Laches., Ledum, Merc. viv., Opium, *Petrol.*, Phosphor., Phosph. ac., *Pulsat.*, Ran. bulb., *Rheum*, Rhus tox., SAMBUC., Sepia, Silic., Stramon., Sulphur, *Viol. tr.*

— **siesta,** after (after dinner): Anac., Phosphor., Pulsat., *Selen.*, Staphis., Sulphur.

— **when awaking** from: Anac., Arnic., Arsen., Bellad., *Borax*, Calad., Calc. carb., Caustic., Cina, Coccul., Conium, *Ferr.*, Hepar, Ipecac., Kreos., Lycop., Magn. carb., Magn. mur., Merc. viv., *Mosch.*, Nitr. ac., Petrol., *Phosphor.*, Phosph. ac., Pulsat., Ran. scel., *Sambuc.*, Selen., Sepia, Silic., Strontia, *Sulphur*, TARAX., Thuya.

Standing; while: Argent., Conium, *Mangan.*, Pulsat., Rhus tox.

Stool; before: Calc. carb., Cuprum, Magn. carb., Merc. viv., Phosphor., Veratr.

— **during:** Arsen., Chamom., Pulsat., Rhus tox., Sulphur.

— **after:** Arsen., Caustic., Nux vom., Rhus tox., Selen.

Stooping; from: Bryon., *Kali carb.*, MERC. CORR., Sepia.

Sun; in the rays of the: *Ant. crud.*, Natr. carb., Pulsat., Sepia.

Talking; when: *Arsen.*, Mar. ver., Nux vom., Oleand., Scilla, Selen., *Sepia.*

Teething; when (children): Acon., *Arsen.*, Chamom.

Tobacco smoking; from: Cicut., Ignat., *Sepia.*

Uncovering; from: Acon., Hepar, Silic.

Vomiting; during: Ant. crud., *Arnic.*, Arsen., Chamom., Laches., Nux vom., Stramon., Veratr.

Walking in the open air; while: Amm. carb., Amm. mur., Argent., Bellad., Borax, Camphor., Cinchon., Hepar, *Nux vom.*, Phosph. ac., Rhus tox., *Sepia*, Spigel., Staphis., Tarax.

— **after:** Arsen., Caustic., Menyanth., *Petrol.*, RAN. SCEL., *Rhus tox.*, Sabin., SEPIA.

Washing: *Amm. carb.*, Calc. carb., Rhus tox., Sepia, Sulphur.

Work; when at: NUX VOM., *Oleand.*, Silic.

AMELIORATION.

Awaking; after: CALAD., Cinchon., Colchic., Helleb., Nux vom., Phosphor., Sepia.

Bed; in: Agar., Bellad., Canthar., Cicut., Coccul., Conium, Hyosc., Laches., *Lauroc.*, Nux vom., Scilla, Silic., Staphis., Stramon.

— **out** of the: Acon., Agn. cast., Ambra, Amm. carb., Ant. tart., Arsen., Asar., Bellad., Calc. carb., Carb. an., Carb. veg., Chelid., Cinchon., Coloc., Droser., Euphorb., *Helleb.*, Ignat., Iod., Kali carb., Mangan., Merc. viv., Mezer., Petrol., Platin., Rhodod., Selen., Sepia, Spigel., Strontia, Sulphur, Sulph. ac., Valer., Veratr.

Breakfast; after: Baryt., Calc. carb., Crocus, Ignat., Iod., Sabad., Staphis.

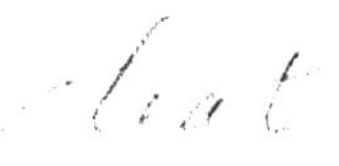

Drinking; **beer,** from: Veratr.

— **coffee,** from: Arsen.

— **water,** from: Bismuth., Caustic., Cuprum, Fluor. ac., *Opium*, Phosphor., Sepia.

— **wine**: Acon., Conium, Opium.

Eating; **while**: ANAC., Ignat., Laches., Mezer., Zinc.

— **after**: Arsen., Cann. sat., *Cinchon.*, Cuprum, Ignat., Iod., Natr. carb., Phosphor., Rhus tox., Strontia.

Exertion of the body; from: Ignat., Sepia, Stann.

Loosening the clothes, from: Bovist., Calc. carb., Lycop., Nux vom.

Mental exertion; from: Natr. carb.

Motion; during (moderate): Ambra, Apis, Asaf., Aurum, Bismuth., Capsic., Conium, Cylcam., Dulcam., Euphorb., Ferr., Lycop., Merc. corr., Pulsat., Rhus tox., Sabad., Sambuc., Selen., Tarax., Valer.

Riding in a wagon; when: Nitr. ac., Nitrum.

Room; in the: Anac., Bellad., Carb. veg., Coccul., Coffea, Conium, Hepar, Guaiac., Laches., Merc. corr., Nux mosch., Nux vom., Silic., Spigel.

Sitting: while: Acon., Ant. tart., Bryon., Colchic., Cuprum, Iod., Merc. viv., Natr. mur., Nux vom., Scilla.

Sleep; during: Helleb.

Standing; while: Bellad., Cann. sat., Iod., Ipecac., Phosphor., Selen.

Stool; after: Bryon., Colchic., Rhus tox., Spigel.

Stooping; from: Colchic., Hyosc.

Supper; after: Anac.

Tobacco smoking; from: Hepar, Sepia.

Uncovering; from: Acon., Calc. carb., Chamom., Cinchon., Ferr., Ignat., Lycop., Mur. ac., Nux vom., Platin., Pulsat., Staphis., Veratr.

Vomiting; after: Acon., Digit., Pulsat., Secal.

Walking in the open air; while: Alum., Asar., Capsic., Lycop., Magn. carb., Mosch., *Phosphor.*, *Pulsat.*, Sabin., Tarax.

Washing; from: Amm. mur., Apis, Asar., Caustic., FLUOR. AC., Pulsat., Spigel.

— **the face:** Asar.

CONCOMITANTS.

Mood; anxious: ACON., Alum., AMBRA, Amm. carb., Anac., Apis, Argent., Arnic., ARSEN., *Asaf.*, *Baryt.*, BELLAD., BOVIST., Bryon., *Calc. carb.*, *Canthar.*, Capsic., Carb. veg., CHAMOM., Cina, Cinchon., COCCUL., Coffea, Colchic., *Conium*, Cyclam., Droser., Euphorb., Ferr., Graphit., Hepar, Hyosc., Ignat., IPECAC., Laches., Lauroc., Lycop., *Magn. carb.*, Magn. mur., MERC. VIV., Mur. ac., Natr. carb., Natr. mur., Nitr. ac., NUX VOM., Opium, Paris, Petrol., PHOSPHOR., PHOSPH. AC., Platin., *Plumbum*, PULSAT., *Rheum*, Rhodod., Rhus tox., *Ruta*, Sabin., *Secal.*, SEPIA, Spigel., SPONG., STANN., Staphis., *Stramon.*, Sulphur, Thuya, Valer., *Veratr.*, *Viol. tr.*, *Zinc.*

— **changeable:** Alum., Ferr., *Ignat.*, Nux mosch., Platin., Valer.

— **complaining and lamenting:** Acon., Bryon., Nux vom., Veratr.

— **crying out:** Acon., *Bellad.*, Bryon., *Capsic.*, Chamom., Coffea, Cuprum, Ipecac., Lycop., Opium, Platin., Pulsat., *Stramon.*, Veratr.

— **dejected:** Apis, Cinchon., *Conium*, Natr. carb., Sulphur.

— **depressed:** Acon., Bellad., Chamom., Ignat., Lycop., Opium, Petrol., *Pulsat.*, Sepia, Stann.

— **despairing:** ACON., Arsen., *Carb. veg.*, Chamom., Conium, Graphit., Ignat., Pulsat., Sepia, *Spong.*, Stann., Sulphur, Veratr.

— **discontented:** *Acon.*, *Bellad.*, Bryon., Petrol., *Phosph. ac.*

— **disinclination to talk** (taciturn): Arnic., *Bellad.*, Chamom., Ignat., Lycop., *Mur. ac.*, Nux vom., *Opium*, Phosphor., *Phosph. ac.*, Pulsat., Veratr.

Mood; excitable: ACON., Alum., Apis, BELLAD., Bryon., CHAMOM., Coccul., *Coffea*, CONIUM, Ignat., Kali carb., Magn. carb., MAR. VER., Mosch., *Nux vom.*, Opium, *Petrol.*, *Sarsap.*, Stramon., Valer.

— **fear of death:** Acon., *Arsen.*, Bryon., Coccul., Ipecac., Mosch., *Nitr. ac.*, *Nux vom.*, Phosphor., *Platin.*, PULSAT.,Rhus tox., RUTA, *Veratr.*

— **impatient:** *Acon.*, Apis, *Arsen.*, Bellad., *Chamom.*, Ignat., *Ipecac.*, Lycop., *Merc. viv.*, *Natr. mur.*, *Nux vom.*, Pulsat., *Rhus tox.*, Viol. tr.

— **impetuous:** *Chamom.*, Coffea, Nux vom.

— **inclination to work:** Opium, Sarsap., *Thuya*, Verbas.

— **listless:** ARNIC., Cinchon., Conium, Opium, Phosphor., *Phosph. ac.*, *Pulsat.*, Sepia, Viol. tr.

— **melancholy:** Arsen., Graphit., Lycop., *Nux mosch.*, Phosph. ac., Sepia.

— **oversensitive:** Acon., Bellad., Carb. veg., Chamom., *Coffea*, Lycop., Mar. ver., Natr. mur., Nitr. ac., NUX VOM., PULSAT., Sepia, Valer.

— **restless:** ACON., Amm. carb., Ant. tart., Apis, *Arnic.*, *Arsen.*, *Baryt.*, BELLAD., *Bovist.*, Bryon., Calc. carb., Chamom., Coffea, Conium, Ignat., Ipecac., Laches., *Lycop.*, Magn. carb., Magn. mur., Merc. viv., Merc. corr., Mosch., Mur. ac., Nux vom., *Opium*, Phosphor., *Phosph. ac.*, Pulsat., Rheum, RHUS TOX., *Ruta*, Sabad., Sabin., Sepia, Silic., Spong., Stann., Staphis., Stramon., Sulphur, Thuya, Valer., Veratr.

— **sensibility to noise:** Acon., Bellad., Calc. carb., *Capsic.*, CONIUM, Ipecac., Lycop., Nux vom.

— **serene:** Acon., Coffea, Natr. carb., Opium, Platin., *Sarsap.*

— **shy:** Conium, Hyosc., *Pulsat.*

— **sighing and groaning:** Acon., *Arnic.*, Arsen., Bellad., Bryon., *Chamom.*, Coccul., Coffea, *Ignat.*, Ipecac., Nux vom., Pulsat., *Rhus tox.*, Sepia, Thuya.

— **singing and trilling:** Bellad., *Mar. ver.*, *Sarsap.*, Stramon., Veratr.

— **sorrowful:** ACON., *Arsen.*, *Bellad.*, Bryon., Coccul., Graphit., Ignat. Lycop., *Natr. carb.*, NATR. MUR., *Phosphor.*, Phosph. ac., Platin., Pulsat., *Rhus tox.*, Sepia, *Silic.*, Staphis., Sulphur.

Mood; startled easily: Acon., *Bellad.*, Calc. carb., Capsic., Ignat., Natr. mur., Nux vom., *Opium*, Petrol., Phosphor., Pulsat., Sepia, Sulphur, *Veratr.*

— **taciturn:** Arnic., *Bellad.*, Chamom., Ignat., Lycop., *Mur. ac.*, Nux vom., *Opium*, Phosphor., *Phosph. ac.*, Pulsat., Veratr.

— **talkative:** Coffea, *Laches.*, MAR. VER., Podophyl., Stramon.

— **tearful:** ACON., BELLAD., Calc. carb., Chamom., Coffea, Graphit., Ignat., *Lycop.*, *Petrol.*, Platin., PULSAT., *Spigel.*, SPONG., Sulphur.

— **vexatious:** Acon., *Arsen.*, Bellad., Calc. carb., *Chamom.*, Conium, Lycop., Mosch., NATR. CARB., Nux vom., Psorin., Pulsat., *Rheum*, Staphis., Thuya.

— **weariness of life:** ARSEN., Laches., Nux vom., Pulsat., Rhus tox., Sepia, *Spong.*, Thuya, Valer.

— **whimpering and whining:** Bellad., Chamom., *Pulsat.*, Rheum.

— **whistling:** Capsic.

Confusion; of the mind: Arsen., *Bellad.*, Bryon., Cinchon., Ipecac., Natr. carb., *Nux vom.*, Pulsat., Rhus tox.

— **of ideas:** Baptis.

Delirium: ACON., *Ant. crud.*, APIS, *Arsen.*, *Baptis.*, BELLAD., *Bryon.*, Calc. carb., Canthar., Capsic., *Carb. veg.*, *Chamom.*, *Cina*, *Cinchon.*, Coccul., COFFEA, Crocus, Cuprum, DULCAM, Hepar, HYOSC., *Ignat.*, Iod., Kali carb., Laches., Lachnanth., Menyanth., *Natr. mur.*, *Nitr. ac.*, *Nux vom.*, OPIUM, Oxal. ac., Phosphor., *Phosph. ac.*, Platin., Podophyl., PULSAT., *Sabad.*, *Sambuc.*, Sanguin., Spong., STRAMON., *Sulphur*, VERATR.

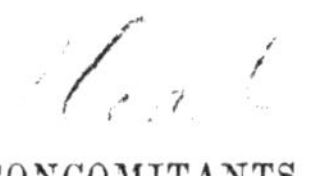

Delirium; anxious: Acon., Bellad., Crocus, *Hyosc.*, Nux vom., *Opium*, Pulsat., Silic., *Stramon.*

— **calm:** *Bellad.*, Crocus, Cuprum, *Hyosc.*, Spong., Stramon., Veratr.

— **imagines herself in pieces** and cannot get herself together: BAPTIS.

— **loquacious:** Bellad., Cuprum, Laches., Podophyl., Rhus tox., *Stramon.*, Veratr.

— **muddled:** Alum., Arsen., *Bryon.*, Calc. carb., Ipecac., Kali carb., Natr. mur., Phosphor., *Rhus tox.*, Veratr.

— **muttering:** APIS, Bellad., Hyosc., Mur. ac., *Opium*, Phosph. ac., Stramon., Tarax.

— **raving:** Acon., Bellad., *Bryon.*, *Hyosc.*, Lycop., Opium, *Stramon.*

— **taciturn:** Ant. crud., Bellad., *Hyosc.*, Mur. ac., Veratr.

— **spitting,** with: Bellad., Capsic.

Dullness of the head: Acon., ANGUST., *Argent.*, ARSEN., *Bellad.*, Borax, BRYON., Calc. carb., *Capsic.*, Carb. veg., *Chamom.*, Conium, Droser., *Ignat.*, Ipecac., *Kali carb.*, Kali hydr., Merc. viv., *Natr. carb.*, Natr. mur., *Nux vom.*, Opium, PHOSPHOR., Phosph. ac., *Pulsat.*, Rhus tox., Ruta, SEPIA, Silic., *Valer.*, VERATR.

Excited fancy: Acon., Bellad., Cinchon., Coffea, Laches., Lauroc., *Opium*, Phosphor., Pulsat., Sabad., Stramon., *Thuya*, Valer.

Frenzy: Ant. crud., Arsen., *Bellad.*, Canthar., CICUT., Dulcam., Hyosc., *Opium*, Stramon., Veratr.

Illusions: Bellad., Bryon., Carb. veg., Hyosc., Magn. mur., Merc. viv., *Opium*, Phosph. ac., Rhus tox., Sambuc., Stramon.

Intellect brightened: Bellad., Coffea, Laches., Opium, Stramon., *Thuya.*

Rage: *Bellad.*, Lycop., Stramon., VERATR.

Stupefaction: *Apis*, *Arnic.*, Arsen., *Bellad.*, Calc. carb., *Camphor.*, *Chamom.*, HYOSC., *Lauroc.*, Natr. mur., NUX VOM., OPIUM, Phosphor., *Phosph. ac.*, PULSAT., *Rhus tox.*, Sepia, Stramon., *Veratr.*

Suicidal mania: *Arsen.*, Bellad., *Nux vom.*, Pulsat., Rhus tox., Stramon.

Unconsciousness: *Acon.*, APIS, *Arnic.*, ARSEN., BELLAD., Borax, Bryon., Calc. carb., Camphor., Chamom., *Coccul.*, *Dulcam.*, *Helleb.*, *Hyosc.*, Lauroc., MUR. AC., NATR. MUR., Nux vom., OPIUM, Phosphor., PHOSPH. AC., *Pulsat.*, Rhus tox., SEPIA, *Stramon.*, Sulphur, *Veratr.*

Vertigo: ACON., *Alum.*, Angust., *Apis*, Argent., Arnic., ARSEN., *Bellad.*, BRYON., *Calc. carb.*, CARB. VEG., Chelid., Cinchon., Corn. flor., Crocus, *Ignat.*, *Ipecac.*, Lauroc., Ledum, LYCOP., *Magn. mur.*, MERC. VIV., Mosch., Natr. carb., Natr. mur., NUX VOM., PHOSPHOR., Phosph. ac., PULSAT., Rhus tox., *Sepia*, *Stramon.*, *Sulphur*, *Veratr.*

Reeling: Alum., *Bellad.*, Bryon., Capsic., Magn. mur., Nux vom., *Opium*, Phosph. ac., Stramon., Sulphur, Veratr.

Staggering: Alum., Argent., Bellad., Camphor., Carb. veg., *Coccul.*, Laches., Lauroc., Ledum, NUX VOM., Opium, *Pulsat.*, Rhus tox.

Headache; in general: Acon., Æsc. hip., Agar., Amm. carb., Angust., Ant. tart., *Apis*, Argent., Arnic., *Arsen.*, Baptis., *Bellad.*, Borax, Bryon., Cact. grand., Calc. carb., Camphor., Capsic., Carb. veg., Chamom., Cina, Cinchon., Coloc., Conium, Corn. cir., Corn. flor., Droser., Dulcam., Eup. perf., Graphit., Helleb., Hepar, Hyosc., Ignat., Ipecac., *Kali carb.*, *Laches.*, Ledum, Lycop., Mangan., Menyanth., Mezer., Mosch., Natr. carb., NATR. MUR., Nitrum, *Nux vom.*, Opium, Oxal. ac., Petrol., Phosphor., Podophyl., Psorin., *Pulsat.*, Rhodod., Rhus tox., Ruta, *Sabad.*, *Sepia*, Silic., Spigel., Staphis., Stramon., Sulphur, Thuya, Valer., Veratr.

— **forehead and temples,** in the: Oxal. ac.

— **occiput,** in the: Acon., *Bellad.*, Helleb., Sepia.

— **congestion,** with: Acon., Apis, Arsen., Bellad., *Cinchon.*, *Ferr.*, HYOSC., Natr. mur., Nux vom., Phosphor., Pulsat., *Rhus tox.*, Sepia, SULPHUR, Thuya.

— **heaviness,** with sensation of: Calc. carb., Caustic.

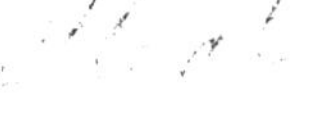

Head; sweat on the: Anac., Baryt., Calc. carb., CHAMOM., Graphit., Hepar, *Magn. carb.*, MAGN. MUR., Paris, Pulsat., Sarsap., Silic., Sulphur, Valer., Veratr.

— — **forehead,** on the: Sarsap.

— — **cold:** Hepar, Veratr.

— **tension:** *Sabad.*

Eyes; pain in the: Acon., Apis, Arsen., Bellad., Borax, Calc. carb., *Canthar.*, Carb. an., Carb. veg., Cicut., *Coloc.*, Digit., Hepar, Hyosc., Ipecac., Laches., *Ledum*, LYCOP., Natr. carb., *Natr. mur.*, Nux vom., Opium, Phosph. ac., Pulsat., *Rhodod.*, Rhus tox., Ruta, Sabad., Seneg., Sepia, Spigel., Stramon., Sulphur, VALER., Veratr.

— **blue rings** around the: *Cina.*

— **brilliant:** *Lachnanth.*

— **burning:** *Petrol.*

— **dryness** of the: *Spigel.*

— **injected:** Baptis.

— **protruding:** *Spigel.*

— **puffed up** around the: *Ferr.*

— **pupils contracted:** *Acon.*

— — **dilated:** *Apis*, *Cina.*

— **red:** *Hyosc.*

— **squinting:** *Apis.*

Sight; aversion to light: Acon., Bellad., Conium, *Hepar*, Sulphur.

— **dark (black)** before the eyes: *Carb. veg.*, *Natr. mur.*, *Pulsat.*, Sepia.

— **fire;** before the eyes, like: Bellad., *Opium.*

— **flickering** before the eyes: Sepia.

— **green,** before the eyes: *Cinchon.*

— **impaired:** Carb. veg., *Natr. mur.*, Sepia.

Ears; pain in the: *Calad.*, Graphit.

— **cold:** *Ipecac.*

Hearing; dullness of: *Rhus tox.*

— **humming and roaring** in the ears: *Arsen.*, *Nux vom.*

Nose; pains in the: Rhodod.

— **coldness** of the: *Colchic.*

— **itching** of the: *Cina.*

Facial pains: Mezer., *Spigel.*

Face; besotted expression of the: Baptis.

— **cold:** Calc. carb., Carb. veg., *Cina,* Cinchon., CYCLAM., Hyosc., IPECAC., Lycop., Nitr. ac., Platin., Ran. scel., RHEUM, *Spong.*, Veratr.

— — **cheeks,** on the: Bellad., *Colchic.*, Natr. carb.

— — **forehead,** on the: Bellad., Cina, Cinchon.

— **color, brownish red:** *Capsic.*

— — **earthy:** *Laches.*

— — **pale:** Acon., *Arsen.*, Bellad., CINA, Coccul., CROCUS, *Ipecac.*, *Lycop.*, Natr. mur., Pulsat., Rhus tox., *Sepia,* Spong., Thuya, Veratr.

— — **red:** ACON., Agar., Alum., *Amm. mur.*, Apis, Argent., Arnic., Arsen., Baptis., BELLAD., *Bryon.*, Camphor., Canthar., Capsic., Carb. veg., *Chamom.*, Chin. sulph., *Cinchon.*, COCCUL., Coffea, Conium, *Crocus,* Cyclam., *Digit.*, Dulcam., *Euphras.*, FERR., HEPAR, Hyosc., Ignat., *Kreos.*, *Laches.*, Lachnanth., *Lycop.*, Merc. viv., Merc. corr., *Nux vom.*, OPIUM, Paris, *Plumbum,* Psorin., *Pulsat.*, *Rhus tox.*, *Ruta,* Scilla, *Sepia,* *Silic.*, Spigel., *Spong.*, STRAMON., *Sulphur,* Valer, *Veratr.*, VIOL. TR., Zinc.

— — — **circumscribed:** ACON., Bryon., *Calc. carb.*, CINCHON., Crocus, Droser., Dulcam., *Ferr.*, Iod., *Kali carb.*, *Kreos.*, Laches., Lachnanth., Ledum, *Lycop.*, Nux vom., *Phosphor.*, Phosph. ac., *Pulsat.*, Sambuc., Sanguin., Sepia, Stann., Stramon., *Sulphur.*

— — — **one side,** on: Acon., Arnic., Bellad., Cann. sat.,

CHAMOM., Coloc., Droser., IGNAT., Ipecac., MOSCH., Natr. mur., *Nux vom.*, Phosphor., *Ran. bulb.*, *Rheum*, Sanguin., Stramon., Sulph. ac., Thuya, Veratr., Viol. tr.

Face; color red, uncovered side, on the: Thuya, *Viol. tr.*

— — — **upper part,** especially: Lachnanth.

— — **yellow:** *Arsen.*, Laches., *Natr. mur.*, Nux vom., *Rhus tox.*

— **puffed up:** *Amm. mur.*, Apis, Arsen., Digit., Ferr., LYCOP.

— **sweat** of the: AMM. MUR., *Ant. tart.*, Bellad., Carb. veg., *Chamom.*, Ignat., Lycop., Opium, Pulsat., Sambuc., Spong., *Valer.*

— — **cold:** *Ant. tart.*, Arsen., CAPSIC., Carb. veg., Cina, *Digit.*, Ipecac., Laches., Spong., Sulphur, Valer., Veratr.

Lips; dryness of the: Arsen., Cinchon., Nux vom., Phosphor., *Rhus tox.*, Veratr.

— **eruption** on the: *Arsen.*, Ignat., *Natr. mur.*, Nux vom., Rhus tox., Sulphur.

— **swelling** of the: *Arsen.*

Submaxillary glands; swelling of the: Calad., Kali carb., Merc. viv.

Teeth; pain in the, in general: *Apis*, Carb. veg., Graphit., Hyosc., *Kali carb.*, Laches., Natr. carb., Pulsat., *Rhus tox.*, SEPIA, Staphis.

— **chattering** of the: *Phosphor.*, Zinc.

Gums; bleeding of the: Carb. veg., Graphit., *Staphis.*

— **swelling** of the: Carb. veg., Graphit., *Staphis.*

— **pain** in the: *Apis*, Hyosc., Rhus tox., Staphis.

Mouth; burning in the: Arsen., Mezer., *Petrol.*

— **dryness** of the: *Arsen.*, *Asar.*, *Bellad.*, Bryon., Cinchon., Coccul., Coffea, Kali bichr., Laches., Lycop., Mur. ac., *Nitr. ac.*,

NUX MOSCH., *Nux vom.*, Opium, Petrol., *Phosphor.*, *Phosph. ac.*, Sabad., Sepia, Spigel., Stramon., Sulphur, Thuya, Valer., Veratr.

Mouth; offensive odor from the: Arnic.

— **soreness** of the: Arum tr.

— **yellowness** of the: *Plumbum.*

Saliva; increased flow of: Acon., Alum., Bellad., Brom., Carb. veg., Cicut., *Droser.*, Hepar, Ignat., Ipecac., Lycop., Merc. viv., Natr. mur., Nitr. ac., *Nux vom.*, Opium, *Pulsat.*, *Rhus tox.*, Seneg., Sepia, Silic., Stramon., Sulphur, Veratr.

Tongue; coated: *Ant. crud.*, Ant. tart., Apis, Arnic., ARSEN., Baptis., Bellad., BRYON., *Chamom.*, Cinchon., Coloc., Ignat., (Ipecac)., Laches., Merc. viv., Nux mosch., NUX VOM., Opium, PHOSPHOR., Phosph. ac., *Pulsat.*, Rhus tox., Ruta, Sabad., Sepia, Silic., Sulphur, Veratr.

— **dryness** of the: Ant. tart., Apis, ARSEN., Asaf., Baptis., BELLAD., Bryon., Calc. carb., Carb. an., Carb. veg., Chamom., Dulcam., Hyosc., Laches., Lycop., Mezer., *Mur. ac.*, *Natr. mur.*, Nitr. ac., OPIUM, Paris, Petrol., PHOSPHOR., PHOSPH. AC., Rhus tox., Stramon., Sulphur, Veratr.

— **redness** of the: Arsen., Arum tr., Kali bichr., Laches., Tart. em.

Speech; difficult: Arsen., BELLAD., Bryon., Calc. carb., Carb. veg., Caustic., Dulcam., *Euphras.*, Hepar, *Hyosc.*, Ignat., Laches., Lycop., Mezer., Mur. ac., Natr. mur., *Nux vom.*, Opium, Phosph. ac., Pulsat., Rhus tox., Stramon., Veratr.

Throat; pains in the: Acon., Apis, Bellad., Bovist., Droser., Ignat., Kali carb., LACHES., Merc. viv., Nitr. ac., Nux vom., Phosphor., Phosph. ac., Pulsat., *Sepia*, Sulphur.

— **burning** in the: *Euphorb.*

— **dryness** of the: Acon., Bellad., Ignat., Nitr. ac., *Nux mosch.*, Nux vom., Opium, Phosphor., Pulsat., Rhus tox., Sepia, Stramon., Sulphur.

Throat; inflammation of the: Acon., Amm. mur., *Apis*, Bellad., Brom., Conium, Merc. viv., Nitr. ac., Nux vom., Phosphor., Sulphur.

Uvula; inflammation of the: Bellad., Coffea, Merc. viv., Nux vom., Sulphur.

Œsophagus; constriction of the: Cimex.

Aversion; to food, in general: Alum., Anac., ANT. CRUD., Ant. tart., *Apis*, Arnic., ARSEN., Baryt., Bellad., Bryon., Calc. carb., *Canthar.*, Cicut., CINCHON., Coccul., *Conium*, Cyclam., Ignat., IPECAC., *Kali carb.*, Laches., Merc. viv., Mezer., Natr. mur., NUX VOM., Opium, Phosphor., Platin., PULSAT., Rheum, Rhus tox., Ruta, *Sabad.*, *Sepia*, *Silic.*, Staphis., Sulphur, Thuya.

— **to drink:** Bellad., Canthar., Coccul., *Helleb.*, Hyosc., Ignat., Stramon., (see thirstlessness).

Loathing; of food: *Amm. carb.*, *Ant. crud.*, Ant. tart., Apis, Arnic., ARSEN., Asar., Bellad., *Bryon.*, Canthar., *Chamom.*, Cinchon., Coccul., Colchic., Cuprum, Cyclam., Digit., Euphorb., Guaiac., Helleb., *Ipecac.*, KALI CARB., Laches., Lycop., Merc. viv., Mosch., Natr. mur., Nux vom., Opium, Petrol., Platin., Plumbum, Pulsat., *Rheum*, Ruta, Sarsap., Secal., Seneg., Sepia, Silic., Sulph. ac.

— **of drink:** Bellad., Canthar., Coccul., Conium, *Helleb.*, Hyosc., Ignat., Laches., Natr. mur., Nux vom., Stramon., Sulphur.

Canine hunger: Agar., Angust., Argent., ARSEN., Aurum, Bellad., *Bryon.*, Calc. carb., *Capsic.*, *Chamom.*, Cicut., CINA, CINCHON., Coffea, Graphit., Helleb., Hyosc., Ignat., Laches., Lycop., Natr. mur., Nux mosch., Nux vom., Oleand., Opium, PHOSPHOR., Pulsat., Sabad., Secal., Sepia, Spigel., Stann., Staphis., Sulphur, Veratr.

Desire for beer: Nux vom.

Desire for; cold things: ACON., Ant. tart., Arsen., Bellad., Bismuth., Borax., *Bryon.*, Calc. carb., Chamom., CINCHON., Crocus, Cuprum, Ignat., MERC. VIV., Oleand., Pulsat., Rhus tox., Ruta, Sabad., Scilla, Silic., Sulphur, Thuya, Veratr.

— **cold water:** ACON., Angust., *Arsen.*, Bellad., Bismuth., Calc. carb., *Chamom.*, CINCHON., Cuprum, *Ignat.*, MERC. VIV., Nux vom., Oleand., Phosphor., Plumbum, Pulsat., Rhus tox., Sabad., Scilla, Thuya, Veratr.

— **sour things:** *Arsen.*, Corn. flor.

— **sweet things:** Corn. flor.

— **water,** yet will not take it: BRYON.

— **wine:** *Cicut.*

Thirst; in general: ACON., Agar., Amm. mur., Anac., Angust., Ant. crud., Ant. tart., Apis, ARNIC., ARSEN., Asar., Bellad., Borax, Bovist., BRYON., Cact. grand., Calad., Calc. carb., CANTHAR., CAPSIC., *Carb. an.*, Carb. veg., CHAMOM., Chelid., *Cina*, Cinchon., Cist. can., Coccul., Coffea, COLCHIC., Coloc., Corn. flor., CROCUS, *Diadem.*, Digit., Droser., Dulcam., *Eup. perf.*, *Eup. purp.*, Guaiac., HEPAR, HYOSC., Ignat., IPECAC., Kali bichr., Kali carb., *Kreos.*, Laches., Lauroc., Lobel. inf., LYCOP., *Magn. mur.*, MERC. VIV., Mosch., *Natr. carb.*, NATR. MUR., *Nitr. ac.*, Nux mosch., *Nux vom.*, Opium, Petrol., Phosphor., Phosph. ac., Platin., PLUMBUM, Podophyl., Psorin., Pulsat., RAN. SCEL., Rhodod., RHUS TOX., Ruta, Sabad., SECAL., *Sepia*, SILIC., *Spigel.*, *Spong.*, Stann., STAPHIS., STRAMON., *Strontia*, *Sulphur*, Sulph. ac., THUYA, VALER., *Veratr.*, Zinc.

— **between chill and heat:** *Amm. mur.*, Arsen., Bryon., *Canthar.*, CINCHON., Droser., Helleb., Kreos., Natr. carb., Nux vom., Psorin., PULSAT., SABAD., *Sepia.*

— **between heat and sweat:** Agn. cast., *Amm. mur.*, Ant. tart., Bryon., CINCHON., *Coffea*, CYCLAM., NUX VOM., Opium, Pulsat., Rhus tox., Stann., *Stramon.*

— **with aversion to drink:** Agn. cast., Arnic., Arsen., *Bellad.*, *Canthar.*, Caustic., HELLEB., *Hyosc.*, Laches, Lycop.,

Merc. viv., Natr. mur., *Nux vom.*, Rhus tox., Sambuc., *Stramon.*, VERATR.

Thirst; drinking little at a time: ARSEN., *Carb. veg.*, *Cinchon.*, *Corn. flor.*, Crocus, *Eup. perf.*, Helleb., *Hyosc.*, LYCOP., Mezer., Pulsat., *Rhus tox.*, *Scilla*, Stramon.

— — **much** at a time: BRYON., Canthar., Stramon.

Thirstlessness: *Agn. cast.*, Amm. mur., Anac., Angust., *Ant. crud.*, Ant. tart., Apis, *Argent.*, Arnic., *Arsen.*, ASAF., Bellad., Brom., Bryon., Calc. carb., *Camphor.*, Canthar., *Capsic.*, CARB. VEG., Chamom., CHELID., Cimex., *Cina*, CINCHON., Coccul., *Coffea*, Coloc., *Conium*, CYCLAM., Digit., Droser., DULCAM., Euphorb., Graphit., Guaiac., HELLEB., Hepar, IGNAT., IPECAC., Kali carb., Kreos., *Laches.*, Lauroc., LEDUM, Magn. carb., Mangan., *Menyanth.*, Merc. viv., MUR. AC., Natr. carb., Natr. mur., *Nitrum*, Nitr. ac., NUX MOSCH., NUX VOM., *Oleand.*, Opium, *Phosphor.*, *Phosph. ac.*, Plumbum, *Pulsat.*, *Rheum*, *Rhodod.*, Rhus tox., RUTA, *Sabad.*, Sabin., SAMBUC., *Scilla*, SEPIA, *Spigel.*, Spong., Staphis., Stramon., *Sulphur*, *Tarax.*, Thuya, Valer., Veratr., *Viol. tr.*

— **with desire to drink:** *Arsen.*, Calad., Camphor., Coccul., *Coloc.*, Graphit., Nux mosch., Phosphor., Phosph. ac.

Taste; bitter: Acon., Alum., *Ant. crud.*, Arnic., *Arsen.*, *Bryon.*, Carb. veg., *Chamom.*, Cinchon., Coccul., *Coloc.*, Droser., Hepar, Ignat., Lycop., Merc. viv., *Natr. mur.*, Nitr. ac., *Nux vom.*, *Phosphor.*, *Pulsat.*, Sabad., Sarsap., *Sepia*, Sulphur, Veratr.

— **putrid:** Acon., Arnic., Bellad., Calc. carb., Carb. veg., Chamom., Conium, HYOSC., Merc. viv., Mur. ac., Natr. mur., Nux vom., Petrol., Phosph. ac., PULSAT., *Rhus tox.*, Sepia, *Staphis.*, Sulphur.

— **offensive:** *Capsic.*, Kali carb., *Staphis.*

— **salty:** Bellad.

Eructations; in general: Alum., Amm. carb., *Ant. crud.*, BRYON., *Carb. veg.*, Cicut., Cinchon., Conium, Ignat., *Laches.*,

NUX VOM., Phosphor., Rhus tox., *Sabad.*, Sepia, Sulphur, Thuya.

Nausea; in general: Acon., Anac., *Ant. crud.*, Ant. tart., Argent., ARSEN., Asar., Bellad., Borax, *Bryon.*, Calc. carb., CARB.VEG., Chamom., *Chelid.*, Cicut., Cina, Cinchon., Coccul., Conium, Cuprum, Cyclam., Diadem., Digit., Droser., Graphit., Helleb., Hepar, IPECAC., Kali bichr., Kali carb., *Lycop.*, *Merc. viv.*, Mosch., *Natr. mur.*, *Nitr. ac.*, NUX VOM., Paris, *Phosphor.*, PULSAT., Rhus tox., Scilla, SEPIA, Silic., Stann., Sulphur, Sulph. ac., Valer., *Veratr.*

Gagging: Cimex.

Running together of water in the mouth: Bryon., Calc. carb., Carb. veg., Coccul., Lycop., *Natr. mur.*, Nitr. ac., NUX VOM., Petrol., *Rhus tox.*, Sabad., SILIC., Sulphur.

Vomit; disposition to: Arsen., Chamom., Cina, Cinchon., *Droser.*, Ipecac., *Nux vom.*, Pulsat., Rhus tox., Sabad., Sepia, Veratr.

Vomiting; in general: *Ant. crud.*, *Arnic.*, ARSEN., Asar., Bellad., Borax, Bryon., Carb. veg., *Chamom.*, *Cina*, Cinchon., Conium, Cuprum, Ferr., Hepar, Ignat., *Ipecac.*, Kali carb., Laches., Lycop., Natr. carb., *Nux vom.*, Phosphor., Pulsat., Scilla, Silic., *Stramon.*, Sulphur, *Veratr.*

— **bitter** (bilious): Ant. crud., *Arsen.*, Bryon., *Chamom.*, Cina, Cinchon., Cuprum, Droser., Ignat., Ipecac., Merc. viv., *Nux vom.*, Phosphor., Psorin., *Pulsat.*, Secal., Sepia, Sulphur, Veratr.

— **ingesta,** of the: Ant. tart., Arnic., *Arsen.*, Bryon., Calc. carb., Chamom., CINA, Coloc., Droser., FERR., IGNAT., Ipecac., Lycop., Merc. viv., Mezer., *Natr. mur.*, *Nux vom.*, Phosphor., *Pulsat.*, Sepia, Silic., Sulphur, Veratr.

— **mucus**: Acon., Arsen., Bellad., CHAMOM., Cina, Cinchon., Conium, Droser., Dulcam., IGNAT., Ipecac., Lycop., Merc. viv., *Nux vom.*, PULSAT., Rheum, Secal., Sepia, Sulphur, Veratr.

— **sour**: Alum., ARNIC., *Arsen.*, *Bellad.*, Calc. carb.,

Chamom., Ipecac., LYCOP., *Nux vom.*, Phosphor., PULSAT., Sepia, Sulphur, Veratr.

Stomach; pains in the, general: Acon., Amm. carb., Ant. crud., *Arnic.*, ARSEN., Baryt., Bellad., BRYON., Calc. carb., *Carb. veg.*, CHAMOM., *Cina*, *Cinchon.*, *Coccul.*, Coloc., Cuprum, *Ferr.*, *Ignat.*, *Ipecac.*, Kali carb., *Lycop.*, Merc. viv., NATR. MUR., NUX VOM., Phosphor., Phosph. ac., PULSAT., *Rhus tox.*, Sabad., SEPIA, Silic., Sulphur, Sulph. ac., Veratr.

— **burning** in the: *Arsen.*, Nux vom., Sepia.

— **cramp** in the: Bellad., Carb. veg., *Coccul.*, Nux vom., Pulsat.

— **pressure** in the: *Amm. carb.*, Arsen., *Cinchon.*, *Ferr.*, Nux vom., Sabad., *Sepia*, Silic.

— **trembling sensation** in the: Capsic., Ignat., IOD., Lycop.

Liver; pains in the: Acon., Alum., ARSEN., Aurum, BORAX, Bryon., Calc. carb., Capsic., CINCHON., Graphit., Kali carb., Laches., Lycop., Magn. mur., Merc. viv., Natr. carb., Nux mosch., *Nux vom.*, Sepia, Stann., Sulphur.

Spleen; pains in the: Agn. cast., Arnic., *Arsen.*, Asaf., *Borax*, Brom., Capsic., CARB. VEG., Chamom., Cinchon., Fluor. ac., Ignat., Mezer., *Natr. mur.*, Nitr. ac., *Nux vom.*, Ran. bulb., Stann., Sulphur.

— **swelling** of the: Agn. cast., *Arsen.*, Brom., Capsic., CARB. VEG., Chamom., *Diadem.*, Ignat., NATR. MUR., Nitr. ac., Sulphur.

Abdomen; pains in the, in general: Acon., ANT. CRUD., Ant. tart., Apis, ARSEN., Baryt., Bellad., *Bovist.*, *Bryon.*, *Calc. carb.*, Canthar., Capsic., CARB. VEG., CHAMOM., Cicut., CINA, *Cinchon.*, Coffea, Coloc., *Ferr.*, Hepar, Ignat., Kali bichr., *Kali carb.*, Leptand., Lycop., Merc. viv., *Mosch.*, Natr. mur., *Nitr. ac.*, Nux vom., Phosphor., *Pulsat.*, *Ran. bulb.*, RHUS TOX., *Sepia*, Silic., Spong., Strontia, *Sulphur*, *Valer.*

Abdomen; beating (pulsating) in the: Acon., Calc. carb., Capsic., *Kali carb.*, Lycop., Phosphor., Sepia.

— **cold feeling** in the: Arsen., Calc. carb., *Menyanth.*, Petrol., Sepia.

— **distention** of the: Arsen., *Carb. veg.*, Cinchon., Colchic., Cuprum, Ferr., Nux vom., Rhus tox., Sepia, *Silic.*, *Stramon.*, Sulphur, Veratr.

— **heaviness in the hypogastrium:** Diadem.

— **labor-like pains** in the: Acon., Bellad., Chamom., Ferr., Ignat., Nux vom., Opium, *Pulsat.*, Sabin., Secal.

— **pinching pains** in the: Ambra, Coloc., Ignat., Phosph. ac., *Zinc.*

— **rumbling in the bowels:** Lachnanth.

— **tension** of the: Arsen., Bellad., Calc. carb., Carb. veg., Colchic., *Ferr.*, Lycop., Merc. viv., *Nux vom.*, Pulsat., SILIC., Strontia, Veratr.

Flatulence; affections from: Agar., *Arsen.*, *Carb. veg.*, Cinchon., Colchic., Graphit., Kali carb., Mar. ver., Nitr. ac., NUX VOM., Phosphor., Phosph. ac.

Diarrhœa: *Acon.*, Amm. mur., *Ant. crud.*, Ant. tart., APIS, Arnic., ARSEN., Asaf., Baptis., Borax, Brom., *Bryon.*, Calad., Calc. carb., Capsic., CHAMOM., CINA, Cinchon., *Coffea*, Coloc., CONIUM, Digit., Dulcam., Ferr., Hyosc., Ipecac., *Laches.*, MERC. VIV., Natr. mur., Nitr. ac., Nux vom., Petrol., *Phosphor.*, *Phosph. ac.*, PULSAT., Oxal. ac., Rheum, RHUS TOX., RUTA, Scilla, Secal., Sepia, SILIC., Stann., *Sulphur*, Sulph. ac., VERATR.

Constipation: Alum., Ambra, Amm. carb., *Ant. crud.*, *Apis*, Arnic., *Bellad.*, *Bryon.*, Calad., Calc. carb., Cann. sat., Canthar., Carb. veg., Caustic., Cinchon., *Coccul.*, Conium, CUPRUM, *Dulcam.*, Fluor. ac., Graphit., Guaiac., Kali carb., Kreos., Laches., Lauroc., LYCOP., Magn. mur., Menyanth., Merc. viv., Mezer., Natr. mur., Nitr. ac., NUX VOM., *Opium*,

Phosphor., Platin., Plumbum, Podophyl., Pulsat., Rhus tox., Sabad., Sarsap., Selen., Sepia, Silic., Stann., STAPHIS., Sulphur, Sulph. ac., Thuya, *Veratr.*, Verbas., Zinc.

Urging to stool: Arnic., Arsen., CAUSTIC., Hyosc., Laches., Merc. viv., *Nux vom.*, Pulsat., *Sulphur.*

— **ineffectual:** Acon., Arnic., *Arsen.*, *Capsic.*, *Coccul.*, LYCOP., Nux vom., Rheum, RHUS TOX., Staphis., *Sulphur*, Veratr.

Urine; brown: *Acon.*, Arnic., *Bellad.*, Bryon., Carb. veg., Ipecac., Lycop., *Nux vom.*, Pulsat., Rhus tox., SEPIA, VERATR.

— **cloudy:** Arsen., Bellad., Bryon., Lycop., *Phosphor.*, Phosph. ac., Pulsat., Rhus tox., Sabad., Sarsap., Sepia.

— **stinking:** Arsen., Baptis., Carb. veg., Dulcam., Phosph. ac., Pulsat., *Sepia*, Viol. tr.

Urination; too frequent: Argent., Bellad., Kreos., *Lycop.*, Merc. viv., *Phosph. ac.*, Rhus tox., Scilla, Staphis., Sulphur.

— **painful:** Ant. crud., Cann. sat., Canthar., *Chamom.*, Colchic., Dulcam., Nitr. ac., Nux vom., Staphis., Sulphur.

— **profuse,** too: Ant. crud., Argent., *Chamom.*, Dulcam., Mur. ac., *Phosphor.*, Scilla, Stramon.

— **scanty,** too: Apis, Cann. sat., Canthar., Colchic., Nitr. ac., Nux vom., Opium, *Pulsat.*, Ruta, Staphis.

— **seldom,** too: *Arsen.*, Cinchon., Colchic., Hyosc., *Opium*, *Pulsat.*, Stramon.

Urging to urinate: Acon., *Ant. tart.*, Bellad., Bryon., Canthar., Caustic., Dulcam., Graphit., Helleb., Hyosc., Kali carb., Lycop., Nux vom., Phosph. ac., *Pulsat.*, Rhus tox., Sabin., Sarsap., Scilla, Staphis., Sulphur.

— **ineffectual:** *Arsen.*, Canthar., Digit., Hyosc., Nux vom., *Pulsat.*, Sarsap., Sulphur.

Sneezing: Arnic., Bellad., Bryon., CARB. VEG., Caustic., *Chamom.*, CINA, *Cinchon.*, Cyclam., Mar. ver., Merc. viv., Pulsat., *Rhus tox.*, SABAD., Silic., Staphis.

Coryza; fluent: Amm. mur., ARSEN., *Aurum.*, Calc. carb., *Carb. veg.*, Chamom., Conium, Euphras., KALI CARB., *Laches.*, *Merc. viv.*, *Mezer.*, Nux vom., Phosphor., PULSAT., RHUS TOX., *Selen.*, Sepia, Silic., Spigel., Sulphur.

— **dry:** *Amm. carb.*, Bellad., Bryon., *Calad.*, Calc. carb., Dulcam., Hepar, Ipecac., LYCOP., Mur. ac., Natr. mur., Nitr. ac., NUX VOM., Petrol., Phosphor., Pulsat., Rhodod., Sambuc., Sepia, SILIC, Spigel., *Sulphur.*

Dryness of the nose: Apis, Arsen., *Bellad.*, Calc. carb., Droser., Graphit., Merc. viv., Natr. mur., Phosphor., *Rhodod.*, Sepia, Silic., *Spigel.*, Sulphur.

Breathing; anxious: ACON., *Apis*, Arnic., Arsen., Bellad., BRYON., Camphor., Chamom., Coffea., Hepar, Ignat., IPECAC., Kali carb., Laches., *Phosphor.*, Platin., *Pulsat.*, Rhus tox., Sambuc., Scilla, Secal., Spong., Stann., Stramon., Viol. tr.

— **deep:** Aurum, *Borax*, Bryon., Capsic., Cuprum, Ipecac., Mur. ac., Opium, *Phosph. ac.*, Platin., Selen., Silic., Stann.

— **oppressed:** ACON., Ambra, *Anac.*, Ant. tart., *Apis.*, Arnic., ARSEN., Aurum, Bellad., *Bovist.*, Brom., BRYON., Cact. grand., *Calc. carb.*, CARB. VEG., Chamom., Cinchon., Coccul., Cuprum, Dulcam., Graphit., Hepar, Ignat., IPECAC., Kali carb., Laches., Lycop., *Merc. viv.*, Mezer., Nitrum, Nux vom., Opium, Phosphor., Platin., Pulsat., Ran. bulb., Rhodod., Rhus tox., RUTA, Sambuc., Seneg., SEPIA, Silic., Spigel., Stann., Sulphur, Thuya, Veratr., VIOL. TR., Zinc.

— **rattling:** *Acon.*, *Arsen.*, Carb. veg., Chamom., Hepar, Ipecac., Lycop., NUX MOSCH., OPIUM, Scilla, Spong., Stann.

— **short:** ACON., Ambra, Amm. carb., *Anac.*, Ant. tart., APIS, Arnic., ARSEN., Aurum, Bellad., BRYON., *Calc. carb.*, *Camphor.*, Carb. veg., Caustic., *Cina*, Cinchon., *Coccul.*, Conium, Cuprum, *Ferr.*, Hepar, *Ignat.*, Ipecac., *Kali carb.*, Laches., LYCOP., Merc. viv., Natr. carb., Natr. mur., Nitr. ac., Nux mosch., Nux vom., PHOSPHOR., Phosph. ac., Platin.,

PULSAT., Rhus tox., RUTA, Sabad., Sambuc., Scilla, Seneg., *Sepia*, Silic., Spigel., Stann., Sulphur, ZINC.

Breath; cold: Camphor., *Carb. veg.*, Cinchon., Mur. ac., Rhus tox., VERATR.

— **hot:** Acon., *Anac.*, Asar., Calc. carb., CHAMOM., COFFEA, Ferr., Mangan., Natr. mur., *Nux vom.*, Rhus tox., Sabad., Strontia, ZINC.

— **fetid:** Baptis.

Cough; with expectoration: Alum., Anac., Argent., ARSEN., Bellad., Bismuth., *Bryon.*, CALC. CARB., Carb. veg., Cicut., *Cinchon.*, Digit., Droser., Dulcam., Ferr., Iod., KALI CARB., Kreos., Lycop., PHOSPHOR., Phosph. ac., PULSAT., Ruta, SCILLA, Seneg., Sepia, *Silic.*, Spong., Stann., Staphis., *Sulphur*, Thuya.

— **without expectoration:** ACON., Angust., Ant. crud., *Apis*, *Arnic.*, *Arsen.*, Bellad., Brom., *Bryon.*, Calc. carb., Carb. veg., Caustic., Chamom., Cina, Cinchon., Coffea., CONIUM, Cuprum, Droser., Hepar, *Hyosc.*, Ignat., IPECAC., *Kali carb.*, Laches., Lycop., NATR. MUR., Nitr. ac., Nux mosch., NUX VOM., Opium, Petrol., PHOSPHOR., Platin., Pulsat., Rhus tox., SABAD., Sambuc., Scilla, Sepia, Spigel., Spong., Staphis., *Sulphur*, Sulph. ac., Veratr., Verbas.

Larynx; pains in the: *Acon.*, Amm. mur., Ant. crud., Apis, Argent., Baryt., *Bellad.*, Brom., Bryon., Canthar., Carb. veg., Caustic., Chamom., *Droser.*, *Hepar*, IOD., Laches., Mangan., Merc. viv., MOSCH., NUX VOM., OPIUM, Paris, *Phosphor.*, PULSAT., Sabad., Sambuc., Seneg., *Spong.*, Sulphur, Veratr., Zinc.

— **dryness** of the: Arsen., Droser., Hepar, Iod., Mangan., Nux vom., *Opium*, Paris, *Petrol.*, Phosphor., *Spong.*, Thuya, Zinc.

Voice hoarse: *Pulsat.*, Sepia.

Throat; external, pains in the: *Laches.*

— **sensitiveness** of the: *Laches.*

— **swelling of the glands** of the: *Bellad.*

Nape of the neck; pains in the: Bryon., Rhus tox.

— **stiffness** of the: *Acon.*

Chest; internal pains: ACON., *Amm. carb.*, Apis, Arnic., *Arsen.*, Bellad., Borax, *Bovist.*, BRYON., Calad., Calc. carb., *Capsic.*, *Carb. veg.*, *Cina*, CINCHON., Coccul., Conium, Dulcam., *Ipecac.*, KALI CARB., Lycop., *Merc. viv.*, Mezer., Mur. ac., Nitr. ac., NUX VOM., *Phosphor.*, Phosph. ac., Psorin., PULSAT., Ran. bulb., *Rhus tox.*, Ruta, Sabad., Seneg., Sepia, *Spigel.*, Stann., Sulphur, Thuya, Zinc.

— **burning in the left:** Seneg.

— **congestion to the:** *Acon.*, Aurum, *Bellad.*, Bryon., Cinchon., Merc. viv., NITR. AC., *Nux vom.*, Phosphor., *Pulsat.*, Scilla, Seneg., Spong., Sulphur, Thuya.

— **contraction** of the: *Acon.*, Arnic., *Arsen.*, Asaf., Cuprum, *Ipecac.*, Kali carb., MERC. VIV., *Mosch.*, Nitrum, Nitr. ac., *Nux vom.*, *Phosphor.*, Phosph. ac., *Platin.*, *Pulsat.*, Rhus tox., Sepia, Spigel., Spong., *Stann.*, Staphis., Stramon., *Sulphur*, Sulph. ac., Thuya, Veratr.

— **rising in the,** sensation of: Amm. mur., Merc. viv., *Nux vom.*, Phosphor.

— **spasm** of the: ARSEN., Asaf., Camphor., Caustic., Coccul., Colchic., Cuprum, Hyosc., Ignat., *Ipecac.*, Mosch., *Nux vom.*, PULSAT., Sepia, Stann., Sulphur.

— **stitches** in the: ACON., *Amm. carb.*, Apis, Arnic., Arsen., Asaf., Bellad., Borax, BRYON., Calc. carb., Carb. veg., Cinchon., Ignat., KALI CARB., Merc. viv., *Natr. mur.*, Nitrum, *Phosphor.*, Psorin., *Pulsat.*, *Rhus tox.*, Scilla, Sepia, Silic., Spigel., Stann., Sulphur, Valer.

Mammæ; swelling of the: Apis, Bryon., *Calc. carb.*, Conium, Lycop., Phosphor., *Pulsat.*

Suppression of milk: *Agn. cast.*, Bellad., *Bryon.*, *Calc. carb.*, Chamom., Dulcam., *Hyosc.*, Ignat., *Pulsat.*, RHUS TOX., Zinc.

Palpitation of the heart: ACON., *Alum.*, Ant. tart., Arnic., ARSEN., Aurum, Bellad., Bryon., Calad., CALC. CARB., Cinchon., *Colchic.*, Cuprum, Hepar, *Ignat.*, Iod., Lycop., *Merc. viv.*, Natr. mur., NITR. AC., Nux vom., *Phosphor.*, Phosph. ac., *Pulsat.*, *Rhus tox.*, SARSAP., SEPIA, Silic., *Spigel.*, Spong., *Sulphur*, Thuya, Viol. od., Zinc.

— **with anxiety:** ACON., *Arsen.*, *Aurum*, CALC. CARB., Cinchon., *Lycop.*, *Natr. mur.*, Nitr. ac., Nux vom., *Phosphor.*, Platin., PULSAT., Sepia, SPIGEL., Sulphur, Thuya, Viol. od.

Scapulæ; pains in the: *Arsen.*, Baryt., Bellad., *Cinchon.*, Kali carb., Kreos., Menyanth., *Merc. viv.*, Nux vom., *Rhus tox.*, SEPIA, Silic., Sulphur, *Veratr.*, Viol. tr.

Back; pains in the: Acon., Ant. tart., Apis, ARNIC., *Arsen.*, BELLAD., Calc. carb., Camphor., Capsic., Carb. veg., *Caustic.*, *Cinchon.*, Coccul., Ignat., Kali carb., *Lycop.*, Merc. viv., NATR. MUR., Nux vom., Petrol., Phosphor., *Pulsat.*, RHUS TOX., *Sepia*, Silic., *Sulphur*, Veratr., Zinc.

Small of the back; pains in the: *Acon.*, Apis, Arnic., *Arsen.*, Bryon., CALC. CARB., *Caustic.*, *Chamom.*, Cinchon., Coccul., *Ignat.*, Kali carb., Lycop., Merc. viv., *Natr. mur.*, NUX VOM., Phosphor., PULSAT., *Rhus tox.*, Ruta, SEPIA, Silic., Strontia, *Sulphur.*

Os Coccygis; pains in the: Agn. cast., Arnic., *Arsen.*, Borax, Calc. carb., Carb. veg., Cinchon., *Hepar*, Ignat., Merc. viv., Phosph. ac., Platin., *Rhus tox.*, Ruta, Sulphur.

Upper limbs; pains in the, in general: *Acon.*, *Ant. crud.*, Apis, ARNIC., *Arsen.*, BELLAD., Bovist., Bryon., CALC. CARB., Capsic., Carb. veg., Caustic., Cinchon., Coccul., *Colchic.*, Cyclam., Euphras., Ferr., *Ignat.*, Ipecac., Kali carb., Lycop., Menyanth., Merc. viv., Nitrum, NUX VOM., Phosphor.,

PULSAT., Ran. bulb., *Rhodod.*, *Rhus tox.*, Ruta, Sabin., Sambuc., SCILLA, *Sepia*, Stann., Staphis., Stramon., Sulphur, THUYA, *Veratr.*, Zinc.

Upper limbs; joints, pains in the: *Calc. carb.*, Kali carb., Rhus tox.

Hands; blue: Amm. carb., Apis, Calc. carb., Camphor., *Cuprum*, Sambuc., *Veratr.*

— **cold:** Arnic., Aurum, Bellad., Camphor., Caustic., Conium, CYCLAM., Droser., EUPHRAS., Helleb., *Ignat.*, IPECAC., Lycop., *Menyanth.*, Mezer., Nux vom., Phosphor., PULSAT., *Ran. bulb.*, Rhus tox., RUTA, SABIN., *Sambuc.*, SCILLA, Selen., *Stramon.*, Sulphur, Thuya, Veratr.

— **dead,** as if: Calc. carb., Nux vom., Secal., *Sepia*, Zinc.

— **distention of the blood vessels:** Amm.carb., ARNIC., Baryt., Calc. carb., *Cinchon.*, Nux vom., *Phosphor.*, PULSAT., Rhus tox., *Sulphur*, THUYA.

— **hot and dry:** Æsc. hip.

— **jerking** of the: *Viol. tr.*

— **sweat** of the: *Amm. carb.*, Kali bichr., *Nitr. ac.*, Thuya.

— **trembling** of the: Valer.

Thumbs; turned in: Bellad., Sulphur, *Viol. tr.*

Fingers; dead, as if: Amm. carb., Ant. tart., *Calc. carb.*, Chelid., Hepar, Pulsat., *Secal.*, Sepia, Sulphur, THUYA.

— **coldness** of the: Ant. tart., Chamom., Tarax., *Thuya.*

Lower limbs; pains in general: Acon., Agn. cast., Amm. carb., Ant. crud., Arnic., ARSEN., Bellad., *Calc. carb.*, Canthar., CAPSIC., CARB. VEG., Caustic., Cinchon., Colchic., Ferr., Ignat., Ipecac., *Lycop.*, Magn. carb., Magn. mur., Natr. mur., Nitrum, *Nux vom.*, Phosphor., *Pulsat.*, Rhodod., Rhus tox., Sambuc., *Sepia*, Spong., *Sulphur*, Thuya, Veratr.

— **heaviness** of the: Alum., *Calc. carb.*, Canthar., *Cinchon.*, Ignat., *Natr. mur.*, *Nux vom.*, *Pulsat.*, Sepia, Stann., Sulphur, Thuya.

— **restlessness** of the: Nitr. ac., Phosphor., RHUS TOX., Scilla, Sepia.

Hips; pains in the: *Arnic.*, Bellad., Lycop., Natr. mur., Pulsat., *Rhus tox.*, *Sepia.*

Thighs; pains in the: Arnic., ARSEN., Carb. veg., Cinchon., Merc. viv., NATR. MUR., Nux vom., Sepia, Staphis., *Thuya.*

— **coldness** of the: Calc. carb., *Ignat.*, Nux vom., SPONG., Sulphur, Thuya.

— **numbness** of the: Ferr., Graphit., *Spong.*

— **sweat** on the: Kali bichr.

Knees; pain in the: CALC. CARB., Cinchon., *Lycop.*, NATR. MUR., Nux vom., Petrol., *Pulsat.*, Rhus tox., *Sepia*, Sulphur, Thuya.

— **coldness** of the: AGN. CAST., Arsen., *Pulsat.*, Sepia.

Legs; pain in the: AMM. CARB., Calc. carb., *Lycop.*, *Pulsat.*, Sepia, Silic., Staphis.

Feet; cold: *Agn. cast.*, AMM. CARB., ANGUST., ANT. CRUD., Calc. carb., Caustic., COCCUL., *Colchic.*, Conium, *Ignat.*, IPECAC., KREOS., LACHES., *Lycop.*, *Magn. carb.*, MENYANTH., Nitr. ac., *Nux vom.*, PETROL., Phosphor., *Phosph. ac.*, PULSAT., (Ran. bulb)., RHODOD., RUTA, SABIN., SAMBUC., SCILLA, *Sepia*, Silic., STRAMON., SULPHUR, Thuya, *Veratr.*, ZINC.

— **coldness of one foot:** *Lycop.*

— **dead,** as if: Ant. crud., *Calc. carb.*, Coffea, Nux vom., Secal., *Sulphur.*

— **sweat** on the: AMM. MUR., Calc. carb., Kali bichr., Lycop., NATR. MUR., Nitr. ac., Phosphor., *Pulsat.*, *Sepia*, Silic., Staphis., Sulphur, Thuya.

— **swollen:** *Arsen.*, Bryon., Caustic., Cinchon., FERR., LYCOP., *Pulsat.*, Secal., Silic.

Limbs; pains in general: *Acon.*, Alum., *Ant. crud.*, (Apis), *Arnic.*, Arsen., Bellad., BRYON., Calc. carb., Capsic., Carb. veg., Caustic., Chamom., *Cinchon.*, *Colchic.*, Dulcam., Ferr., *Helleb.*, IGNAT., Kali carb., *Lycop.*, *Nux vom.*, Pulsat.,

Rhodod., RHUS TOX., Sepia, Silic., Sulphur, Tarax., Thuya, Veratr., *Zinc.*

Limbs; bending and stretching of the: Æsc. hip., Alum., Bellad., *Borax*, Bryon., CALC. CARB., Caustic., Chamom., Natr. mur., *Nux vom.*, RHUS TOX., SABAD., Sepia, Spong., Sulphur.

— **beaten,** feel as if: *Arnic.*, *Arsen.*, *Bellad.*, Bryon., Calc. carb., CINCHON., *Coccul.*, Ignat., Magn. carb., *Mosch.*, NATR. MUR., NUX VOM., Phosphor., PULSAT., RHODOD., *Ruta*, Sepia, Silic., *Spigel.*, Sulphur, Thuya, Valer., *Veratr.*

— **crawling** in the, sensation of: *Acon.*, Arnic., Colchic., Platin., RHUS TOX., Secal., *Sepia*, Spigel., Stramon.

— **heaviness** of the: Apis, *Bellad.*, CALC. CARB., Diadem., Helleb., Merc. viv., NUX VOM., RHUS TOX., Stann., Staphis., *Sulphur.*

— **lameness** of the: *Arnic.*, ARSEN., *Bellad.*, Cina, Coccul., Cyclam., *Ignat.*, *Nux vom.*, *Phosph. ac.*, Pulsat., SABAD., Sabin.

— **go "to-sleep"**: Apis, Calc. carb., Carb. veg., Chamom., Cinchon., *Coccul.*, Crocus, Graphit., Ignat., *Kali carb.*, LYCOP., Merc. viv., *Natr. mur.*, *Nux vom.*, Petrol., Phosphor., *Pulsat.*, Rhodod., Rhus tox., Sepia, Silic., Thuya, Veratr.

Sleeplessness: Alum., Amm. carb., Amm. mur., ANAC., APIS, Arnic., Arsen., Baryt., Bellad., Borax, *Bryon.*, *Calc. carb.*, Cann. sat., Carb. veg., *Caustic.*, *Chamom.*, Cinchon., Clemat., Coccul., Coffea, Conium, Graphit., *Hepar*, Ignat., Kali bichr., Kreos., Lauroc., Ledum, *Magn. carb.*, *Magn. mur.*, Mangan., Merc. viv., Merc. corr., Mosch., Natr. mur., Nitrum, NITR. AC., Nux mosch., *Nux vom.*, *Petrol.*, PHOSPHOR., *Phosph. ac.*, *Pulsat.*, Ran. bulb., *Ran. scel.*, RHODOD., RHUS TOX., Sabad., *Sabin.*, Sarsap., Sepia, *Silic.*, *Staphis.*, Strontia, SULPHUR, THUYA, Veratr.

Yawning: Æsc. hip., Arnic., *Arsen.*, Bryon., *Caustic.*, Cina, Crocus, *Ignat.*, KALI CARB., Kreos., NITR. AC.,

NUX VOM., *Opium*, *Phosphor.*, Platin., *Rhus tox.*, SABAD., Sepia.

Stretching and bending; limbs, of the: Æsc. hip., Alum., Bellad., *Borax.*, Bryon., CALC. CARB., Caustic., Chamom., Natr. mur., *Nux vom.*, RHUS TOX., SABAD., Sepia, Spong., Sulphur.

Sleepiness: *Acon.*, Ant. crud., ANT. TART., *Apis*, Arnic., *Arsen.*, ASAF., Bellad., Borax, CALAD., Capsic., *Chamom.*, Crocus, Cyclam., HEPAR, IGNAT., Kali carb., Laches., Mezer., Mosch., Natr. carb., *Natr. mur.*, *Nux mosch.*, Nux vom., OPIUM, Petrol., PHOSPHOR., PHOSPH. AC., PLUMBUM, Psorin., PULSAT., Rhus tox., Sabad., *Sepia*, Stramon., Sulphur, *Veratr.*, Viol. tr.

Sleep: Anac., ANT. TART., *Apis*, *Arnic.*, *Bellad.*, *Calad.*, CAPSIC., Dulcam., *Hepar*, *Ignat.*, *Laches.*, Merc. viv., Merc. corr., NATR. CARB., *Natr. mur.*, OPIUM, *Petrol.*, Sabad., *Stramon.*, *Veratr.*

— **between chill and heat:** *Nux vom.*

— **restless:** Psorin.

Somnolence: *Acon.*, ANT. TART., APIS, *Bellad.*, Calc. carb., Cact. grand., *Camphor.*, Cicut., Conium, Crocus, Hepar, Hyosc., Ignat., Lachnanth., Ledum, *Nux mosch.*, OPIUM, *Phosphor.*, *Phosph. ac.*, Pulsat., Secal., *Spong.*, Stramon., Valer., *Veratr.*

During sleep; dreaming: *Acon.*, Bryon., Cinchon., NUX VOM., Phosphor., *Phosph. ac.*, *Pulsat.*, *Rhus tox.*, Sabad., Sepia, Silic., SPIGEL., Staphis., Sulphur, Thuya.

— **moaning and lamenting:** *Acon.*, *Arnic.*, Baryt., *Bellad.*, Bryon., Calc. carb., *Chamom.*, Coccul., *Ignat.*, *Ipecac.*, Mur. ac., Nux vom., *Pulsat.*, Silic., Thuya.

— **murmuring:** Apis, *Bellad.*, MUR. AC., Opium, Phosphor., *Phosph. ac.*, Rhus tox., Silic.

— **sliding down** in bed: Arsen., *Mur. ac.*

— **snoring:** Anac., Cinchon., Graphit., *Ignat.*, Mur. ac., *Nux. vom.*, OPIUM, Silic., Stramon.

During sleep; starting: ACON., *Apis*, Arnic., *Bellad.*, Bryon., CHAMOM., Cinchon., Ipecac., LYCOP., Phosphor., PULSAT., Sambuc., Sepia, Silic., Sulphur.

Apoplexy: *Acon.*, *Bellad.*, Calc. carb., Coccul., Hyosc., *Laches.*, Lycop., NUX VOM., OPIUM, *Sepia*, Silic., Stramon., Thuya.

Blood vessels; distention of the: Amm. carb., Arnic., Bellad., CAMPHOR., CINCHON., *Coccul.*, CROCUS., *Cyclam.*, *Ferr.*, Hyosc., Mosch., PHOSPH. AC., *Pulsat.*, RAN. SCEL., *Rhus tox.*, Staphis., Thuya.

— **burning** in the: *Arsen.*, Bryon.

— **beating** in the: ACON., ARSEN., Bellad., *Calad.*, Cinchon., (Opium), Zinc.

Burning pains: Hydrast.

Clothing unbearable: Acon., BOVIST., Calc. carb., EUPHORB., Ferr., *Lycop.*, Spigel., Veratr.

Excitability; nervous: Apis, *Bellad.*, Capsic., *Chamom.*, COCCUL., COFFEA, CONIUM, Kali carb., MAR. VER., *Nux vom.*, Petrol., Phosph. ac., Sepia, Valer.

Faintness: Arnic., Eup. perf., *Ignat.*, NUX VOM., PETROL., Sulphur, Thuya,

Floccillation: Arnic., Arsen., BELLAD., Chamom., Cinchon., Hepar, *Hyosc.*, Iod., MUR. AC., OPIUM, Phosphor., PHOSPH. AC., Rhus tox., Stramon., Sulphur.

Insensibility to touch: *Bellad.*, Calc. carb., Cann. sat., *Hyosc.*, Ignat., *Lycop.*, OPIUM, *Phosphor.*, PHOSPH. AC., *Pulsat.*, Rhus tox., Stann., Stramon., THUYA.

Jerkings: Arsen., Bellad., BRYON., Chamom., Coloc., Cuprum, Hyosc., Ignat., Menyanth., Merc. viv., *Natr. mur.*, *Opium*, *Pulsat.*, *Rhus tox.*, *Secal.*, Stramon., Sulphur, Thuya, Veratr., *Viol. tr.*

— **muscles,** of the: *Bellad.*, Coloc., Cuprum, IOD., KALI CARB., *Mezer.*, Natr. carb., Platin., *Secal.*, Spong., Viol. tr.

Lassitude (weakness): Anac., *Apis*, Argent., ARSEN.,

Bellad., Borax., *Bryon.*, *Calc. carb.*, Camphor., Canthar., Caustic., *Cinchon.*, CUPRUM, Digit., Droser., Eup. perf., *Ferr.*, IGNAT., Iod., Ipecac., Kali carb., Kreos., Lauroc., LYCOP., *Menyanth.*, Merc. viv., NATR. CARB., *Natr. mur.*, NITR. AC., Nux mosch., NUX VOM., *Phosphor.*, *Phosph. ac.*, Plumbum, Psorin., *Pulsat.*, Rheum, Rhodod., RHUS TOX., Sabad., SEPIA, Silic., Spigel., *Stann.*, *Sulphur*, Thuya, VERATR.

Lie down; desire to: *Acon.*, ARSEN., *Bryon.*, Calad., Canthar., Chamom., *Coccul.*, Cyclam., Droser., NUX VOM., Sepia.

Prostration: Apis, Baptis., *Cinchon.*, Eup. perf., LYCOP., Mar. ver., PETROL., *Phosph. ac.*, Rhodod., Spong., Valer.

Restlessness; bodily: ACON., Amm. carb., Anac., Ant. tart., *Arnic.*, *Arsen.*, BARYT., *Bellad.*, BOVIST., *Bryon.*, *Calc. carb.*, Cann. sat., Carb. veg., Chamom., Cinchon., Coffea, Ferr., Gelsem., *Hyosc.*, Ignat., Ipecac., Lachnanth., *Lycop.*, MAGN. CARB., Magn. mur., *Merc. viv.*, Merc. corr., MOSCH., MUR. AC., Natr. sulph., Nitr. ac., Nux vom., Opium, Phosphor., Phosph. ac., Platin., Pulsat., Rheum, RHUS TOX., RUTA, SABIN., Sambuc., Sepia, Silic., Spong., Staphis., Stramon., Thuya, Valer., Veratr.

Sinking: Psorin.

Spasms; clonic: BELLAD., *Chamom.*, Cicut., Coccul., Cuprum, *Hyosc.*, OPIUM, *Sepia*, Stramon., Thuya, *Veratr.*

— **tonic:** *Bellad.*, Cicut., *Coccul.*, Petrol., Platin., Sepia, *Veratr.*

Stitches; bones, in the: *Bellad.*, Calc. carb., Caustic., Conium, *Helleb.*, Merc. viv., *Pulsat.*, Sarsap., Sepia.

— **joints,** in the: Baryt., *Calc. carb.*, HELLEB., Kali carb., Merc. viv., RHUS TOX., Silic., Spigel., Tarax., Thuya.

— **muscles**; in the: *Bellad.*, BRYON., Calc. carb., Merc. viv., *Pulsat.*, RHUS TOX., Spigel., Staphis., Sulphur, Tarax., Thuya.

Tearing (drawing); bones, in the: Argent., *Cinchon.*, Cyclam., *Eup. purp.*, Kali carb., Merc. viv., Rhodod., Sabin., Staphis.

Tearing (drawing); joints, in the: Agn. cast., *Calc. carb.*, *Caustic.*, HELLEB., Kali carb., *Lycop.*, Merc. viv., Nux vom., Phosphor., Phosph. ac., RHUS TOX., Strontia, *Sulphur*, Thuya, Zinc.

— **muscles,** in the: *Acon.*, Ant. crud., ARNIC., *Arsen.*, Bellad., *Bryon.*, CALC. CARB., Capsic., CARB. VEG., Caustic., Chamom., Chelid., CINCHON., Colchic., Dulcam., Ferr., Hepar, Ignat., Kali carb., Ledum, LYCOP., *Merc. viv.*, Nitrum, Nitr. ac., *Nux vom.*, Phosphor., Pulsat., *Rhodod.*, Rhus tox., SEPIA, *Silic.*, Staphis., Strontia, *Sulphur*, Tarax., Veratr., Zinc.

Trembling: Arnic., ARSEN., Bellad., *Borax*, Bryon., *Calc. carb.*, *Camphor.*, Cicut., Coccul., Conium, IGNAT., Lycop., *Magn. carb.*, Merc. viv., NATR. MUR., *Opium*, Platin., PULSAT., *Rhus tox.*, Ruta, SEPIA, Stramon., Sulphur, Thuya, Valer., Veratr., ZINC.

Uncover; desire to: ACON., *Apis*, Arsen., Asar., Bovist., Calc. carb., Chamom., CINCHON., Coffea, EUPHORB., FERR., FLUOR. AC.. *Ignat.*, Iod., *Lycop.*, MOSCH., MUR. AC., NITR. AC., Nux vom., OPIUM, Phosphor., Phosph. ac., *Platin.*, *Pulsat.*, Rhus tox., Secal., Seneg., Spigel., STAPHIS., Sulphur, Thuya, *Veratr.*

— **aversion to:** *Clemat.*, *Hepar*, *Graphit.*, MAGN. CARB., NUX VOM., *Pulsat.*, Rhus tox., SAMBUC., SCILLA.

Uncovering, unbearable: Amm. carb., Arsen., *Aurum*, Carb. an., Carb. veg., Cicut., Cinchon., Clemat., Coccul., Coffea, *Colchic.*, Conium, HEPAR, Kali carb., Kreos., Laches., *Merc. viv.*, Nux mosch., NUX VOM., *Petrol.*, Pulsat., Rhodod., *Rhus tox.*, Sabad., *Sambuc.*, SCILLA, Sepia, *Silic.*, Spigel., Stramon., Strontia.

Bone-pains: *Arnic.*, Cinchon., Ignat., Natr. mur., *Pulsat.*

Glands; swelling of the: *Bellad.*, Lycop., Merc. viv., Nitr. ac., Phosphor., Rhus tox., *Sepia*, SILIC., Sulphur.

Skin; burning, in the: See burning heat.

Skin; crawling and prickling, in the: CROCUS, Platin., *Pulsat.*, Rhus tox., Sepia, Spigel., Sulphur, Thuya.

— **dryness** of the: See dry heat.

— **eruptions** on the: Arsen., Bryon., Calc. carb., *Conium*, Ipecac., Lycop., Natr. mur., Pulsat., RHUS TOX., Sepia, Sulphur.

— **itching** on the: AMM. CARB., *Ant. crud.*, Bryon., *Chamom.*, Lycop., MANGAN., Merc. viv., *Pulsat.*, Rhus tox., Silic., SPONG., Staphis., Sulphur.

— **paleness** of the: Coccul., Ferr., *Lycop.*, MOSCH., Nitr. ac., *Pulsat.*, Sulphur.

— **parchment,** like: *Arsen.*, Cinchon., IPECAC., Lycop., Silic.

— **redness** of the: *Apis*, ARSEN., Bellad., Canthar., IGNAT., Merc. viv., *Nux vom.*, *Opium*, Phosph. ac., *Pulsat.*, Rhus tox.

— **smarting** on the: *Chamom.*, Pulsat.

— **stitching** in the: Bryon., CINCHON., MERC. CORR., Nitr. ac., *Oleand.*, Pulsat., *Rhus tox.*, *Sabad.*, *Spong.*, Viol. tr.

— **yellowness** of the: Ambra, *Ant. crud.*, APIS, Arsen., Bryon., CHAMOM., *Cinchon.*, Coccul., Conium, Digit., FERR., Ignat., Laches., MERC. CORR., NUX VOM., Opium, *Pulsat.*, Rhus tox., Sepia, Sulphur.

SWEAT.

Sweat; in general: ACON., Act. rac., Æsc. hip., Agar., Agn. cast., Alum., Ambra, AMM. CARB., Amm. mur., Anac., Angust., *Ant. crud.*, *Ant. tart.*, Apis, Argent., Arnic., ARSEN., Asar., Aurum, Baptis., *Baryt.*, *Bellad.*, (Bismuth)., Borax, Bovist., Brom., BRYON., Cact. grand., Calad., CALC. CARB., Camphor., (Cann. sat)., Canthar., Capsic., *Carb. an.*, CARB. VEG., *Caustic.*, CHAMOM., Chelid., *Chin. sulph.*, Cicut., Cimex, Cina, CINCHON., Cist. can., Clemat., *Coccul.*, *Coffea*, (Colchic.), Coloc., CONIUM, Corn. cir., Corn. flor., Crocus, Cuprum, Cyclam., Diadem., Digit., Droser., Dulcam., Eup.

perf., Eup. purp., Euphorb., Euphras., FERR., Fluor. ac., *Gelsem.*, GRAPHIT., Guaiac., Helleb., HEPAR, Hydr. ac., HYOSC., Ignat., IOD., *Ipecac.*, *Kali bichr.*, KALI CARB., Kali hydr., Kreos., LACHES., Lachnanth., Lauroc., Ledum, Lobel. inf., LYCOP., Magn. carb., Magn. mur., *Mangan.*, MERC. VIV., Merc. corr., Mezer., Mosch., Mur. ac., NATR. CARB., NATR. MUR., Natr. sulph., Nitrum, *Nitr. ac.*, Nux mosch., NUX VOM., OPIUM, Oxal. ac., Paris, *Petrol.*, PHOSPHOR., PHOSPH. AC., Platin., Plumbum, Podophyl., Psorin., *Pulsat.*, Ran. bulb., Ran. scel., Rheum, *Rhodod.*, RHUS TOX., Ruta, SABAD., Sabin., SAMBUC., Sarsap., Secal., SELEN., (Seneg)., SEPIA, *Silic.*, Spigel., Spong., Stann., *Staphis.*, STRAMON., Strontia, SULPHUR, *Sulph. ac.*, TARAX., Therid., *Thuya*, *Valer.*, VERATR., Viol. od., Viol. tr., Zinc.

Sweat; excited too easily: *Agar.*, Ambra, Amm. carb., Amm. mur., Anac., *Ant. tart.*, Arsen., ASAR., Bellad., Borax, *Brom.*, BRYON., CALC. CARB., Canthar., *Carb. an.*, *Carb. veg.*, Caustic., Chin. sulph., CINCHON., Coccul., Coloc., Conium, Dulcam., FERR., Fluor. ac., Gelsem., *Graphit.*, Guaiac., HEPAR, *Hyosc.*, Ignat., Iod., *Ipecac.*, KALI CARB., Kreos., LACHES., Ledum, Lobel. inf., LYCOP., Magn. carb., Magn. mur., *Merc. viv.*, NATR. CARB., NATR. MUR., Nitrum, Nitr. ac., Nux vom., Opium, *Petrol.*, Phosphor., PHOSPH. AC., Psorin., PULSAT., *Rheum*, *Rhodod.*, Rhus tox., Sabad., Sarsap., SELEN., Seneg., SEPIA, *Silic.*, Spigel., Spong., *Stann.*, STAPHIS., Stramon., SULPHUR, *Sulph. ac.*, *Thuya*, Valer., Veratr., ZINC.

— **want of** (inability to sweat): Acon., *Alum.*, Ambra, Amm. carb., Apis, Arnic., Arsen., BELLAD., Bismuth., Bryon., Calc. carb., Cann. sat., *Chamom.*, *Cinchon.*, Coffea, COLCHIC., *Dulcam.*, Eup. purp., GRAPHIT., Hyosc., Iod., Ipecac., KALI CARB., Ledum, Lycop., Magn. carb., Mar. ver., Merc. viv., Merc. corr., Natr. carb., Nitr. ac., Nux mosch., Nux vom., Oleand., Opium, Phosphor., Phosph. ac., Platin., Psorin., Pulsat., *Rhus tox.*, Sabad., *Sambuc.*, SCILLA, Secal., Seneg., Sepia, SILIC., Spong., *Staphis.*, Sulphur, Thuya, Verbas., Viol. od.

Sweat; suppressed: Acon., Apis, Arsen., *Bellad.*, Bryon., Calc. carb., Carb. veg., CHAMOM., *Cinchon.*, COLCHIC., Cuprum, DULCAM., Graphit., Hepar, *Kali carb.*, Ledum, Lycop., Mar. ver., Merc. viv., Natr. carb., Natr. mur., Nux mosch., Nux vom., Oleand., Opium, Phosphor., Phosph. ac., Pulsat., Rhus tox., Sabad., Secal., Selen., Seneg., SEPIA, *Silic.*, Sulphur, Verbas.

— **sensation as from breaking out of:** Alum., Asar., Calc. carb., Crocus, Iod., IGNAT., *Pulsat.*, Sarsap., STANN., Sulphur, Sulph. ac.

— **anxious:** Acon., *Alum.*, Ant. crud., Arnic., ARSEN., *Baryt.*, Bellad., Bovist., Bryon., CALC. CARB., Canthar., *Carb. veg.*, Caustic., CHAMOM., Cicut., CINCHON., *Coffea*, Crocus, FERR., Graphit., Hepar, Ignat., Kreos., Lycop., MANGAN., *Merc. viv.*, *Merc. corr.*, Mezer., Mur. ac., NATR. CARB., Natr. mur., Nitrum, Nitr. ac., *Nux vom.*, Phosphor., PHOSPH. AC., *Plumbum*, *Pulsat.*, Rheum, *Rhus tox.*, Sabad., *Selen.*, SEPIA, *Spong.*, *Stann.*, Staphis., Stramon., SULPHUR, THUYA, *Veratr.*

— **attracting the flies:** *Calad.*, Bryon., Pulsat., Thuya.

— **bloody:** Arnic., LACHES., *Nux mosch.*

— **burning:** *Merc. viv.*, NATR. CARB., Veratr.

— **clammy:** Acon., *Anac.*, *Ant. tart.*, Arnic., *Arsen.*, Bryon., *Calc. carb.*, *Camphor.*, Carb. an., Carb. veg., CHAMOM., Cinchon., Coloc., *Digit.*, *Ferr.*, *Fluor. ac.*, *Helleb.*, *Hepar*, Iod., Laches., LYCOP., *Merc. viv.*, Mezer., *Mosch.*, *Nux vom.*, Oxal. ac., PHOSPHOR., PHOSPH. AC., *Plumbum*, Psorin., *Secal.*, *Spigel.*, *Sulph. ac.*, VERATR.

— **cold:** Acon., Act. rac., Ambra, Amm. carb., *Anac.*, ANT. TART., *Arnic.*, ARSEN., Asaf., Aurum, Baryt., Bellad., *Bryon.*, Calc. carb., CAMPHOR., *Cann. sat.*, *Canthar.*, *Capsic.*, CARB. VEG., *Cina*, CINCHON., COCCUL., Coffea, Crocus., *Cuprum*, *Digit.*, Dulcam., *Euphorb.*, Ferr., *Graphit.*, *Helleb.*, *Hepar*, *Hyosc.*, Ignat., IPECAC., *Laches.*, Lobel. inf., *Lycop.*, Mangan., *Merc. viv.*, MERC. CORR., Mur. ac., *Natr. carb.*,

Nitr. ac., *Nux vom.*, Opium, Oxal. ac., Petrol., Phosphor., Phosph. ac., *Plumbum*, *Pulsat.*, Ran. scel., *Rheum*, Rhus tox., *Ruta*, Sabad., SECAL., Sepia, *Spigel.*, *Spong.*, *Staphis.*, *Stramon.*, *Sulphur*, Sulph. ac., Therid., *Thuya*, VERATR.

Sweat; crawling sensation, causing a: *Rhodod.*

— **debilitating:** Acon., Ambra, *Ant. crud.*, Arnic., ARSEN., *Baryt.*, BRYON., *Calad.*, *Calc. carb.*, CAMPHOR., Canthar., *Carb. an.*, Caustic., Chin. sulph., CINCHON., *Coccul.*, Crocus, Digit., FERR., Graphit., *Hyosc.*, IOD., Lycop., MERC. VIV., *Natr. mur.*, NITRUM, Nux vom., PHOSPHOR., Phosph. ac., Psorin., *Rhodod.*, SAMBUC., SEPIA, *Silic.*, *Stann.*, *Sulphur*, *Tarax.*, Veratr.

— **not debilitating:** *Arsen.*, *Bovist.*, Bryon., CALAD., Calc. carb., Carb. an., Cicut., *Coloc.*, CUPRUM, Helleb., LYCOP., Natr. carb., *Phosphor.*, PULSAT., RHUS TOX., SEPIA, *Spigel.*, Tarax., THUYA.

— **greasy:** *Agar.*, Aurum, *Bryon.*, *Cinchon.*, Fluor. ac., MAGN. CARB., *Merc. viv.*, *Natr. mur.*, Plumbum, Rhus tox., *Selen.*, Stramon., THUYA.

— **hot:** Act. rac., Anac., Ant. crud., Asar., *Bellad.*, Bryon., Camphor., Canthar., Carb. veg., *Chamom.*, Cinchon., Digit., Droser., Helleb., IGNAT., IPECAC., Kreos., Laches., Ledum, OPIUM, Paris, Phosphor., Podophyl., Pulsat., *Sabad.*, SEPIA, Silic., *Stann.*, Staphis., *Stramon.*, Thuya, Veratr., VIOL. TR.

— **inodorous:** Ant. crud., Rhus tox., Sepia.

— **itching,** causing: Calc. carb., Cann. sat., *Coloc.*, Fluor. ac., Ipecac., LEDUM, *Lycop.*, MANGAN., *Opium*, PARIS, RHODOD., RHUS TOX., Sabad., Spong., *Sulphur.*

— **odor, acrid:** Rhus tox.

— — **aromatic:** *Rhodod.*, Sepia.

— — **bitter:** Veratr.

— — **blood,** like: *Lycop.*

— — **cadaverous:** Thuya.

— — **camphor,** like: Camphor.

— — **cheese,** like: Conium, Hepar, *Plumbum*, Sulphur.

Sweat; odor, elder flowers, like: *Sepia.*

— — **empyreumatic:** BELLAD., *Bryon.*, Magn. carb., Sulphur, Thuya.

— — **honey,** like: *Thuya.*

— — **horse urine,** like: *Nitr. ac.*

— — **mouldy:** Merc. viv., Nux vom., *Pulsat.*, Rhus tox., *Stann.*

— — **musk,** like: Mosch., *Pulsat.*, Sulphur.

— — **musty:** Merc. viv., Nux vom., PULSAT., RHUS TOX., *Stann.*

— — **offensive** (stinking): Amm. carb., Amm. mur., *Arnic.*, *Arsen.*, Baptist., BARYT., Bellad., Canthar., *Carb. an.*, *Carb. veg.*, Coloc., *Conium*, *Cyclam.*, DULCAM., *Euphras.*, *Ferr.*, Fluor. ac., GRAPHIT., Guaiac., HEPAR, *Kali carb.*, Laches., *Ledum*, *Lycop.*, Magn. carb., *Merc. viv.*, Merc. corr., NITR. AC., NUX VOM., PHOSPHOR., Plumbum, Psorin., PULSAT., *Rhodod.*, Rhus tox., SELEN., *Sepia*, *Silic.*, Spigel., STAPHIS., Sulphur, THUYA, *Veratr.*, *Zinc.*

— — **onions,** like: Bovist., *Lycop.*

— — **putrid,** *Carb. veg.*, Nux vom., *Rhus tox.*, Silic., Staphis., *Stramon.*

— — **rhubarb,** like: Rheum.

— — **rotten eggs,** like: Plumbum, *Staphis.*, Sulphur.

— — **sour:** *Acon.*, *Arnic.*, ARSEN., ASAR., Bellad., *Bryon.*, Calc. carb., *Carb. veg.*, Caustic., *Chamom.*, Cinchon., Ferr., Fluor. ac., *Graphit.*, *Hepar*, *Hyosc.*, Ignat., IOD., *Ipecac.*, *Kali carb.*, *Ledum*, LYCOP., Magn. carb., *Merc. viv.*, *Natr. mur.*, NITR. AC., *Nux vom.*, Psorin., Pulsat., Rheum, *Rhus tox.*, SEPIA, SILIC., Spigel., Staphis., SULPHUR, *Sulph. ac.*, Thuya, VERATR.

— — **sulphur,** like: *Phosphor.*

— — **sulphuretted hydrogen,** like: Plumbum, *Staphis.*, Sulphur.

— — **sweetish:** *Thuya.*

— — **sweetish-sour:** Bryon., *Pulsat.*

Sweat; odor, urine, like: CANTHAR., *Coloc.*, Nitr. ac.

— — **wheat-bread,** like: Ignat.

— **phosphorescent:** Phosphor.

— **red:** Arnic., *Carb. veg.*, Dulcam., LACHES., NUX MOSCH.

— **shrivelling the fingers:** Ant. crud., *Merc. viv.*, Phosph. ac.

— **smarting:** CHAMOM., *Conium*, Fluor. ac., Ipecac., Paris, *Tarax.*

— **soreness,** causing: Coffea, FLUOR. AC., *Helleb.*, Iod., Lycop., Ran. bulb., Silic., Zinc.

— **staining; the linen:** Arsen., BELLAD., Carb. an., *Graphit.*, Laches., Magn. carb., *Merc. viv.*, Rheum, *Selen.*

— — — **yellow:** Arsen., Bellad., *Carb. an.*, GRAPHIT., LACHES., *Magn. carb.*, *Merc. viv.*, *Rheum*, SELEN., Thuya, *Veratr.*

— — **red:** Thuya.

— — **skin and eyes yellow:** Arsen.

— **stiffening the linen:** Merc. viv., *Selen.*

— **viscous:** *Plumbum.*

— **weakening:** see debilitating.

PARTIAL SWEAT.

Sweat; head, only on the: Chamom., Phosphor., *Pulsat.*, Sabad., Sepia, *Silic.*, Spigel., Stann.

— — **except** on the: *Bellad.*, Merc. viv., Nux vom., RHUS TOX., SAMBUC., *Sepia*, Thuya.

— **upper body,** on the: Acon., Agar., Anac., Ant. tart., Argent., Arnic., ASAR., Baryt., Bellad., Bovist., *Camphor.*, Canthar., *Carb. veg.*, Caustic., Chamom., Cina, Cinchon., Coccul., Euphras., *Fluor. ac.*, Graphit., Guaiac., Ipecac., KALI CARB., Lauroc., Magn. carb., Magn. mur., Merc. corr., Mosch., Mur. ac., Natr. carb., Nitr. ac., *Nux vom.*, OPIUM, PARIS, Petrol., Phosphor., Phosph. ac., Plumbum, Pulsat., Rheum, Rhus tox.,

Ruta, Sabad., *Secal.*, Selen., SEPIA, Silic., *Spigel.*, SULPH. AC., Valer., Veratr.

Sweat; lower body, on the: Apis, *Arsen.*, Asaf., Bryon., Calc. carb., *Coloc.*, Conium, CROCUS, Droser., Euphorb., *Hyosc.*, Mangan., Merc. viv., Nitrum, Nitr. ac., Nux vom., Rhodod., Sepia, Silic., Thuya, Zinc.

— **one side,** on, in general: Alum., Ambra, Anac., BARYT., Bellad., Bryon., Carb. veg., Chamom., *Cinchon.*, Coccul., Fluor. ac., Ignat., NUX VOM., *Phosphor.*, PULSAT., Ran. bulb., Rheum, Rhus tox., Sabin., Spigel., Stann., *Sulphur*, Thuya.

— **left side,** on the: Anac., BARYT., *Cinchon.*, Fluor. ac., Phosphor., Pulsat., Rhus tox., Spigel., Stann., Sulphur.

— **right side,** on the: Bellad., Bryon., Fluor. ac., Nux vom., *Phosphor.*, *Pulsat.*, Ran. bulb., Sabin.

— **anterior body,** on the: Agar., Ambra, Anac., ARGENT., Arnic., *Asar.*, *Bellad.*, Bovist., *Calc. carb.*, *Canthar.*, Cina, COCCUL., Droser., Euphras., Graphit., Ipecac., Lauroc., Merc. viv., Merc. corr., Natr. mur., *Nitrum*, PHOSPHOR., Plumbum, Rheum, Ruta, Sabad., Secal., SELEN., Staphis.

— **posterior body,** on the: Arsen., Calc. carb., Caustic., *Cinchon.*, *Dulcam.*, Ferr., Guaiac., Laches., Ledum, Mangan., Mosch., *Mur. ac.*, Natr. carb., Paris, Petrol., *Phosph. ac.*, Pulsat., Sabin., SEPIA, *Stann.*, Stramon., Sulphur.

— **affected parts,** on the: AMBRA, ANT. TART., Arsen., Bryon., *Caustic.*, *Coccul.*, Fluor. ac., MERC. VIV., Natr. carb., Nitr. ac., Nux vom., RHUS TOX., Sepia, Stramon., STRONTIA.

— **covered parts,** on the: ACON., BELLAD., Chamom., Cinchon., Ledum, Nitr. ac., Nux vom., *Pulsat.*, Spigel., Thuya.

— **itching parts,** on the: Amm. carb., Bryon., Calc. carb., Cann. sat., *Chamom.*, Coloc., Ipecac., Ledum, *Lycop.*, MANGAN., Opium, *Paris*, *Rhodod.*, RHUS TOX., *Sabad.*, Spong., Sulphur.

— **joints,** only on the: AMM. CARB., Arsen., Bellad., Bryon., *Calc. carb.*, Droser., Ledum, *Lycop.*, Mangan., Nux vom., Phosph. ac., *Rhus tox.*, Stann., *Sulphur.*

Sweat; part on which one lies, of the: Acon., *Bellad.*, CINCHON., NITR. AC., Nux vom., Pulsat.

— **single (small) spots,** on: Merc. viv.

— **uncovered parts,** on the: THUYA.

— **head,** on the: Acon., Ambra, ANAC., Ant. tart., Apis, *Bellad.*, Borax, Bovist., Bryon., CALC. CARB., Camphor., Carb. an., Carb. veg., *Caustic.*, CHAMOM., Cimex, Cina, *Cinchon.*, *Coloc.*, Digit., *Graphit.*, GUAIAC., Hepar, Ipecac., *Kali carb.*, Lauroc., Ledum, *Magn. carb.*, *Magn. mur.*, MERC. VIV., Merc. corr., Mezer., Mosch., MUR. AC., Natr. mur., Nitr. ac., *Nux vom.*, Opium, Paris, Petrol., PHOSPHOR., *Phosph. ac.*, Plumbum, PULSAT., RHEUM, Rhus tox., Ruta, Secal., Sepia, SILIC., *Spigel.*, Sulphur, Sulph. ac., Thuya, *Valer.*, Veratr.

— — **one side** of the: Ambra, *Baryt.*, *Nux vom.*, PULSAT. *Sulphur.*

— — **occiput,** on the: Arsen., *Anac.*, Calc. carb., *Cinchon.*, Ferr., Magn. carb., Mosch., Nitr. ac., Nux vom., PHOSPH. AC., *Sepia*, *Silic.*, Spigel., Stann., SULPHUR.

— — **clammy:** *Chamom.*, Merc. viv., Nux vom.

— — **cold:** Bryon., Cina, Digit., *Hepar*, Merc. viv., Merc. corr., Podophyl., *Veratr.*

— **ears,** on the: Pulsat.

— **nose,** on the: Bellad., *Cina*, Lauroc., *Natr. mur.*, Rheum, *Ruta.*

— **face,** on the: *Acon.*, *Alum.*, Ambra, *Amm. mur.*, ANGUST., *Ant. tart.*, Argent., *Arnic.*, Arsen., Asaf., BELLAD., Borax, *Bryon.*, Calc. carb., Camphor., Cann. sat., *Capsic.*, Carb. an., *Carb. veg.*, CHAMOM., Cicut., CINA, *Cinchon.*, *Coccul.*, *Coffea*, Conium, Crocus, *Cuprum*, *Digit.*, *Droser.*, Dulcam., Guaiac., Helleb., Hepar, *Hyosc.*, IGNAT., *Ipecac.*, *Kali carb.*, Lauroc., Ledum, LYCOP., Magn. carb., *Merc. viv.*, Mosch., Natr. carb., *Natr. mur.*, Natr. sulph., NUX VOM., OPIUM, Paris, Petrol., Platin., Plumbum, Psorin., PULSAT., Ran. scel., *Rheum*, Rhus tox., Ruta, *Sabad.*, SAMBUC., Sarsap., Sepia, SILIC.,

Spigel., SPONG., Stann., Staphis., Stramon., Sulphur, Sulph. ac., *Thuya*, VALER., *Veratr.*, Viol. tr.

Sweat; face, spreading from the: *Sambuc.*

— — **one side** of the: Alum., *Ambra*, *Baryt.*, NUX VOM., PULSAT., Sulphur.

— — **cold,** on the: Ant. tart., Arnic., *Arsen.*, Bellad., *Bryon.*, *Calc. carb.*, *Capsic.*, CARB. VEG., CINA, Cinchon., *Coccul.*, Crocus, Cuprum, *Digit.*, *Ipecac.*, MERC. CORR., Natr. mur., *Nux vom.*, *Opium*, Oxal. ac., Platin., *Rheum*, Rhus tox., Ruta, *Spigel.*, Spong., Staphis., *Sulphur*, VERATR.

— **forehead,** on the: *Angust.*, Cina, *Guaiac.*, LEDUM, Merc. corr., NATR. CARB., OPIUM, *Ran. scel.*, Rheum, SARSAP., Staphis., *Valer.*, VERATR.

— — **cold,** on the: *Cina*, *Merc. corr.*, OPIUM, Staphis., VERATR.

— **upper lip,** on the: Acon., Coffea, Kali carb., Nux vom., *Rheum.*

— **pit of stomach,** on the: *Bellad.*, Nux vom., Secal.

— **abdomen,** on the: AMBRA, ANAC., *Argent.*, Asar., Canthar., CICUT., Droser., Ipecac., Merc. viv., Nux vom., Phosphor., Plumbum, *Rhus tox.*, Selen., Staphis.

— **umbilicus, spreading** from the: *Rhus tox.*

— **groins,** in the: Ambra, Canthar., *Selen.*, Sepia, *Thuya.*

— **anus,** at the: *Thuya.*

— **pubes,** on the: *Selen.*, Sepia, Thuya.

— **perinæum,** on the: *Alum.*, *Aurum*, Calc. carb., *Carb. an.*, Carb. veg., Conium, *Hepar*, Nux vom., THUYA.

— **male genitals,** on the: Agn. cast., Alum., Amm. carb., *Arsen.*, AURUM, Baryt., Bellad., *Calad.*, *Calc. carb.*, *Canthar.*, Carb. an., *Carb. veg.*, Conium, FLUOR. AC., *Hepar*, *Ignat.*, *Lycop.*, Magn. mur., Merc. viv., Mezer., Phosph. ac., *Pulsat.*, Rhodod., SELEN., SEPIA, Silic., Staphis., *Sulphur*, THUYA.

— — **smelling sweetish** (like honey): *Thuya.*

— — **offensive smelling:** Fluor. ac., Sulphur.

— **scrotum,** on the: Agn. cast., Amm. carb., *Aurum*, Baryt.,

Bellad., *Calc. carb.*, Carb. an., Carb. veg., *Conium*, Hepar, *Ignat.*, *Lycop.*, Magn. mur., Merc. viv., Mezer., Natr. sulph., *Rhodod.*, *Selen.*, SEPIA, *Silic.*, Staphis., Sulphur, THUYA.

Sweat; scrotum, on one side of the: *Thuya.*

— **female genitals,** on the: *Alum.*, *Aurum*, Bellad., *Calc. carb.*, *Canthar.*, Cicut., Conium, Fluor. ac., Hepar, Ignat., *Merc. viv.*, *Pulsat.*, SELEN., SEPIA, Silic., *Sulphur*, THUYA.

— **throat,** on the: Alum., *Bellad.*, Cann. sat., Chamom., *Clemat.*, *Coffea*, Euphorb., Ipecac., Kali carb., MANGAN., Nux vom., Paris, RHUS TOX., Spigel., STANN., Sulphur.

— **nape of the neck,** in the: *Anac.*, Arsen., CALC. CARB., *Cinchon.*, Ferr., Magn. carb. Mosch., Nitr. ac., Nux vom., PHOSPH. AC., *Sepia*, *Silic.*, Spigel., Stann., SULPHUR.

— **chest,** on the: *Agar.*, Anac., ARGENT., *Arnic.*, Asar., Bellad., BOVIST., CALC. CARB., Canthar., Cimex, Cinchon., COCCUL., Droser., EUPHRAS., Graphit., Hepar, Ipecac., *Lycop.*, Merc. viv., Merc. corr., NITRUM, Nitr. ac., *Phosphor.*, *Phosph. ac.*, Plumbum, Rhus tox., Sabad., Secal., SELEN., *Sepia*, Silic., Spigel.

— — **cold:** *Coccul.*, Hepar, *Lycop.*, *Merc. corr.*

— — **offensive smelling:** *Arnic.*, Graphit., Hepar, LYCOP., *Phosphor.*, SELEN., *Sepia.*

— **axillæ,** in the: *Asar.*, *Bovist.*, BRYON., *Calc. carb.*, Capsic., Carb. an., *Carb. veg.*, DULCAM., *Hepar*, Kali carb., Laches., Merc. corr., Natr. mur., Nitr. ac., Petrol., *Phosphor.*, RHODOD., Sabad., *Scilla*, SELEN., SEPIA, SULPHUR, Sulph. ac., *Thuya*, Veratr., Zinc.

— — **offensive smelling:** Carb. veg., *Dulcam.*, HEPAR, Merc. corr., *Nitr. ac.*, Phosphor., *Rhodod.*, *Selen.*, *Sepia*, *Sulphur*, Thuya.

— **back,** on the: Acon., ANAC., Arsen., *Calc. carb.*, Caustic., CINCHON., Coffea, *Dulcam.*, Guaiac., Hepar, *Ipecac.*, Kali bichr., Laches., Ledum, *Lycop.*, *Mur. ac.*, Natr. carb., *Nux vom.*, Paris, *Petrol.*, Phosphor., *Phosph. ac.*, Pulsat., Rhus tox., Sabin., SEPIA, Silic., Stann., Stramon., Sulphur.

Sweat; arm (whole), on the: Asaf., Asar., Ipecac., Petrol., *Strontia.*

— **forearm,** on the: *Petrol.*

— **hands,** on the: Acon., AGN. CAST., Ambra, Amm. mur., Anac., Ant. tart., ARSEN., Baryt., Bellad., Bryon., CALC. CARB., Camphor., *Canthar.*, Capsic., Carb. veg., Chamom., *Cina,* Cinchon., Coccul., Coffea, *Coloc.*, *Conium,* Digit., Dulcam., Fluor. ac., Helleb., Hepar, Ignat., Iod., *Ipecac.*, Kali bichr., Kreos., Lauroc., *Ledum,* Lycop., *Merc. viv.*, Merc. corr., Natr. carb., *Natr. mur.*, *Nitr. ac.*, *Nux vom.*, Petrol., PHOSPHOR., Phosph. ac., Pulsat., Rheum, Rhodod., Rhus tox., Sarsap., *Sepia,* *Silic.*, *Spigel.*, SULPHUR, THUYA, Veratr., Zinc.

— — **cold:** *Arsen.*, Bellad., CANTHAR., Chamom., *Cina,* Hepar, Iod., *Ipecac.*, Merc. corr., Nux vom., Oxal. ac., *Rheum,* *Sepia,* Spigel., *Sulphur,* *Thuya.*

— — **clammy:** Anac., *Arsen.*, Calc. carb., Coloc., Merc. viv., *Nux vom.*, PHOSPHOR., Spigel.

— **palms of the hands,** in the: *Acon.*, *Amm. mur.*, *Anac.*, Baryt., Bryon., *Calc. carb.*, Camphor., Capsic., *Chamom.*, *Conium,* Digit., DULCAM., *Fluor. ac.*, Helleb., *Ignat.*, Kali carb., Kreos., Lauroc., *Ledum,* Lycop., *Merc. viv.*, Nitr. ac., NUX VOM., Phosphor., Psorin., *Rheum,* Rhus tox., Spigel., SULPHUR.

— **fingers,** on the: Agn. cast., *Ant. crud.*, Baryt., Carb. veg., Ignat., Rhodod., *Sulphur.*

— **lower limbs** (whole) on the: Arsen., Asaf., *Borax,* *Calc. carb.*, *Coloc.*, Conium, Crocus, Hepar, HYOSC., Mangan., Merc. viv., NITRUM, *Phosphor.*, Rhodod., Secal., *Sepia,* Zinc.

— **thighs,** on the: AMBRA, ARSEN., *Carb. an.*, *Coloc.*, Droser., Euphorb., Hyosc., Kali bichr., Merc. viv., *Nux vom.*, Rhus tox., Sepia, *Thuya.*

— **knees,** on the: Amm. carb., Arsen., Bryon., *Calc. carb.*, Droser., Ledum, *Lycop.*, Spong.

Sweat; leg, on the: Arsen., Bryon., Coloc., EUPHORB., Hyosc., MANGAN., Merc. viv., Mezer., Nux vom., PETROL., Podophyl., Rhodod., *Sulphur.*

— **feet,** on the: Acon., Amm. carb., Amm. mur., *Angust.*, Apis, Arnic., Arsen., BARYT., Bellad., Bryon., CALC. CARB., Camphor., *Cann. sat.*, *Canthar.*, Carb. an., CARB. VEG., Chelid., COCCUL., Coffea, *Coloc.*, *Cuprum*, Cyclam., Droser., Euphorb., *Fluor. ac.*, *Graphit.*, Helleb., Hepar, IOD., Ipecac., Kali bichr., *Kali carb.*, Kreos., Laches., *Ledum*, *Lycop.*, *Magn. mur.*, Mangan., Merc. viv., Mezer., Mur. ac., Natr. carb., *Natr. mur.*, Nitr. ac., Petrol., PHOSPHOR., *Phosph. ac.*, Plumbum, PULSAT., Ran. bulb., Rhus tox., Sabad., Sabin., *Scilla*, Secal., Selen., SEPIA, SILIC., *Staphis.*, SULPHUR, THUYA, Zinc.

— — **ascending** from the: Bellad.

— — **cold:** *Angust.*, Cann. sat., *Canthar.*, CARB. VEG., Coccul., *Cuprum*, Droser., Graphit., *Hepar*, Ipecac., LYCOP., *Magn. mur.*, Merc. viv., Mezer., MUR. AC., Nitr. ac., Oxal. ac., PULSAT., *Scilla*, Secal., *Silic.*, STAPHIS., *Sulphur*, Thuya.

— — **offensive smelling:** Amm. carb., Amm. mur., Arsen., BARYT., Cyclam., *Graphit.*, KALI CARB., *Nitr. ac.*, *Phosphor.*, *Plumbum*, PULSAT., *Sepia*, SILIC., Sulphur, THUYA, Zinc.

— — **suppressed:** Apis, *Cuprum*, *Kali carb.*, Lycop., *Merc. viv.*, Natr. carb., *Natr. mur.*, Nitr. ac., *Phosphor.*, Phosph. ac., Rhus tox., *Selen.* SEPIA, SILIC., Sulphur, Thuya.

— — **corroding:** Coffea, FLUOR. AC., *Helleb.*, Iod., Lycop., Ran. bulb., Silic., Zinc.

— **soles of the feet:** Acon., AMM. MUR., Arnic., Chelid., Kali carb., *Merc. viv.*, *Natr. mur.*, Nitr. ac., Petrol., *Plumbum*, Sabad., *Silic.*, Sulphur.

— **toes, on and between** the: *Acon.*, Arnic., Clemat., *Cyclam.*, Ferr., Helleb., *Kali carb.*, Ran. bulb., *Scilla*, *Sepia*, SILIC., Tarax., *Thuya.*

AGGRAVATION.

ACCORDING TO TIME.

Morning (morning-sweat): Acon., *Alum.*, Ambra, *Amm. carb.*, *Amm. mur.*, *Angust.*, *Ant. crud.*, Apis, Argent., Arnic., Arsen., *Aurum*, Bellad., *Borax*, *Bovist.*, BRYON., CALC. CARB., Canthar., Capsic., *Carb. an.*, *Carb. veg.*, *Caustic.*, Chamom., *Chelid.*, *Cicut.*, CINCHON., *Clemat.*, *Coccul.*, *Coffea*, Coloc., *Conium*, Digit., *Droser.*, *Dulcam.*, *Euphorb.*, Euphras., FERR., Graphit., Guaiac., HELLEB., HEPAR, Ignat., IOD., *Kali carb.*, *Kreos.*, Laches., Lachnanth., Lauroc., Ledum, *Lycop.*, MAGN. CARB., *Magn. mur.*, *Merc. viv.*, *Merc. corr.*, MOSCH., *Mur. ac.*, NATR. CARB., NATR. MUR., *Nitrum*, Nitr. ac., NUX VOM., OPIUM, *Paris*, Petrol., PHOSPHOR., PHOSPH. AC., PULSAT., *Ran. bulb.*, *Ran. scel.*, Rhodod., RHUS TOX., *Ruta*, *Sabad.*, SAMBUC., *Selen.*, SEPIA, SILIC., Spigel., *Spong.*, STANN., *Strontia*, *Sulphur*, *Sulph. ac.*, Tarax., Thuya, VERATR., Zinc.

Forenoon: Acon., Carb. veg., Cicut., FERR., HEPAR, Merc. viv., *Natr. carb.*, Natr. mur., Phosphor., Sabad., *Selen.*, *Sepia*, Silic., Staphis., Strontia, *Sulph. ac.*, *Valer.*

Afternoon: Agar., Alum., Amm. mur., *Bellad.*, Calad., Capsic., FLUOR. AC., HEPAR, Kali bichr., Lauroc., Lycop., *Magn. mur.*, Nitrum, Nux vom., Phosphor., Pulsat., *Selen.*, Stann., Staphis., Thuya, Zinc.

Evening: Acon., Agar., Amm. mur., *Anac.*, Ant. tart., Apis, ARSEN., Asar., *Baryt.*, *Bellad.*, Borax, Bovist., Bryon., *Calc. carb.*, Capsic., Caustic., CHAMOM., CINCHON., Coloc., *Conium*, *Fluor. ac.*, Graphit., *Helleb.*, *Hepar*, Hyosc., Ipecac., Kali carb., Laches., Lycop., Magn. carb., MENYANTH., *Merc. viv.*, *Mur. ac.*, Nitrum, Opium, Phosph. ac., Psorin., Pulsat., Rhus tox., Sambuc., *Sarsap.*, *Selen.*, *Sepia*, Silic., Spigel., *Spong.*, Stramon., *Sulphur*, Sulph. ac., *Tarax.*, Thuya, VERATR., Zinc.

Night: *Acon.*, Act. rac., *Agar.*, *Alum.*, *Ambra*, AMM. CARB., *Amm. mur.*, *Anac.*, Ant. crud., *Ant. tart.*, Apis, Argent., Arnic., ARSEN., *Asar.*, *Aurum*, BARYT., Bellad.,

Borax, Bovist., BRYON., CALC. CARB., Canthar., Capsic., Carb. an., CARB. VEG., *Caustic.*, *Chamom.*, *Chelid.*, *Cicut.*, CINCHON., *Clemat.*, COCCUL., Coffea, *Coloc.*, *Conium*, *Crocus*, *Cuprum*, *Cyclam.*, *Digit.*, *Droser.*, *Dulcam.*, Euphorb., *Euphras.*, FERR., GRAPHIT., *Guaiac.*, Helleb., HEPAR, Hyosc., Ignat., IOD., IPECAC., KALI CARB., LACHES., *Lauroc.* LEDUM, Lobel. inf., LYCOP., MAGN. CARB., Magn. mur., *Mangan.*, *Menyanth.*, MERC. VIV., *Merc. corr.*, *Mur. ac.*, NATR. CARB., *Natr. mur.*, Natr. sulph., *Nitrum*, NITR. AC., NUX VOM., Oxal. ac., PETROL., PHOSPHOR., *Phosph. ac.*, Platin., Psorin., PULSAT., Rhodod., RHUS TOX., Sabad., *Sabin.*, SAMBUC., SELEN., SEPIA, SILIC., *Spigel.*, *Spong.*, STANN., STAPHIS., *Stramon.*, *Strontia*, SULPHUR, Sulph. ac., TARAX., Thuya, *Valer.*, VERATR., *Viol. od.*, *Viol. tr.*, ZINC.

Midnight; before: Amm. mur., Ant. tart., ARSEN., Asar., Bellad., Bryon., Calc. carb., Canthar., *Carb. an.*, CARB. VEG., Chamom., Cinchon., *Conium*, HEPAR, *Laches.*, Lauroc., Ledum, *Lycop.*, Magn. carb., *Menyanth.*, *Merc. viv.*, MUR. AC., Natr. carb., Natr. mur., Nitrum, Opium, Phosph. ac., Ran. bulb., Rhus tox., Sabad., Sambuc., Sarsap., *Sepia*, Staphis., *Sulphur*, TARAX., Thuya, Valer., *Veratr.*

— **after:** Act. rac., *Alum.*, AMBRA, *Amm. mur.*, Argent., *Arsen.*, *Aurum*, Bellad., *Bryon.*, *Calc. carb.*, Capsic., *Chelid.*, *Cinchon.*, *Clemat.*, Conium, *Droser.*, *Ferr.*, Graphit., HELLEB., HEPAR, Hyosc., KALI CARB., Lachnanth., Lauroc., Lycop., MAGN. CARB., MAGN. MUR., Merc. viv., Natr. mur., NUX VOM., PHOSPHOR., Phosph. ac., Plumbum, Pulsat., Ran. scel., *Rhus tox.*, *Sabad.*, *Sambuc.*, *Silic.*, STANN., Staphis., SULPHUR, *Tarax.*, Thuya.

Predominating during the day: Agar., Ambra, *Amm. carb.*, *Amm. mur.*, Bellad., Bryon., CALC. CARB., *Carb. an.*, Carb. veg., Caustic., *Cinchon.*, *Dulcam.*, FERR., Graphit., *Hepar*, KALI CARB., LYCOP., Merc. viv., NATR. CARB., NATR. MUR., Nux vom., *Phosphor.*, PHOSPH. AC., Pulsat.,

Rhus tox., *Selen.*, SEPIA, Silic., Staphis., SULPHUR, Sulph. ac., *Veratr.*, ZINC.

Periodically; returning: Alum., ANT. CRUD., *Arsen.*, BARYT., *Bovist.*, Calc. carb., Capsic., Carb. veg., CINCHON., *Ferr.*, *Ipecac.*, Laches., Lycop., Mur. ac., NATR. MUR., Nitrum, *Nitr. ac.*, Rhus tox., *Sepia*, Silic., Staphis., Sulphur, Veratr.

Attacks; frequent, short: Chamom., Cuprum, *Ipecac.*, *Natr. carb.*, Spigel., *Stann.*, *Sulph. ac.*, *Valer.*

Every other (third) day: Ant. crud., Baryt., FERR., *Nitr. ac.*

Hour; returning at a certain: Act. rac., *Ant. crud.*, *Bovist.*, Cina, Ignat., SABAD., Spigel.

ACCORDING TO CIRCUMSTANCE.

Air; in the cold: Arsen., BRYON., CALC. CARB., Carb. an., Caustic., Cinchon., Guaiac., Hepar, Kali carb., *Lycop.*, Nux vom., Rhus tox., Sepia, Veratr.

— **in the open:** Agar., Anac., Bellad., *Bryon.*, CALC. CARB., Capsic., *Carb. an.*, Carb. veg., *Caustic.*, Chamom., Cinchon., Ferr., *Guaiac.*, Hepar, Kali carb., Laches., Lycop., Nux vom., Petrol., Phosph. ac., *Rhodod.*, Selen., Sepia, *Silic.*, Stramon., Sulph. ac., Thuya, Valer.

Anger; after: Acon., Bryon., *Chamom.*, Lycop., *Petrol.*, SEPIA, Staphis.

Arising from bed; when: Apis, *Bryon.*, CALC. CARB., Carb. veg., Chamom., Hepar, *Laches.*, Lycop., Natr. mur., Nux vom., Phosphor., Phosph. ac., Rhodod., RHUS TOX., *Sambuc.*, *Selen.*, Sepia., Silic., Staphis., Sulphur, Sulph. ac., Thuya.

Attacks of indisposition; before the: *Merc. viv.*

— **during** the: Calc. carb., Camphor., Chamom., MERC. VIV., *Nux vom.*, Rhus tox., Selen., SEPIA, Sulphur, *Veratr.*

— **after** the: Arsen., Bellad., Bryon., Calc. carb., Caustic., Chamom., Cinchon., CUPRUM, Ferr., Hepar, Ignat., Magn.

carb., Merc. viv., Nux vom., *Oleand.*, Plumbum, Sambuc., Secal., Selen., *Sepia*, Silic., Stramon., *Sulphur*, Veratr.

Awake; while: Arsen., Bellad., Bryon., Carb. an., Cinchon., Hepar, *Merc. viv.*, *Nux vom.*, *Phosphor.*, Phosph. ac., PULSAT., SAMBUC., Sepia, Thuya.

Awaking; when: Alum., Ambra, Amm. mur., ANT. CRUD., Arnic., *Arsen.*, Baryt., Borax., *Calc. carb.*, Capsic., Carb. an., Carb. veg., *Caustic.*, Chamom., *Chelid.*, Cicut., *Cinchon.*, *Clemat.*, Coloc., Conium, Crocus, Cyclam., Droser., Dulcam., Euphras., Ferr., Hepar, Ipecac., Kali carb., Kreos., Lauroc., Ledum, Lycop., Magn. carb., *Merc. viv.*, Mezer., Natr. carb., Natr. mur., Nitr. ac., *Nux vom.*, PARIS, *Phosphor.*, Phosph. ac., Pulsat., *Ran. bulb.*, Sabad., SAMBUC., SEPIA, Silic., Spong., Staphis., SULPHUR, *Tarax.*, Thuya.

— **after**: Bellad., *Bryon.*, Carb. an., Cinchon., Hepar, Nux vom., *Phosphor.*, Phosph. ac., SAMBUC., Sepia.

Bed; in: *Alum.*, Ambra, Amm. mur., Ant. crud., Ant. tart., *Arsen.*, Asar., Bellad., Bryon., CALC. CARB., Carb. an., Carb. veg., Caustic., CHAMOM., Cinchon., EUPHORB., Ferr., HELLEB., Hepar, Kali carb., Lycop., Magn. carb., MENYANTH., MERC. VIV., MUR. AC., Nitrum, Nux vom., Opium, Phosphor., Phosph. ac., *Pulsat.*, Ran. bulb., RHUS TOX., RUTA, Sabad., *Sambuc.*, Sarsap., SELEN., *Sepia*, Silic., Staphis., *Sulphur*, Tarax., Thuya, Valer., *Veratr.*

Closing the eyes; when: Bellad., BRYON., *Calc. carb.*, *Carb. an.*, Caustic., Cinchon., CONIUM, Graphit., Laches., Magn. mur., Pulsat., Sepia, Sulphur, Thuya.

Coition; after: *Agar.*, CALC. CARB., *Cinchon.*, Kali carb., Laches., Petrol., *Selen.*, SEPIA, Sulphur.

Climacteric years; during the: *Calc. carb.*, SULPH. AC.

Convulsions: See Epileptic attacks.

— **after**: See Epileptic attacks.

Coryza; during the: Arsen., *Calc. carb.*, Chamom., Kali carb., Lycop., MERC. VIV., Natr. mur., *Silic.*

Coughing; while: Acon., Ant. tart., ARSEN., Bellad., Bryon., Calc. carb., Capsic., Carb. veg., Cinchon., Digit.,

Droser., HEPAR, *Ipecac.*, Kali carb., Lycop., Natr. carb., Natr. mur., *Nitrum*, *Nux vom.*, PHOSPHOR., Phosph. ac., *Rhus tox.*, *Sabad.*, Sambuc., Selen., SEPIA, *Spong.*, Sulphur, *Veratr.*

Covering; from: *Acon.*, BELLAD., Calc. carb., Chamom., Cinchon., Ledum, Lycop., *Nitr. ac.*, *Pulsat.*, *Spigel.*, *Staphis.*, Sulphur, *Thuya*, Veratr.

Discharges; from suppression of natural: BELLAD., *Bryon.*, Calc. carb., Caustic., *Chamom.*, CINCHON., Hepar, *Ipecac.*, Kali carb., Laches., Lycop., Natr. carb., *Nux vom.*, Opium, Phosph. ac., RHUS TOX., Selen., *Sepia*, *Sulphur*, Thuya, Veratr.

Dreaming; while: Ledum.

Drinking; while: Arsen., Cinchon., Ferr., Hepar, *Pulsat.*, Rhodod., Rhus tox., *Selen.*, Silic., Stramon., Sulphur, Tarax., *Veratr.*

— **warm things:** Bryon., *Kali carb.*, MERC. VIV., Phosphor., *Sulph. ac.*

Driving; after: Therid.

Eating; while: Amm. carb., Ant. tart., Arsen., *Baryt.*, Bryon., Calc. carb., *Carb. an.*, CARB. VEG., Caustic., Chamom., *Conium*, Graphit., Hepar, *Ignat.*, KALI CARB., Lauroc., Lycop., Magn. mur., Mar. ver., MERC. VIV., Natr. carb., *Natr. mur.*, NITR. AC., Nux vom., Phosphor., *Pulsat.*, Sarsap., *Sepia*, Silic., Spigel., Sulph. ac., Valer.

— **after:** Alum., Arsen., Borax, BRYON., CALC. CARB., Carb. an., *Carb. veg.*, CAUSTIC., Chamom., Cinchon., *Conium*, Graphit., KALI CARB., LAUROC., *Lycop.*, Natr. carb., *Natr. mur.*, NITR. AC., *Nux vom.*, Paris, Petrol., PHOSPHOR., *Phosph. ac.*, Rhus tox., *Selen.*, SEPIA, *Silic.*, SULPHUR, Sulph. ac., Thuya, Veratr., VIOL. TR.

— — **warm food:** Bellad., *Bryon.*, Carb. an., Carb. veg., Chamom., Euphorb., Ferr., Kali carb., Laches., PHOSPHOR., Phosph. ac., Pulsat., Sepia, SULPH. AC., *Thuya.*

Epileptic attacks; during: Bellad., Camphor., Carb. an., Nux vom., *Sepia.*

Epileptic attacks; after: CUPRUM, *Ferr.*, Ignat., Magn. carb., Plumbum, Secal., Silic., Stramon.

Exertion; bodily, from: Acon., Agar., Arsen., Asar., Bellad., *Brom.*, *Bryon.*, CALC. CARB., Caustic., Chamom., *Cinchon.*, Graphit., *Hepar*, IOD., *Kali carb.*, Kreos., Laches., Ledum, LYCOP., Merc. viv., NATR. CARB., *Natr. mur.*, NITRUM, Nux vom., *Rheum*, RHUS TOX., Sabad., Selen., SEPIA, Silic., Spigel., *Stann.*, SULPHUR, Sulph. ac., Thuya, Veratr.

— **mental,** (reading, writing) from: Bellad., Borax, *Calc. carb.*, Graphit., HEPAR, Hyosc., *Kali carb.*, Laches., Lycop., Natr. mur., Nux vom., *Sepia*, Silic., Staphis., Sulphur.

Fever; after the: Ant. tart., ARSEN., Bellad., Bovist., Bryon., *Calad.*, Calc. carb., Carb. veg., Coloc., *Cinchon.*, CUPRUM, Helleb., Hepar, *Lycop.*, Natr. carb., Natr. mur., *Nux vom.*, *Phosphor.*, Pulsat., *Rhus tox.*, Spigel., Thuya.

Fright; after: Acon., *Bellad.*, Lycop., *Opium*, Silic.

Itching of the skin; after: Chamom., Coloc., Lycop., Rhus tox.

Lying; while: Arsen., Bryon., *Capsic.*, Chamom., *Ferr.*, Hepar, Hyosc., *Lycop.*, Natr. carb., Phosph. ac., Rhodod., RHUS TOX., SAMBUC., *Sepia*, Silic., *Tarax.*, Valer.

— **in bed:** see Bed.

Lying down; after: Arsen., Asar., Lycop., MENYANTH., *Merc. viv.*, *Pulsat.*, Rhus tox., Sambuc., Selen., *Tarax.*, Veratr.

Menses; before the: *Calc. carb.*, Lycop., Mangan., Sepia, Sulphur, *Thuya*, *Veratr.*

— **at the beginning** of the: Acon., Caustic., Chamom., *Hyosc.*, *Phosphor.*, Sepia.

— **during** the: Calc. carb., Caustic., Chamom., Cinchon., GRAPHIT., *Hyosc.*, Kali carb., Kreos., Lycop., *Magn. mur.* Phosphor., *Sepia*, Silic., Sulphur, Veratr.

Motion; during: Acon., *Agar.*, AMBRA, Amm. mur., Anac., Ant. tart., Arsen., Asar., Baryt., *Bellad.*, *Brom.*, BRYON., CALC. CARB., *Canthar.*, CARB. AN., *Carb. veg.*,

Caustic., Chamom., CINCHON., *Coccul.*, Dulcam., FERR., *Fluor. ac.*, Gelsem., GRAPHIT., Guaiac., HEPAR, Iod., Ipecac., KALI CARB., Laches., *Ledum*, LYCOP., Magn. carb., MERC. VIV., NATR. CARB., NATR. MUR., *Nitrum*, *Nitr. ac.*, *Nux vom.*, Opium, Petrol., Phosphor., Phosph. ac., *Pulsat.*, *Rheum*, Rhodod., Rhus tox., Sabad. *Sambuc.*, SELEN., SEPIA, SILIC., Spigel., STANN., Staphis., Stramon., SULPHUR, *Sulph. ac.*, Thuya, *Valer.*, VERATR., ZINC.

Motion; after: Agar., *Arsen.*, Carb. veg., Caustic., Hyosc., Kali carb., RHUS TOX., SEPIA, Stann., Stramon., *Sulph. ac.*, *Valer.*

Pains; with the: Acon., *Ant. tart.*, Bellad., *Bryon.*, Calc. carb., Caustic., *Chamom.*, Cinchon., *Coloc.*, Dulcam., Hepar, Hyosc., LACHES., Lycop., MERC. VIV., NATR. CARB., *Rhus tox.*, Selen., SEPIA, Spigel., Stramon., *Sulphur*, Thuya, Veratr.

Reading: See Exertion; mental.

Rest; during: Anac., Apis, *Arsen.*, *Asar.*, *Calc. carb.*, Capsic., *Conium*, *Ferr.*, Lycop., Phosph. ac., Rhus tox., *Sambuc.*, SEPIA, Silic., Spong., Staphis., *Sulphur*, Sulph. ac., Tarax., Valer.

Riding in a carriage; when: Psorin.

Room; in the: Acon., Agn. cast., *Apis*, Bryon., Caustic., *Fluor. ac.*, *Ipecac.*, *Nux vom.*, *Phosphor.*, Pulsat., Rhodod., Rhus tox., Sepia, Sulphur, Valer.

Sitting; while: *Anac.*, ARSEN., *Asar.*, *Calc. carb.*, Capsic., Caustic., Cinchon., *Conium*, *Ferr.*, Lycop., Mangan., Natr. carb., Phosphor., Phosph. ac., Rhodod., *Rhus tox.*, SEPIA, Spong., *Staphis.*, Sulphur, *Sulph. ac.*, Tarax., Valer.

Sleep; before falling asleep: Arsen., Calc. carb., MERC. VIV., *Phosphor.*, *Rhus tox.*, Sarsap., Sepia, Tarax., Veratr.

— **when falling asleep:** Ant. crud., *Arsen.*, *Calc. carb.*, Carb. an., Conium, Lycop., Magn. carb., MERC. VIV., Mezer., Mur. ac., Opium, *Phosphor.*, Rhus tox., Sarsap., *Sepia*, SULPHUR, *Tarax.*, Thuya, Veratr.

Sleep; before: Bryon., Cinchon., Hepar, *Merc. viv.*, Nux vom., *Phosphor.*, Phosph. ac., SAMBUC., Sepia.

— **at the beginning** of: ARSEN., Bryon., *Calc. carb.*, *Carb. an.*, Carb. veg., Cinchon., *Conium*, Graphit., *Lycop.*, Merc. viv., MUR. AC., Phosphor., Rhus tox., *Sepia*, *Sulphur*, TARAX., THUYA, Veratr.

— **during:** Acon., Act. rac., *Agar.*, *Ant. crud.*, Ant. tart., *Arsen.*, Baryt., *Bellad.*, *Borax*, Bryon., Calc. carb., *Carb. an.*, Carb. veg., CHAMOM., *Chelid.*, Cicut., CINCHON., *Conium*, *Cyclam.*, Digit., *Euphras.*, *Ferr.*, Hepar, HYOSC., Ignat., Kali carb., Lycop., *Merc. viv.*, Mezer., *Natr. mur.*, Nitr. ac., Nux vom., *Opium*, *Phosphor.*, *Phosph. ac.*, PLATIN., Podophyl., PULSAT., Rhodod., Rhus tox., *Sabad.*, SELEN., Sepia, *Silic.*, *Stramon.*, *Sulphur*, Tarax., Thuya, Veratr., Zinc.

— **after:** Lachnanth.

Stool; before: *Acon.*, Ant. tart., Bellad., Bryon., Calc. carb., Capsic., Caustic., Kali carb., MERC. VIV., Opium, Phosphor., Rhus tox., Veratr.

— **during:** Acon., *Arsen.*, Bellad., Calc. carb., Carb. veg., Chamom., Cinchon., *Dulcam.*, Ferr., Hepar, Ipecac., MERC. VIV., Natr. carb., Natr. mur., Rhus tox., Sepia, *Stramon.*, *Sulphur*, VERATR.

— **after:** ACON., Arsen., Calc. carb., Camphor., Carb. veg., CAUSTIC., Cinchon., Kali carb., Laches., *Merc. viv.*, Phosphor., Rhus tox., *Selen.*, Sepia, Sulphur, Veratr.

Strangers; among: Ambra, BARYT., Lycop., *Sepia*, Stramon.

Talking; from: Alum., Anac., Bryon., *Calc. carb.*, Carb. an., Carb. veg., Chamom., Cinchon., *Fluor. ac.*, *Graphit.*, Hepar, IOD., *Merc. viv.*, Natr. carb., Natr. mur., Nux vom., *Phosph. ac.*, RHUS TOX., SELEN., Sepia, SULPHUR, Sulph. ac., Veratr.

Tobacco smoking; from: Arsen., Ipecac., Laches., *Natr. mur.*, Selen., Spigel., Staphis., Tarax., Thuya.

Toothache; during: Hyosc., *Merc. viv.*, Rhus tox., Sepia, Veratr.

Urination; before: Ant. tart., Bryon., Coloc., Phosph. ac., *Rhus tox.*

— **during:** Bellad., *Hepar*, Ipecac., Lycop., MERC. VIV., Phosph. ac., Sepia, Sulphur, *Thuya.*

— **after:** Bellad., Coloc., *Hepar*, Merc. viv., Natr. mur., Selen., Staphis., Sulphur, Thuya.

Vertigo; during: Bellad., Ignat., *Ipecac.*, Rhus tox., Selen., *Thuya*, Veratr.

Walking; when: Agar., *Ambra*, Amm. mur., Anac., Ant. tart., Asar., Baryt., *Bellad.*, Brom., BRYON., Calad., *Calc. carb.*, Canthar., *Carb. an.*, Carb. veg., *Caustic.*, Cinchon., COCCUL., Dulcam., *Ferr.*, Fluor. ac., *Graphit.*, *Guaiac.*, *Hepar*, IOD., Ipecac., *Kali carb.*, Laches., *Ledum*, LYCOP., Magn. carb., MERC. VIV., *Natr. carb.*, *Natr. mur.*, Nitrum, Nitr. ac., Nux vom., Opium, Petrol., Phosphor., Phosph. ac., Psorin., *Pulsat.*, *Rheum*, *Rhodod.*, Rhus tox., *Selen.*, Seneg., SEPIA, *Silic.*, Spigel., *Stann.*, Staphis., Stramon., SULPHUR, Sulph. ac., Thuya, Valer., *Veratr.*, Zinc.

— **open air,** in the: AGN. CAST., Amm. mur., Bellad., BRYON., CALC. CARB., *Carb. an.*, Carb. veg., CAUSTIC., Chamom., CINCHON., Coloc., Ferr., *Guaiac.*, *Hepar*, Kali carb., Ledum, *Lycop.*, *Merc. viv.*, Nitr. ac., *Nux vom.*, Phosphor., *Phosph. ac.*, Psorin., RHODOD., Rhus tox., *Selen.*, Sepia, Spigel., Stramon., *Sulphur*, Zinc.

— — **after:** Alum., Ant. crud., Bryon., Canthar., Ferr., Ledum, Menyanth., *Petrol.*, Phosphor., *Rhodod.*, Rhus tox., *Ruta*, SEPIA, Therid.

Wind, in the: Arsen., BELLAD., Chamom., Cinchon., Lycop., Phosphor.

Work; during manual: Amm. mur., Kali carb., Laches., *Natr. mur.*, Sepia, Silic., Sulphur.

AMELIORATIONS.

Awaking; after: Ant. crud., *Arsen.*, Bellad., Chamom., CHELID., Cinchon., Cyclam., *Euphras.*, Ferr., *Helleb.*,

Hyosc., NUX VOM., Opium, PHOSPHOR., PLATIN., PULSAT., Selen., *Sepia*, Silic., Stramon., *Sulphur*, THUYA.

Drinking; water, after: Apis, Bryon., CAUSTIC., *Cuprum*, Ipecac., *Nux vom.*, *Opium*, *Phosphor.*, Pulsat., Sepia, *Silic.*, Spigel., Tarax., Thuya.

— **wine, after:** Acon., Apis, Conium, Laches., *Opium*, Sulph. ac., Thuya.

Eating; while: Anac., *Ignat.*, Laches., Mezer., PHOSPHOR., Zinc.

— **after:** Alum., *Cinchon.*, Cuprum, *Ferr.*, Fluor. ac., Ignat., Kali carb., *Natr. carb.*, Petrol., Phosphor., *Rhus tox.*, Sepia, Veratr.

Exertion; bodily, from: *Ignat.*, Sepia, Stann.

— **mental,** from: Ferr., Natr. carb.

Lying in bed; while: Arsen., BELLAD., BRYON., Calc. carb., Caustic., Conium, Hepar, Kali carb., Laches., Lycop., NUX VOM., Rhus tox., Scilla, Silic., Staphis., *Stramon.*, Sulphur.

Motion; during: Anac., ARSEN., Asar., Bellad., Calc. carb., *Capsic.*, *Conium*, Cyclam., Dulcam., *Ferr.*, Lycop., *Merc. viv.*, Phosph. ac., *Pulsat.*, RHUS TOX., *Sabad.*, SAMBUC., Selen., Sepia, Silic., Spong., Sulphur, SULPH. AC., Tarax., Thuya, *Valer.*, Veratr.

— **after:** see during rest.

Rest; during: Acon., Ant. tart., *Bellad.*, *Bryon.*, Calad., Camphor., Carb. an., Hepar, Ipecac., *Ledum*, Merc. viv., Natr. carb., Natr. mur., NUX VOM., Phosphor., Platin., *Selen.*, Staphis.

Rising from bed; after: Alum., Ambra, Ant. crud., Ant. tart., *Arsen.*, *Bellad.*, Bryon., CALC. CARB., Capsic., Carb. an., Caustic., *Cinchon.*, Conium, Cyclam., Dulcam., Ferr., Helleb., Ignat., Iod., Kali carb., *Lycop.*, Menyanth., Merc. viv., Mur. ac., Nux vom., *Pulsat.*, RHUS TOX., Ruta, Sabad., *Selen.*, SEPIA, *Spigel.*, Staphis., *Sulphur*, Tarax., Thuya, *Valer.*, Veratr., *Viol. tr.*

Room; in the: *Bellad.*, Calc. carb., Capsic., Carb. an., Carb. veg., *Chamom.*, Cinchon., *Conium*, Ferr., Laches., *Merc. viv.*, NUX VOM., Petrol., Rhus tox., SELEN., Sepia, SILIC., Spigel., Stramon., Thuya, Valer.

Sleep; falling asleep, when: Bryon., *Merc. viv.*, Nux vom., Phosphor., Phosph. ac., SAMBUC.

— **during**: Arsen., Bellad., Bryon., Carb. an., Cinchon., Hepar, *Merc. viv.*, *Nux vom.*, *Phosphor.*, Phosph. ac., PULSAT., SAMBUC., Sepia, Thuya.

— **after**; see after awaking.

Stool; after: Borax, BRYON., Pulsat., RHUS TOX., *Spigel.*, Sulphur, Thuya, Veratr.

Talking; from: Ferr., *Hepar*, Natr. carb.

Uncovering; from: *Acon.*, Bellad., *Calc. carb.*, CHAMOM., *Cinchon.*, Ferr., *Ignat.*, LYCOP., Nitr. ac., Nux vom., Pulsat., Spigel., *Staphis.*, Sulphur, Thuya, Veratr.

Walking in the open air: Alum., ARSEN., *Capsic.*, Conium, Dulcam., Lycop., Nux vom., Phosphor., *Pulsat.*, Rhus tox., Sepia, Tarax., *Thuya*, Viol. tr.

Washing; after: Apis, *Asar.*, *Calc. carb.*, Caustic., *Euphras.*, FLUOR. AC., NUX VOM., *Pulsat.*, Rhodod., Sabad., Spigel.

Cessation of all complaints during the sweat: Psorin.

Sweat relieves the pains: Gelsem.

CONCOMITANTS.

Mood; anxious: Acon., *Alum.*, Ant. crud., Arnic., ARSEN., *Baryt.*, Bellad., Bovist., Bryon., CALC. CARB., Canthar., Carb. veg., Caustic., CHAMOM., Cicut., CINCHON., *Coffea*, Crocus, FERR., Graphit., Hepar, Ignat., Kreos., Lycop., MANGAN., *Merc. viv.*, *Merc. corr.*, Mezer., Mur. ac., NATR. CARB., Natr. mur., Nitrum, Nitr. ac., *Nux vom.*, Phosphor., *Phosph. ac.*, *Plumbum*, *Pulsat.*, Rheum, *Rhus tox.*, Sabad., *Selen.*, SEPIA, *Spong.*, *Stann.*, Staphis., Stramon., SULPHUR, THUYA, *Veratr.*

Mood; changeable: Alum., *Aurum*, Crocus, *Ferr.*, IGNAT., *Platin.*, Stramon., Sulph. ac., Valer., Zinc.

— **complaining and lamenting:** *Acon.*, Bryon., Ignat., Nux vom., Veratr.

— **crying out:** Arnic., BELLAD., Calc. carb., *Camphor.*, *Chamom.*, CUPRUM, Lycop., OPIUM, Platin., Phosphor., Rheum, Stramon.

— **dejected:** Acon., *Apis*, Arsen., Bellad., *Calc. carb.*, Cinchon., CONIUM, Hepar, Nux vom., Rhus tox., Sabin., SEPIA, *Sulphur*, Thuya.

— **depressed:** Apis, Bellad., *Cinchon.*, Conium, *Sepia*, Spigel., Sulphur.

— **despairing:** Acon., *Arsen.*, Aurum, Bryon., *Calc. carb.*, CARB. VEG., *Chamom.*, *Graphit.*, Lycop., Nux vom., Rhus tox., *Sepia*, Stann., Veratr.

— **discontented:** Bellad., Bryon., Natr. mur., *Phosph. ac.*, Thuya.

— **disinclined to talk:** Arnic., *Bellad.*, Bryon., Calc. carb., Cinchon., *Ignat.*, Merc. viv., Mur. ac., Opium, PHOSPHOR., *Phosph. ac.*, *Veratr.*

— **exciteable:** *Acon.*, *Bellad.*, CHAMOM., *Coccul.*, COFFEA, *Conium*, Lycop., MAR. VER., Nux vom., Phosph. ac., *Sepia.*

— **fear of death:** *Acon.*, Arsen., Bryon., Nitrum, *Nitr. ac.*, Nux vom., Phosphor., Platin., Pulsat., Rhus tox., *Veratr.*

— **impatient:** *Acon.*, Apis, Aurum, *Chamom.*, Ignat., Merc. viv., Rhus tox., Sulph. ac., Zinc.

— **impetuous:** *Acon.*, *Arsen.*, *Bryon.*, Carb. veg., CHAMOM., *Coffea*, Ferr., *Hepar*, Hyosc., Natr. mur., NUX VOM., Phosphor., Stramon., Sulphur, Thuya.

— **listless:** Apis, *Arsen.*, Bellad., *Calc. carb.*, *Cinchon.*, Laches., PHOSPHOR., PHOSPH. AC., *Pulsat.*, Selen., *Sepia.*

— **melancholy:** Arsen., *Aurum*, *Calc. carb.*, Conium, Ignat., Lycop., Natr. mur., Selen.

— **oversensitive:** *Acon.*, Aurum, Baryt., Bellad., *Chamom.*, Cinchon., COFFEA, Conium, Nux vom., Selen., *Sepia.*

Mood; restless: Acon., *Amm. carb.*, *Arnic.*, ARSEN., BELLAD., Bovist., BRYON., *Calc. carb.*, *Chamom.*, Cinchon., *Ignat.*, LYCOP., Merc. viv., *Nux vom.*, PHOSPH. AC., Pulsat., *Rhus tox.*, Ruta, Sabad., Sambuc., SEPIA, Silic., Stann., Sulphur, *Veratr.*

— **sensitiveness to noise:** Arnic., CAPSIC., CHAMOM., Cinchon., *Coffea*, Lycop., Natr. carb., NUX VOM., Sabad., Zinc.

— **serene:** Apis, Arsen., Bellad., *Coffea*, Crocus, OPIUM, *Sarsap.*

— **sighing and groaning:** *Acon.*, Arsen., Baryt., BRYON., *Chamom.*, Cinchon., *Coccul.*, Cuprum, IGNAT., *Ipecac.*, Nux vom., Phosphor., Rhus tox., *Sepia*, Stramon., Veratr.

— **singing and trilling:** *Bellad.*, Crocus, Kali carb., Spong., *Stramon.*, Veratr.

— **shy:** Arsen., *Bellad.*, Laches., Lycop., Pulsat., Sepia.

— **sorrowful:** *Acon.*, Bellad., Bryon., *Calc. carb.*, Graphit., Ignat., *Natr. mur.*, Nitr. ac., Nux vom., Pulsat., *Rhus tox.*, *Sepia*, Sulphur.

— **startled easily:** Acon., Bellad., *Calc. carb.*, Caustic., *Chamom.*, Nux vom., *Petrol.*, *Phosphor.*, Pulsat., Sabad., Sambuc., Sepia, Spong., Sulphur, Veratr.

— **suicidal mania:** see weariness of life.

— **talkative:** Arsen., Bellad., *Calad.*, Coccul., Hyosc., Laches., *Selen.*, Tarax.

— **tearful:** Acon., Aurum, BELLAD., Bryon., *Calc. carb.*, *Chamom.*, Cinchon., Graphit., LYCOP., Nux vom., *Petrol.*, Platin., *Pulsat.*, Rheum, Rhus tox., Sepia, Spong., Sulphur, Veratr.

— **vexatious:** Bellad., Bryon., *Calc. carb.*, *Chamom.*, Cinchon., Conium, *Hepar*, Merc. viv., Nux vom., Pulsat., RHEUM, Rhus tox., Sabad., Sambuc., *Sulphur*, Thuya.

— **weariness of life:** Alum., *Arsen.*, *Aurum*, CALC. CARB., Hepar, *Merc. viv.*, Nux vom., Pulsat., Rhus tox., Sepia Silic., *Spong.*, Thuya.

Mood; whimpering and whining: Acon., Bellad., Bryon., Camphor., *Chamom.*, *Merc. viv.*, Rheum.

Delirium: Acon., Arsen., Aurum, BELLAD., Bryon., Calc. carb., CHAMOM., Cina, Cinchon., Dulcam., *Hyosc.*, Iod., Ignat., Kali carb., Natr. mur., Nux vom., OPIUM, *Phosph. ac.*, Platin., Sambuc., STRAMON., Sulphur, *Veratr.*

Dullness of the head: Acon., Angust., Arsen., BELLAD., *Bryon.*, Calc. carb., *Capsic.*, Cinchon., Droser., Graphit., Ipecac., Kali carb., Merc. viv., Natr. carb., *Natr. mur.*, *Nux vom.*, Opium, *Phosphor.*, Phosph. ac., *Rhus tox.*, Ruta, Sabad., SEPIA, Silic., *Sulphur*, Thuya, *Valer.*, Veratr.

Excited fancy: *Acon.*, Carb. veg., Iod., Nitr. ac., *Opium*, *Phosphor.*, Sulphur.

Frenzy: see Delirium.

Intellect brightened: *Coffea*, Laches., *Opium*, Phosphor., Thuya, Valer., Viol. od.

Muddled (Düseligkeit): *Bellad.*, BRYON., Calc. carb., *Cinchon.*, Ipecac., Lauroc., Nux vom., Opium, Phosph. ac., PULSAT., Rheum, *Rhus tox.*, Stramon., Veratr.

Rage: Acon., *Arsen.*, Bellad., *Canthar.*, Caustic., Hyosc., Nitr. ac., Nux vom., *Opium*, Sabad., *Stramon.*, Veratr.

Stupefaction: *Arnic.*, Arsen., Bellad., Bryon., Calc. carb., Chamom., HYOSC., Lauroc., Nux vom., OPIUM, *Phosphor.*, PHOSPH. AC., *Rhus tox.*, Stramon., Veratr.

Unconsciousness: Arnic., *Arsen.*, Bellad., Camphor., Coccul., Helleb., Hyosc., Mur. ac., Natr. mur., Opium, *Phosph. ac.*, Rhus tox., Sepia, Sambuc., Stramon.

Vertigo: Alum., Apis, ARSEN., Bellad., Bovist., *Bryon.*, CALC. CARB., Cinchon., Ignat., IPECAC., Lachnanth., Lauroc., Merc. corr., Nux vom., PHOSPHOR., Phosph. ac., RHUS TOX., *Selen.*, Sepia, Sulphur, Therid., *Thuya*, *Veratr.*

Head, pains in the: Amm. carb., Angust., *Ant. crud.*, Ant. tart., *Arnic.*, *Arsen.*, *Bellad.*, BRYON., *Calc. carb.*,

Carb.veg.,Caustic.,CHAMOM.,Cinchon.,Conium, Droser., Ferr., Graphit., Helleb., Hepar, Ipecac., Kali carb., Ledum, Lycop., Mangan., Merc. viv., Mezer., Natr. carb., Natr. mur., Nitrum, NUX VOM., Petrol., Phosphor., Rhodod., RHUS TOX., Ruta, Selen., SEPIA, Silic., Spigel., *Sulphur*, *Veratr.*

Head; external pains: ARSEN., CALC. CARB., Graphit., Hepar, MERC. VIV., Mezer., Natr. mur., Phosdhor., *Rhus tox.*, *Sabad.*, *Sepia*, Silic., Staphis., Thuya.

Eyes; pain in the: *Acon.*, Arnic., Arsen., BELLAD., *Bryon.*, *Calc. carb.*, Canthar., Caustic., Chamom., *Hepar*, Ledum, LYCOP., Merc. viv., Natr. carb., Nux vom., Phosphor., Pulsat., Rhodod., RHUS TOX., Sepia, Silic., SPIGEL., *Sulphur*, Thuya, Veratr.

— **pupils contracted:** Camphor., Capsic., *Chamom.*, Coccul., Mezer., Mur. ac., Phosphor., Pulsat., SEPIA, Silic., SULPHUR, Thuya, *Veratr.*

— — **dilated:** Bellad., *Calc. carb.*, Cina, Hepar, Hyosc., Opium, Spigel., Stramon.

Sight; decreased power of vision: Bellad., Calc. carb., Caustic., Conium, Hepar, Hyosc., *Merc. viv.*, NATR. MUR., Phosphor., Pulsat., Silic., STRAMON., Sulphur.

— **fire** before the eyes, like: *Bellad.*, Caustic., Kali carb., Natr. mur., *Nux vom.*, Pulsat., Spigel.

— **flickering** before the: Caustic., *Chamom.*, Graphit., Lycop., *Nux vom.*, SEPIA, Staphis.

— **aversion to light:** Acon., Arnic., *Arsen.*, *Bellad.*, Bryon., *Calc. carb.*, *Chamom.*, Cinchon., Graphit., Hepar, Lycop., *Merc. viv.*, NUX VOM., Phosphor., Pulsat., RHUS TOX., *Sepia*, Stramon., SULPHUR.

Ears; pain in the: ACON., Bellad., CALAD., *Calc. carb.*, Caustic., GRAPHIT., Lycop., Merc. viv., Natr. mur., Nitr. ac., Pulsat., SEPIA, Sulphur, Thuya.

— **humming** in the: ARSEN., Bellad., *Calc. carb.*, *Caustic.*, Graphit., Hepar, Lycop., NUX VOM., Pulsat., Sabad., *Sepia*, SULPHUR.

Nose; pains in the: Caustic., *Merc. viv.*, Phosph. ac., Pulsat., RHODOD., *Rhus tox.*, Thuya.

— **coldness** of the: Nux vom., Phosph. ac., *Veratr.*

— **itching** of the: *Cina*, Laches., Merc. viv., *Selen.*, Silic.

Face; pain in the: Bryon., Calc. carb., Mezer., Nux vom., *Sepia*, SPIGEL., Thuya.

— **bluish red:** Apis, Bellad., Bryon., LACHES., Opium, Sambuc.

— **cold:** Camphor., Chamom., *Cina*, Hyosc., *Lycop.*, VERATR.

— — **cheeks:** Bellad., Chamom.

— — **forehead:** Carb. veg., Cina, *Veratr.*

— **hot:** Acon., Bellad., CALC. CARB., Chamom., Cinchon., Coffea, CONIUM, Ferr., Ignat., NUX VOM., Sabad., Silic., Stramon., *Tarax.*, *Valer.*

— **pale:** Arsen., Bellad., CINA, Cinchon., *Lycop.*, Nux vom., *Pulsat.*, *Rhus tox.*, SELEN., *Sepia*, *Sulphur*, VERATR.,

— **puffed up:** AMM. MUR., Apis, Arsen., Bellad., Bryon., *Chamom.*, LYCOP., *Merc. viv.*, Nux vom., Rhus tox., *Sepia.*

— **red:** Acon., Agar., Alum., *Amm. mur.*, Arsen., Bellad., Bryon., *Chamom.*, CINCHON., Coffea, Conium, Ferr., Hepar, Hyosc., IGNAT., Lycop., Merc. viv., *Nux vom.*, OPIUM, Phosphor., Pulsat., Rhus tox., Sabad., *Sambuc.*, SEPIA, SULPHUR, *Veratr.*, Zinc.

— **shining, greasy** looking: Natr. mur., *Rhus tox.*, Selen.

— **yellow:** CINCHON., Conium, Ferr., NATR. MUR., Nux vom., *Rhus tox.*, *Sepia*, *Sulphur.*

Lips; dryness of the: Acon., Arnic., Arsen., Bellad., *Bryon.*, Cinchon., Ferr., Merc. viv., NUX VOM., *Phosphor.*, Rhus tox., *Sepia*, Veratr.

— **eruption** on the: Ant. crud., *Arsen.*, *Bryon.*, Calc. carb., Caustic., *Ignat.*, Ipecac., Lycop., *Natr. mur.*, *Nux vom.*, Rhus tox., *Sepia*, Silic.

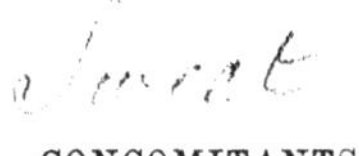

Lips; swelling of the: Apis, *Arsen.*, *Bryon.*, Calc. carb., Conium, Mezer., Natr. mur., *Sulphur.*

Submaxillary glands; swelling of the: Calad., *Kali carb.*

Teeth; pains in the: Bryon., CARB. VEG., *Chamom.*, Cinchon., Graphit., HYOSC., Kali carb., Nux vom., Pulsat., RHUS TOX., *Sepia*, Staphis., Zinc.

Gums; bleeding of the: Arsen., Carb. veg., Merc. viv., Natr. mur., *Sepia*, STAPHIS., Sulphur.

— **swelling** of the: Calc. carb., Carb. veg., Merc. viv., Natr. mur., Nux vom., Phosphor., Rhus tox., *Sepia*, Staphis., *Sulphur.*

Mouth; burning in the: Apis, Arsen., *Chamom.*, Mezer., *Petrol.*

— **dryness** of the: Acon., Amm. mur., Apis, Baryt., Bryon., Chamom., Laches., Lycop., *Nitr. ac.*, *Nux vom.*, Petrol., PHOSPHOR., *Phosph. ac.*, Rhus tox., Sabad., SEPIA, Stramon., *Sulphur*, *Thuya*, Veratr.

— **offensive odor** from the: Acon., ARNIC., Bryon., Carb. veg., *Chamom.*, Ipecac., Laches., MERC. VIV., Nitr. ac., NUX VOM., Pulsat.

— **saliva,** increase of: Bellad., Cinchon., *Droser.*, Dulcam., *Merc. viv.*, Nitr. ac., *Rhus tox.*, Spigel.

Tongue; coated: *Ant. crud.*, Bellad., *Bryon.*, *Chamom.*, Ipecac., Lycop., *Merc. viv.*, Nux mosch., *Nux vom.*, Opium, Phosphor., Phosph. ac., Sulphur.

— **dry:** Arsen., Bellad., *Calc. carb.*, Merc. viv., Mezer., Phosphor., Phosph. ac., *Sulphur.*

Throat; pains in the: Acon., Apis, BELLAD., Bovist., *Chamom.*, Conium, DROSER., Kali carb., Laches., *Merc. viv.*, Nitr. ac., Nux vom., *Phosphor.*, *Phosph. ac.*, Pulsat., Rhus tox., Sabad., SEPIA, Sulphur, Thuya.

Throat; burning: Acon., Apis, *Arsen.*, Bellad., Chamom., Merc. viv., Mezer., Nitr. ac., Nux vom., Rhus tox., Sabad., *Sulphur*, Veratr.

— **dryness** of the: BELLAD., *Chamom.*, Coccul., Hyosc., Laches., *Nitr. ac.*, Nux vom., PHOSPHOR., Pulsat., Sabad., Selen., Staphis, Stramon., Veratr.

— **inflammation** of the: ACON., Amm. mur., Apis, Baryt., BELLAD., Bryon., Chamom., *Conium*, Laches., *Merc. viv.*, Nitr. ac., *Nux vom.*, Pulsat., Sepia, Sulphur.

— — **uvula,** of the: *Acon.*, Bellad., Calc. carb., Cann. sat., Merc. viv., NUX VOM., Sulphur.

Appetite; want of: Alum., Anac., *Ant. crud.*, Ant. tart., Apis, Arsen., Canthar., CINCHON., CONIUM, Cyclam., *Ipecac.*, *Kali carb.*, NUX VOM., Phosphor., Pulsat., Rheum, RHUS TOX., Sabad., SAMBUC., SEPIA, *Silic.*, Staphis., *Stramon.*, Sulphur, Thuya, Veratr.

Loathing of food: Amm. carb., *Ant. crud.*, ARSEN., Bryon., CHAMOM., Ipecac., Kali carb., Rheum.

Hunger; (canine hunger): Arsen., Bryon., CALC. CARB., *Capsic.*, Chamom., Cimex, CINA, *Cinchon.*, Coccul., Ignat., Iod., *Lycop.*, Nux vom., *Phosphor.*, Pulsat., Rhus tox., Ruta, Sabad., SILIC., Staphis., *Veratr.*

Thirst: Acon., Alum., Ant. crud., Arnic., ARSEN., *Bellad.*, Bryon., Calc. carb., CHAMOM., Chelid., CINCHON., *Coffea*, *Diadem.*, *Hepar*, *Iod.*, *Lycop.*, *Magn. mur.*, Merc. viv., Natr. carb., NATR. MUR., Nux vom., Phosph. ac., Pulsat., RHUS TOX., Sabad., Silic., STRAMON., *Sulphur*, Sulph. ac., TARAX., Thuya, *Veratr.*

— **between heat and sweat:** Agn. cast., *Amm. mur.*, Ant. tart., Bryon., CINCHON., *Coffea*, CYCLAM., NUX VOM., Opium, Pulsat., Rhus tox., Stann., *Stramon.*

— **after the sweat:** *Amm. mur.*, Ant. crud., Ant. tart., Arsen., Bellad., Cinchon., Ignat., LYCOP., Natr. mur., *Nux vom.*, Rhus tox.

Thirstlessness: Agn. cast., Amm. mur., Apis, Arnic., *Arsen.*, *Bellad.*, Bryon., Camphor., Capsic., Carb. veg., Caustic., Coffea, Cyclam., Digit., Euphorb., HELLEB., Hepar, IGNAT., Mangan., Menyanth., Merc. viv., Natr. sulph., Nux mosch., Nux vom., *Phosphor.*, PULSAT., Rhodod., RHUS TOX., Sabad., *Sabin.*, SAMBUC., SEPIA, Spigel., *Staphis.*, Stramon., Thuya, VERATR.

Taste; bitter: Acon., Alum., *Ant. crud.*, *Arsen.*, BRYON., Carb. veg., CHAMOM., Cinchon., *Hepar*, Merc. viv., *Natr. mur.*, Nux vom., Phosphor., PULSAT., SEPIA, Silic., Sulphur, Veratr.

— **putrid:** Arnic., Carb. veg., Chamom., Conium, Merc. viv., PULSAT., *Rhus tox.*, *Sepia*, *Staphis.*, Sulphur.

— **offensive:** Ant. crud., Arsen., Bryon., *Calc. carb.*, KALI CARB., *Nux vom.*, Pulsat., Sepia, Stann., *Staphis.*, Valer., Zinc.

— **salty:** Ant. tart., *Arsen.*, BELLAD., Carb. veg., Cinchon., Lycop., MERC. VIV., Phosphor., Pulsat., *Sepia*, Sulphur.

Eructations; in general: Alum., *Ant. crud.*, Arnic., Bellad., BRYON., *Carb. veg.*, Coccul., Conium, Merc. viv., Natr. mur., *Nux vom.*, Phosphor., Pulsat., Rhus tox., SABAD., *Sepia*, Sulphur, Sulph. ac., Thuya, Veratr.

Nausea: *Ant. crud.*, ARSEN., *Bryon.*, Cinchon., Conium, Droser., *Hepar*, IGNAT., IPECAC., Kali carb., *Ledum*, *Lycop.*, *Merc. viv.*, Nitr. ac., *Phosphor.*, Pulsat., Rhus tox., *Selen.*, *Sepia*, Silic., Sulphur, Sulph. ac., THUYA, *Veratr.*

Qualmishness; (water running together in the mouth): Arsen., Bryon., *Calc. carb.*, Caustic., Merc. viv., *Nux vom.*, *Rhus tox.*, Sepia, SILIC., *Sulphur*, Veratr.

Vomit; disposition to: Acon., ARSEN., CHAMOM., *Droser.*, Ipecac., Nux vom., Pulsat., *Rhus tox.*, Sabad., SEPIA, *Veratr.*

Vomiting; in general: Ant. crud., *Arnic.*, Arsen., *Bellad.*, Bryon., *Camphor.*, CHAMOM., CINA, *Cinchon.*, *Conium*, *Ferr.*, *Hepar*, *Hyosc.*, Ignat., IPECAC., Kali carb., Laches., *Lycop.*, Natr. carb., Nux vom., Pulsat., *Selen.*, Sepia, *Silic.*, Stramon., SULPHUR, Therid., *Thuya*, *Veratr.*

— **bitter:** Ant. crud., *Arsen.*, Bryon., CHAMOM., CINCHON., Ignat., Ipecac., Merc. viv., *Nux vom.*, Pulsat., Sepia, Veratr.

— **ingesta,** of the: Arsen., Bryon., *Cina*, FERR., *Ignat.*, Nux vom., Silic.

— **mucus:** Chamom., Ignat., *Pulsat.*

— **sour:** Calc. carb., Cinchon., LYCOP., Nux vom., Phosphor., *Pulsat.*, Sepia, Sulphur.

Stomach; pains in the: Arnic., ARSEN., Bryon., *Calc. carb.*, *Carb. veg.*, Caustic., CHAMOM., Cinchon., *Coccul.*, Ferr., *Ipecac.*, Lycop., Nux vom., *Pulsat.*, RHUS TOX., Sabad., *Sepia*, Silic., *Sulphur*, Sulph. ac., Veratr.

Liver; pains in the: Arnic., *Arsen.*, Bryon., Calc. carb., Chamom., CINCHON., Kali carb., Laches., Magn. mur., *Merc. viv.*, Natr. mur., *Nux vom.*, Sabad., SEPIA, Thuya.

Spleen; pains in the: Arnic., Asaf., Bryon., CARB. VEG., Cinchon., Ferr., *Ignat.*, NATR. MUR., Rhus tox., Selen., Sulph. ac., Thuya.

Abdomen; pains in the, in general: Ant. crud., *Ant. tart.*, *Arsen.*, Baryt., BELLAD., Bovist., *Bryon.*, *Calc. carb.*, CHAMOM., Cina, *Cinchon.*, Coloc., *Ferr.*, *Helleb.*, Kali carb., Lycop., Merc. viv., Nitr. ac., *Nux vom.*, Phosphor., Pulsat., Ran. bulb., RHUS TOX., SEPIA, STRAMON., Strontia, *Sulphur*, Thuya, VERATR.

Flatulence; affections from: Arnic., Carb. veg., CHAMOM., *Cinchon.*, Graphit., Ignat., Lycop., NUX VOM., *Phosphor.*, *Phosph. ac.*, Pulsat., Staphis., *Veratr.*

Diarrhœa: *Acon.*, Ant. crud., Apis, Arnic., *Arsen.*, Bryon., Calc. carb., Capsic., CHAMOM., Cina, Cinchon., Coffea, *Conium*, MERC. VIV., *Merc. corr.*, PHOSPHOR., *Phosph. ac.*, Pulsat., RHUS TOX., Sepia, Silic., STRAMON., Sulphur, Veratr.

Constipation: *Ant. crud.*, APIS, Arnic., *Bellad.*, *Bryon.*, Calc. carb., Carb. veg., Cinchon., COCCUL., Conium, Dulcam., Graphit., *Lycop.*, Merc. viv., Mezer., Nitr. ac., NUX VOM., OPIUM, Sabad., Selen., *Sepia*, *Silic.*, *Staphis.*, *Sulphur*, Sulph. ac., Thuya, Veratr.

Urging to stool: *Arsen.*, Capsic., *Caustic.*, Coccul., *Merc. viv.*, Nitr. ac., *Nux vom.*, Phosphor., Pulsat., Rheum, *Rhus tox.*, Staphis., SULPHUR.

— **ineffectual:** *Arsen.*, Capsic., Coccul., *Merc. viv.*, *Nux vom.*, Rheum, *Rhus tox.*, SULPHUR.

Urine; brown: *Acon.*, Ant. tart., Arnic., ARSEN., Bellad., *Bryon.*, *Calc. carb.*, Canthar., Carb. veg., Hepar, Ipecac., *Merc. viv.*, Pulsat., *Selen.*, SEPIA, Staphis., *Sulphur*, Thuya, *Veratr.*

— **cloudy:** *Cina*, Cinchon., *Conium*, Dulcam., Ignat., IPECAC., MERC. VIV., PHOSPHOR., Pulsat., Rhus tox., Sabad., *Sepia.*

— **pale:** Arnic., *Bellad.*, Cinchon., Conium, Ignat., Phosphor., PHOSPH. AC., Pulsat., Rhus tox., Stramon., Thuya.

— **stinking:** Arsen., Carb. veg., Dulcam., Nitr. ac., Phosph. ac., Pulsat., *Sepia*, Thuya, Viol. tr.

Urination; frequent, too: Ant. crud., Baryt., CALC. CARB., *Caustic.*, Ignat., Kali carb., Laches., LYCOP., *Merc. viv.*, Mur. ac., Natr. carb., Natr. mur., *Phosphor.*, *Phosph. ac.*, RHUS TOX., Scilla, *Selen.*, Staphis., SULPHUR, Thuya.

— **painful:** CANTHAR., CHAMOM., Hepar, Lycop., *Merc. viv.*, Nitr. ac., Pulsat., Sulphur, *Thuya.*

— **profuse,** too: ACON., Ant. crud., Bellad., *Chamom.*, DULCAM., Ignat., Laches., Lycop., *Magn. carb.*, *Mur. ac.*,

Natr. carb., Natr. mur., PHOSPHOR., *Phosph. ac.*, RHUS TOX., Sambuc., Scilla, Seneg., Spigel., Stann., Stramon., Thuya.

Urination; scanty, too: Ant. tart., Apis, Arnic., Bellad., *Bryon.*, CALC. CARB., *Canthar.*, Carb. veg., Caustic., *Cinchon.*, Digit., Dulcam., *Graphit.*, HELLEB., Hepar, Hyosc., *Merc. viv.*, Nitr. ac., *Nux vom.*, OPIUM, Pulsat., Rhus tox., Staphis., SULPHUR, *Veratr.*

— **seldom,** too: Acon., *Arsen.*, Camphor., *Canthar.*, *Cinchon.*, Hepar, Hyosc., *Nux vom.*, Opium, Pulsat., *Sepia*, Stramon.

— **supressed:** Acon., *Apis*, Arnic., Arsen., Camphor., *Canthar.*, Dulcam., Hyosc., *Lycop.*, OPIUM, *Pulsat.*, Stramon., Sulphur.

Urging to urinate: *Ant. tart.*, Apis, Arnic., BRYON., Canthar., *Caustic.*, Dulcam., Graphit., Helleb., Hyosc., Lycop., MERC. VIV., Mur. ac., *Nux vom.*, Phosphor., *Phosph. ac.*, Pulsat., Rhus tox., Scilla, Staphis., *Sulphur*, THUYA.

— **ineffectual:** ARSEN., Camphor., *Canthar.*, Caustic., Digit., Dulcam., Hyosc., *Nux vom.*, Pulsat., *Sulphur.*

Sneezing: Ant. tart., BELLAD., Carb. veg., CHAMOM., Cina, *Cyclam.*, Laches., Pulsat., *Rhus tox.*, *Sabad.*, Silic., Staphis., SULPHUR.

Coryza; fluent: Amm. mur., Ant. tart., *Arsen.*, BELLAD., Calc. carb., Carb. veg., Caustic., CHAMOM., *Cyclam.*, Euphras., *Laches.*, MERC. VIV., Mezer., Natr. carb., *Pulsat.*, RHUS TOX., *Scilla*, *Selen.*, Silic., SULPHUR, Thuya.

— **dry:** *Bryon.*, Calad., Calc. carb., Dulcam., *Ipecac.*, Kali carb., *Lycop.*, Natr. mur., Nitr. ac., NUX VOM., Phosphor., *Rhodod.*, Rhus tox., *Sambuc.*, Silic.

Dryness of the nose: Bellad., *Calc. carb.*, Graphit., Natr. mur., Nitr. ac., Phosphor., Silic.

Breathing; anxious: Acon., *Arsen.*, Bellad., *Bryon.*,

CHAMOM., Ignat., Ipecac., Opium, Phosphor., *Pulsat.*, *Rhus tox.*, Sambuc., Spong., Stramon.

Breathing; deep: *Bryon.*, Ipecac., *Opium*, *Phosphor.*, PHOSPH. AC., Ran. bulb., *Selen.*, Silic., Stramon.

— **oppressed** (oppression of the chest): Acon., ARSEN., *Bellad.*, BRYON., CHAMOM., Ignat., IPECAC., *Merc. viv.*, *Nux vom.*, Opium, Phosphor., Pulsat., RHUS TOX., Sabad., Sambuc., SEPIA, SULPHUR, Thuya, VERATR.

— **rattling:** Ant. tart., CHAMOM., Ferr., Hyosc., Ipecac., *Lycop.*, Opium, Stramon.

Breath; cold: Carb. veg., Cinchon., Mur. ac., *Rhus tox.*, VERATR.

— **hot:** Acon., *Chamom.*, *Rhus tox.*, Sabad., Strontia, *Zinc.*

— **shortness of:** Acon., *Anac.*, ARSEN., Bryon., Cina, Ferr., Ignat., *Ipecac.*, Kali carb., Lycop., *Mangan.*, Natr. carb., NUX VOM., Opium, PHOSPHOR., Pulsat., *Rhus tox.*, Sambuc., SEPIA, SULPHUR, Veratr., *Zinc.*

Cough, with expectoration: Ant. tart., ARSEN., Bellad., *Bryon.*, *Calc. carb.*, *Digit.*, *Droser.*, Ferr., *Merc. viv.*, *Natr. carb.*, Nitrum, PHOSPHOR., Phosph. ac., Pulsat., Scilla, SEPIA, Silic., *Spong.*, *Sulphur.*, Thuya, Veratr.

— **without expectoration:** Acon., Ant. tart., Apis, ARSEN., Bellad., Bryon., *Caustic.*, CHAMOM., Coffea, Conium, *Droser.*, *Hepar*, Hyosc., Ignat., *Ipecac.*, Ledum, Lycop., *Merc. viv.*, Nitrum, Nitr. ac., *Nux vom.*, PHOSPHOR., Pulsat., RHUS TOX., Sabad., *Sambuc.*, SEPIA, *Spong.*, Strontia, SULPHUR, *Veratr.*

Larynx; pains in the: Acon., Apis, BELLAD., Bovist., Conium, *Droser.*, *Hepar*, Kali carb., Laches., Nux vom., *Phosphor.*, Phosph. ac., Pulsat., SEPIA, Spong., *Sulphur.*

— **dryness** of the: *Arsen.*, CALC. CARB., *Caustic.*, Droser., *Hepar*, Mangan., Mezer., Opium, *Phosphor.*, Selen., SPONG., *Sulphur*, Thuya, ZINC.

Voice; hoarse: Acon., Carb. veg., *Chamom.*, Droser., *Hepar*, NUX VOM., Phosphor., Silic., Spong., *Sulphur*, Thuya.

External throat; pains in the: *Bellad.*, *Calc. carb.*, Conium, Laches., Lycop., *Nux vom.*, Phosphor., Sepia, Sulphur, Thuya.

— **sensitiveness** of the: Bellad., Cinchon., *Laches.*, Scilla.

— **swelling of the glands:** BELLAD., *Calc. carb.*, *Chamom.*, Lycop., *Merc. viv.*, *Rhus tox.*, Spong., Staphis., Thuya.

Nape of the neck; pains in the: *Acon.*, Amm. carb., Graphit., Mosch., Sabin., Sulphur.

— **stiffness** of the: *Acon.*, Bellad., *Calc. carb.*, Carb. veg., Ignat., Kali carb., Lycop., Nitr. ac., *Nux vom.*, Pulsat., *Rhus tox.*, *Sepia*, Staphis., Sulphur, Thuya.

Chest; pains in the, in general: Acon., Apis, *Arsen.*, BELLAD., Bovist., BRYON., Calad., Calc. carb., CHAMOM., Cinchon., Dulcam., Ipecac., *Kali carb.*, Lycop., Mezer., Nux vom., Phosphor., Pulsat., Rhus tox., Sabad., *Sepia*, Spigel., *Sulphur*.

— **congestion** to the: Acon., Apis, *Bellad.*, Bryon., *Cinchon.*, NUX VOM., Phosphor., Pulsat., Rhus tox., *Sepia*, *Sulphur*.

— **rising** in the, sensation of: *Merc. viv.*, Nux vom., Phosphor., Spigel., Thuya.

Heart; palpitation of the: Acon., Calc. carb., Cinchon., Hepar, Ignat., Lycop., *Merc. viv.*, Phosphor., Phosph. ac., *Rhus tox.*, Sarsap., SEPIA, Spigel., Sulphur.

Mammæ; swelling of the: Bryon., Calc. carb., Chamom., *Pulsat.*, Silic.

Milk increased: Acon., *Bellad.*, *Bryon.*, Calc. carb., Cinchon., Conium, Phosphor., *Pulsat.*, Rhus tox., Stramon.

— **vanishing** of: Agn. cast., Bryon., *Calc. carb.*, Chamom., Cinchon., *Dulcam.*, Ignat., Pulsat., Rhus tox., *Sepia*, Zinc.

Scapulæ; pains in the: Amm. mur., *Arsen.*, Baryt., Bellad., *Calc. carb.*, Caustic., *Cinchon.*, Kali carb., *Merc. viv.*, Natr. carb., NUX VOM., *Rhus tox.*, SEPIA, Silic., *Sulphur.*

Back; pains in the: Acon., Ant. tart., Apis, *Arnic.*, ARSEN., *Bellad.*, CALC. CARB., Carb. veg., CAUSTIC., *Cinchon.*, Coccul., Ignat., Kali carb., *Lycop.*, Merc. viv., NATR. MUR., NUX VOM., Petrol., Phosphor., Pulsat., RHUS TOX., SEPIA, Silic., SULPHUR, Thuya, Veratr., Zinc.

Small of the back; pains in the: Acon., Apis, Arnic., *Arsen.*, Baryt., Bryon., CALC. CARB., *Caustic.*, *Chamom.*, Cinchon., *Coccul.*, Ignat., Kali carb., *Kreos.*, Lycop., Magn. mur., *Merc. viv.*, Natr. mur., NUX VOM., Phosphor., Pulsat., RHUS TOX., Sabin., SEPIA, Silic., *Sulphur*, Thuya, Veratr.

Os coccygis; pains in the: Arnic., *Arsen.*, Borax, *Calc. carb.*, Carb. veg., Caustic., Cinchon., Graphit., *Hepar*, Ignat., *Merc. viv.*, Phosph. ac., RHUS TOX., *Sulphur.*

Upper limbs; pains in the: Anac., *Ant. tart.*, *Arnic.*, ARSEN., *Bellad.*, *Bryon.*, CALC. CARB., Canthar., Carb. veg., Chamom., *Cinchon.*, *Coffea*, Digit., Helleb., Ignat., Ledum, LYCOP., MERC. VIV., *Merc. corr.*, Nitrum, NUX VOM., Opium, Phosphor., *Pulsat.*, RHODOD., RHUS TOX., Sabad., *Sepia*, SULPHUR, Tarax., Zinc.

— — **joints,** of the: *Calc. carb.*, Caustic., Cinchon., HELLEB., Kali carb., Ledum, Lycop., *Merc. viv.*, Nitrum, *Nux vom.*, Phosphor., Phosph. ac., RHUS TOX., Sarsap., *Sepia*, SULPHUR, *Thuya*, Zinc.

Hands; blue: Amm. carb., Apis, Baryt., *Calc. carb.*, Camphor., SAMBUC., *Veratr.*

— **cold:** Arnic., Bellad., *Camphor.*, *Caustic.*, Chamom., Cinchon., Ipecac., Lycop., Mezer., NITR. AC., *Nux vom.*,

Phosphor., *Rhus tox.*, SAMBUC., Scilla, *Selen.*, *Sepia*, SULPHUR, Thuya, *Veratr.*

Hands; dead, as if: *Calc. carb.*, Lycop., *Nux vom.*, Pulsat., Sepia, Thuya, Zinc.

— **distention of the blood vessels:** Amm. carb., Baryt., Phosphor., *Sulphur*, Thuya.

— **heat,** of the: Acon., *Calc. carb.*, Helleb., Lycop., NUX VOM., Opium, Phosphor., Scilla, SEPIA, Staphis.

— **jerking** of the: Bryon., *Chamom.*, Cina, Cinchon., Cuprum, Ignat., *Opium*, Rheum, RHUS TOX.

— **trembling** of the: Ant. tart., *Bryon.*, Cinchon., Coccul., *Merc. viv.*, Opium, Phosphor., *Rhus tox.*, *Sulphur.*

Thumbs turned in: *Bellad.*, *Chamom.*, Hyosc., Ignat., Stann., Stramon., Viol. tr.

Fingers; cold: Ant. tart., Chamom., *Chelid.*, Tarax., Thuya.

— **dead,** as if: Amm. mur., Ant. tart., *Arsen.*, *Calc. carb.*, *Chamom.*, Chelid., Hepar, NUX VOM., Pulsat., SULPHUR, Thuya, *Veratr.*

— **heat** of the: Sabad., *Thuya.*

— **shrivelling** of the: Ambra, ANT. CRUD., Cuprum, MERC. VIV., *Phosph. ac.*, Veratr.

Nails blue: *Chelid.*, Cinchon., Coccul., Digit., Natr. mur., *Nitr. ac.*, Silic.

Lower limbs; pains in the: Amm. carb., ANT. TART., *Arnic.*, ARSEN., Baryt., Bellad., Bovist., Bryon., *Calc. carb.*, Canthar., Carb. veg., Caustic., *Cinchon.*, *Helleb.*, Ignat., Ledum, *Lycop.*, MERC. VIV., *Merc. corr.*, NATR. MUR., *Nitrum*, NUX VOM., Opium, *Phosphor.*, *Phosph. ac.*, Pulsat., *Rhodod.*, RHUS TOX., Ruta, SABAD., SEPIA, Silic., SULPHUR., *Tarax.*, Thuya, Veratr.

— **heaviness** of the: Bellad., *Calc. carb.*, Canthar., *Cinchon.*, Helleb., Ignat., Mezer., Natr. carb., Natr. mur., NUX VOM., Phosphor., *Pulsat.*, *Rhus tox.*, *Sepia*, Stann., SULPHUR, Thuya.

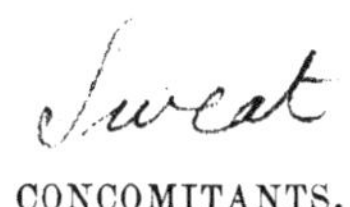

Lower limbs; restlessness of the: Alum., Amm. carb., *Arnic.*, ARSEN., *Bellad.*, Bovist., *Bryon.*, CALC. CARB., Carb. veg., Caustic., Ipecac., LYCOP., *Merc. viv.*, Mosch., *Nitr. ac.*, *Phosphor.*, *Phosph. ac.*, RHUS TOX., Ruta, Scilla, SEPIA, Silic., SULPHUR, Thuya.

Hips; pains in the: Acon., *Arnic.*, Arsen., Bellad., *Calc. carb.*, *Caustic.*, Chamom., Hepar, Merc. viv., Nux vom., Pulsat., RHUS TOX., Ruta, *Sepia*, Staphis., *Sulphur.*

Thighs; pains in the: Arnic., ARSEN., Cinchon., *Merc. viv.*, Mezer., NATR. MUR., Nux vom., Rhus tox., *Sepia*, Staphis., Thuya.

— **coldness** of the: Calad., Calc. carb., Nux vom., *Sulphur*, Thuya.

Knees; pains in the: Baryt., Bryon., CALC. CARB., Caustic., Cinchon., Ferr., HELLEB., Ledum, Lycop., *Merc. viv.*, Natr. mur., *Nux vom.*, Phosphor., Pulsat., RHUS TOX., SEPIA, Stann., Staphis, SULPHUR, Thuya, Veratr.

— **coldness** of the: Agn. cast., *Arsen.*, Cinchon., Pulsat., SEPIA, *Sulphur.*

Legs; pains in the: Acon., *Amm. carb.*, Bellad., Bryon., CALC. CARB., Graphit., Ignat., *Lycop.*, Merc. viv., Mezer., Nux vom., Phosph. ac., Pulsat., SEPIA, Silic., Staphis., *Sulphur.*

Feet; cold: Acon., Ant. crud., Ant. tart., Arnic., *Calc. carb.*, *Caustic.*, Cinchon., Conium, Graphit., Ipecac., Laches., LYCOP., Nitr. ac., NUX VOM., Phosphor., Podophyl., Pulsat., *Rhus tox.*, SAMBUC., Scilla, Selen., SEPIA, Silic., SULPHUR, Thuya, Veratr.

— **dead,** as if: Bellad., *Calc. carb.*, Graphit., *Sulphur.*

— **heat** of the: Acon., Bryon., Ledum, *Nux vom.*, *Phosphor.*, Pulsat., Scilla, Staphis, Sulphur.

— **swelling** of the: *Arsen.*, *Calc. carb.*, Caustic., *Ferr.*, *Lycop.*, Merc. viv., Natr. carb., Natr. mur., Phosphor., Phosph. ac., Pulsat., *Sepia*, Silic., *Sulphur*, Sulph. ac.

Limbs; pains in the, in general: Acon., Alum., Ant. crud., *Ant. tart.*, Apis, Arnic., *Arsen.*, Bellad., *Bryon.*, CALC.

CARB., Capsic., Carb. veg., Caustic., *Chamom.*, *Cinchon.*, Colchic., Dulcam., Ferr., *Helleb.*, *Ignat.*, Kali carb., LYCOP., MERC. VIV., *Merc. corr.*, Nitrum, NUX VOM., Phosphor., Pulsat., *Rhodod.*, RHUS TOX., Sabad., SEPIA, Silic., SULPHUR, Tarax., Thuya, Veratr, Zinc.

Limbs; bending and stretching the: Alum., Bellad., *Borax*, Bryon., CALC. CARB., Caustic., Chamom., *Natr. mur.*, *Nux vom.*, RHUS TOX., *Sabad.*, Sepia, Spong., Sulphur.

— **beaten, feel** as if: *Arnic.*, Arsen., Bellad., Bryon., Calc. carb., CINCHON., Coccul., *Hepar*, Ignat., Magn. carb., Merc. viv., Mosch., *Natr. mur.*, NUX VOM., Phosphor., Phosph. ac., *Pulsat.*, RHODOD., Rhus tox., Ruta, *Sepia*, Silic., Spigel., *Sulphur*, Thuya, Valer., *Veratr.*

— **crawling** in the: *Acon.*, *Arnic.*, ARSEN., Colchic., Platin., RHUS TOX., Secal., *Sepia*, Silic., Stramon.

— **heaviness** of the: Apis, *Bellad.*, CALC. CARB., Helleb., Merc. viv., NUX VOM., RHUS TOX., Stramon., Staphis., *Sulphur.*

— **lameness** of the: Acon., Arnic., ARSEN., Bellad., Cina, Coccul., Cyclam., *Ignat.*, *Nux vom.*, Phosph. ac., Pulsat., *Sabad.*, Sabin.

— **go "to-sleep"**: Apis, *Calc. carb.*, Carb. an., Carb. veg., *Chamom.*, Cinchon., Coccul., Graphit., Ignat., Kali carb., LYCOP., MERC. VIV., Natr. mur., NUX VOM., Petrol., Phosphor., Pulsat., Rhodod., *Rhus tox.*, Sepia, *Silic.*, Sulphur, *Thuya*, Veratr.

Apoplexy: Acon., *Bellad.*, Calc. carb., Coccul., Hyosc., Laches., Lycop., *Nux vom.*, OPIUM, Sepia, Silic., Stramon., Thuya.

Blood-vessels; beating in the: *Acon.*, *Arsen.*, BELLAD., Calc. carb., Cinchon., Graphit., Hepar, Merc. viv., *Nux vom.*, Opium, Phosphor., Pulsat., *Rhus tox.*, Sabad., *Selen.*, SEPIA, Sulphur, Thuya, Zinc.

— **burning** in the: *Arsen.*, Bryon., Hyosc., Rhus tox.

— **distention** of the: Amm. carb., Arnic., *Bellad.*, *Camphor.*, *Cinchon.*, Coccul., *Crocus*, Cyclam., FERR., Hyosc., Lycop.,

Phosphor., *Phosph. ac.*, Pulsat., *Rhus tox.*, *Sepia*, Staphis., Sulphur, *Thuya.*

Excitability; nervous: Acon., Apis, Bellad., Capsic., CHAMOM., *Cinchon.*, *Coffea*, Ferr., Kali carb., *Mar. ver.*, NUX VOM., Petrol., Phosph. ac., SEPIA, Sulphur, Valer., Veratr.

Fainting: Arnic., *Bryon.*, Ignat., *Nux vom.*, *Petrol.*, *Selen.*, Sulphur, Therid., *Thuya.*

Floccillation: Acon., *Arsen.*, BELLAD., Chamom., Cinchon., *Hepar*, Hyosc., Iod., MUR. AC., *Opium*, *Phosphor.*, *Phosph. ac.*, *Rhus tox.*, Stramon., *Sulphur*, Thuya.

Insensibility: Arsen., *Bellad.*, Calc. carb., Cann. sat., Caustic., *Hyosc.*, Ignat., *Lycop.*, MUR. AC., *Opium*, *Phosphor.*, *Phosph. ac.*, Pulsat., Rhus tox., *Stramon.*, Thuya.

Jerkings: Arsen., Bellad., *Bryon.*, Caustic., *Chamom.*, Coloc., Cuprum, Hyosc., Ignat., Menyanth., Merc. viv., Natr. mur., Nux vom., OPIUM, Pulsat., *Rhus tox.*, Secal., Stramon., Sulphur, Thuya, Veratr., Viol. tr.

Lassitude (weakness): Acon., Ambra, Anac., *Ant. crud.*, Ant. tart., *Apis*, Argent., Arnic., ARSEN., *Baryt.*, Bellad., Borax, BRYON., Calad., CALC. CARB., *Camphor.*, Canthar., *Carb. an.*, *Carb. veg.*, Caustic., CINCHON., COCCUL., Crocus, *Cuprum*, *Digit.*, Droser., FERR., Graphit., *Hyosc.*, *Ignat.*, IOD., *Ipecac.*, Kali carb., Kreos., Lauroc., *Lycop.*, Menyanth., MERC. VIV., *Natr. carb.*, *Natr. mur.*, Nitrum, NITR. AC., Nux mosch., NUX VOM., *Phosphor.*, *Phosph. ac.*, Plumbum, *Pulsat.*, Rheum, *Rhodod.*, *Rhus tox.*, *Sabad.*, SAMBUC., *Sepia*, *Silic.*, Spigel., *Stann.*, SULPHUR, *Tarax.*, Thuya, *Veratr.*

Lie down; desire to: *Acon.*, Apis, ARSEN., *Bryon.*, Calad., Canthar., *Chamom.*, Coccul., Cyclam., NUX VOM., Sepia.

Muscles; jerking of the: *Bellad.*, Coloc., Cuprum, Iod., *Kali carb.*, Mezer., Natr. carb., *Opium*, *Platin.*, RHUS TOX., Secal., Spong., Viol. tr.

Prostration: Apis, Carb. veg., Caustic., CINCHON.,

Lycop., Merc. viv., *Petrol.*, Phosphor., *Phosph. ac.*, Sambuc., *Selen.*, Spong., Stann., Valer.

Restlessness; bodily: *Acon.*, Amm. carb., Anac., Ant. tart., *Arnic.*, ARSEN., *Baryt.*, *Bellad.*, *Bovist.*, BRYON., CALC. CARB., Cann. sat., Carb. veg., *Chamom.*, Cinchon., Coffea, Ferr., *Hyosc.*, Ignat., *Ipecac.*, *Lycop.*, *Magn. carb.*, Magn. mur., MERC. VIV., Merc. corr., *Mosch.*, *Mur. ac.*, Nitr. ac., *Nux vom.*, Opium, Phosphor., *Phosph. ac.*, Platin., Pulsat., Rheum, RHUS TOX., *Ruta*, *Sabin.*, *Sambuc.*, SEPIA, Silic., Spong., Staphis., Stramon., Thuya, Valer., Veratr.

Spasms; clonic: BELLAD., CHAMOM., Cicut., Coccul., *Cuprum*, *Hyosc.*, OPIUM, *Sepia*, Stramon., Thuya, Veratr.

— **tonic:** *Bellad.*, Cicut., *Coccul.*, Nux vom., Petrol., Platin., Sepia, *Veratr.*

Stitches; bones, in the: *Bellad.*, *Calc. carb.*, Caustic., Conium, *Helleb.*, Merc. viv., *Pulsat.*, Sarsap., Sepia.

— **joints,** in the: Baryt., *Calc. carb.*, HELLEB., Kali carb., Merc. viv., RHUS TOX., Silic., Spigel., Tarax., Thuya.

— **muscles,** in the: *Bellad.*, BRYON., Calc. carb., Merc. viv., Pulsat., *Rhus tox.*, Spigel., Staphis., Sulphur, Tarax., Thuya.

Tearing (drawing); bones, in the: Argent., *Cinchon.*, Cyclam., Kali carb., Merc. viv., Rhodod., Sabin., Staphis.

— **joints,** in the: Agn. cast., *Calc. carb.*, *Caustic.*, HELLEB., Kali carb., Lycop., Merc. viv., Nux vom., Phosphor., Phosph. ac., RHUS TOX., Strontia, *Sulphur*, Thuya, Zinc.

— **muscles,** in the: Acon., Ant. crud., *Arnic.*, *Arsen.*, Bellad., *Bryon.*, CALC. CARB., Capsic., *Carb. veg.*, Caustic., *Chamom.*, Chelid., *Cinchon.*, Colchic., Dulcam., Ferr., Hepar, Ignat., Kali carb., Ledum, *Lycop.*, *Merc. viv.*, Merc. corr., Nitrum, Nitr. ac., NUX VOM., Phosphor., Pulsat., Rhodod., *Rhus tox.*, SEPIA, Silic., Staphis., Strontia, *Sulphur*, Tarax., Veratr., Zinc.

Trembling: Arnic., ARSEN., Bellad., Borax, Bryon, *Calc. carb.*, Camphor., Cicut., Coccul., Conium, *Ignat.*, Lycop., *Magn. mur.*, Merc. viv., NATR. CARB., *Natr. mur.*, Opium,

Platin., *Pulsat.*, RHUS TOX., *Ruta*, SEPIA, Stramon., SULPHUR, *Thuya*, Valer., Veratr., *Zinc.*

Uncover; desire to: Acon., Apis, Asar., *Bovist.*, CALC. CARB., Chamom., Coffea, *Euphorb.*, FERR., *Fluor. ac.*, Ignat., Iod., *Ledum*, *Lycop.*, *Mosch.*, MUR. AC., *Nitr. ac.*, OPIUM, Phosphor., Phosph. ac., Platin., *Pulsat.*, Secal., Seneg., Spigel., Staphis., *Sulphur*, Thuya, Veratr.

Uncovering; unbearable: Amm. carb., Aurum, Carb. an., Carb. veg., Cicut., *Cinchon.*, CLEMAT., Coccul., Coffea, Colchic., Conium, GRAPHIT., HEPAR, Kali carb., Kreos., Laches., *Magn. carb.*, Merc. viv., NATR. CARB., Natr. mur., Nux mosch., NUX VOM., *Petrol.*, Rhodod., RHUS TOX., Sabad., SAMBUC., *Scilla*, *Sepia*, Silic., Stramon., STRONTIA, Viol. tr.

Stretching and bending of the limbs: Alum., Bellad., BORAX, Bryon., CALC. CARB., Caustic., Chamom., NATR. MUR., *Nux vom.*, RHUS TOX., *Sabad.*, Sepia, Spong., Sulphur.

Yawning: Arnic., *Arsen.*, Bryon., Caustic., Cina, Crocus, Ignat., *Kali carb.*, Kreos., *Nitr. ac.*, NUX VOM., Opium, Phosphor., Platin., *Rhus tox.*, *Sabad.*, SEPIA.

Sleepiness: *Acon.*, Ant. crud., ANT. TART., *Apis*, Arnic., Arsen., *Asaf.*, BELLAD., Borax, CALAD., Capsic., CHAMOM., *Cina*, Crocus, Cyclam., *Hepar*, *Ignat.*, Kali carb., Laches., Lycop., MEZER., Mosch., Natr. carb., Natr. mur., *Nitr. ac.*, *Nux mosch.*, Nux vom., OPIUM, Petrol., *Phosphor.*, *Phosph. ac.*, *Plumbum*, PULSAT., Rhus tox., SABAD., Sepia, Stramon., Sulphur, Veratr., Viol. tr.

Sleep: Acon., Anac., *Ant. tart.*, *Apis*, Arnic., BELLAD., *Calad.*, Calc. carb., *Camphor.*, *Capsic.*, Cicut., Conium, Crocus, Dulcam., Hepar, Hyosc., IGNAT., Laches., Ledum, Merc. viv., Merc. corr., *Mezer.*, Natr. carb., Natr. mur., NITR. AC., Nux mosch., OPIUM, Petrol., *Phosphor.*, Phosph. ac., Pulsat., *Sabad.*, Secal., Spong., Stramon., Valer., Veratr.

— **after the sweat:** *Ant. tart.*, Arnic., ARSEN., Borax, *Calad.*, *Chamom.*, Ignat., Mezer., Natr. mur., Nux mosch., OPIUM, Plumbum, *Rhus tox.*, Sabad., Sepia.

During sleep; blowing exhalation: *Cinchon.*

— **dreaming:** Acon., ARSEN., Bryon., Cinchon., *Nux vom.*, PHOSPHOR., Phosph. ac., *Pulsat.*, Rhus tox., Sabad., SEPIA, *Silic.*, *Spigel.*, Staphis., *Sulphur*, Thuya.

— **moaning and lamenting:** Acon., Arnic., Baryt., *Bellad.*, Bryon., Calad., Calc. carb., *Chamom.*, Coccul., *Ignat.*, Ipecac., *Mur. ac.*, Nux vom., Pulsat., Silic., Stramon., Thuya.

— **murmuring:** Apis, Bellad., *Mur. ac.*, Opium, *Phosphor.*, Phosph. ac., *Rhus tox.*, Silic.

— **sliding down in bed:** Arsen., *Mur. ac.*

— **snoring:** Anac., *Cinchon.*, Graphit., Hyosc., Ignat., *Mur. ac.*, Nux vom., OPIUM, *Silic.*, Stramon.

— **starting:** *Acon.*, Apis, Arnic., BELLAD., Bryon., *Chamom.*, Cinchon., Ipecac., *Lycop.*, Nux vom., Phosphor., PULSAT., Sambuc., *Sepia*, Silic., Sulphur.

Somnolence: Acon., ANT. TART., *Apis*, Bellad., Calc. carb., Camphor., Cicut., *Cinchon.*, Conium, Crocus, Hepar, Hyosc., Ipecac., Ledum, Nux mosch., OPIUM, Phosphor., Phosph. ac., PULSAT., RHUS TOX., Secal., Spong., Stramon., Valer., Veratr.

Sleeplessness: Alum., Amm. carb., Amm. mur., ANAC., *Apis*, Arnic., *Arsen.*, Baryt., Bellad., Borax, *Bryon.*, *Calc. carb.*, Cann. sat., Carb. veg., Caustic., *Chamom.*, *Chelid.*, Cicut., CINCHON., *Clemat.*, Coccul., COFFEA, Conium, Droser., Graphit., Hepar, Ignat., Kreos., Lauroc., Ledum, Magn. carb., Magn. mur., Mangan., *Merc. viv.*, Merc. corr., Mosch., Natr. mur., Nitrum, *Nitr. ac.*, Nux mosch., Nux vom., Petrol., *Phosphor.*, PHOSPH. AC., *Pulsat.*, *Ran. bulb.*, Ran. scel., *Rhodod.*, RHUS TOX., *Sabad.*, *Sabin.*, Sarsap., *Selen.*, Sepia, Silic., Staphis., Strontia, *Sulphur*, *Tarax.*, *Thuya*, Veratr.

Bone-pains: *Arnic.*, Cinchon., Ignat., Natr. mur., *Pulsat.*

Glands; swelling of the: *Bellad.*, Lycop., Merc. viv., Nitr. ac., Phosphor., Rhus tox., *Sepia*, *Silic.*, Sulphur.

Skin; burning: Acon., ARSEN., Bellad., Bryon., Capsic., Laches., Lycop., MERC. VIV., Mezer., *Natr. carb.*, Petrol., Phosphor., Pulsat., *Rhus tox.*, SEPIA, Silic., Stann., *Veratr.*

— **cold:** Lachnanth.

— **crawling and prickling:** Arnic., ARSEN., *Coccul.*, Colchic., *Crocus*, *Nux vom.*, Platin., *Pulsat.*, RHODOD., RHUS TOX., Selen., *Sepia*, Spigel., Sulphur, *Tarax.*, Thuya.

— **eruptions:** *Apis*, Arsen., Bryon., Calc. carb., *Conium*, Ipecac., Lycop., Natr. mur., OPIUM, Pulsat., RHUS TOX., SEPIA, Sulphur, *Thuya.*

— **itching:** *Amm. carb.*, Ant. crud., Baryt., Bryon., CALC. CARB., Chamom., *Coloc.*, *Fluor. ac.*, Ipecac., *Ledum*, LYCOP., MANGAN., Merc. viv., Opium, Paris, Pulsat., RHODOD., RHUS TOX., *Sabad.*, Silic., SPONG., Staphis., *Sulphur*, Thuya, Viol. tr.

— **pungent heat:** Eup. perf.

— **smarting** on the: CHAMOM., *Conium*, *Ipecac.*, *Paris*, Pulsat., Tarax.

PART III.

RELATION OF THE FEVER STAGES.

---

1. BEGINNING WITH CHILL.

Chill; then heat: ACON., *Alum.*, Ambra, Amm. carb., Amm. mur., Ant. crud., *Ant. tart.*, Apis, *Arnic.*, Arsen., Asar., Baryt., *Bellad.*, Borax, Bryon., Cact. grand., Calc. carb., Canthar., *Capsic.*, Carb. an., *Carb. veg.*, Caustic., Chamom., *Cina*, *Cinchon.*, Coffea, Corn. cir., Crocus, CYCLAM., Diadem.,

Digit., *Droser.*, Dulcam., *Graphit.*, Guaiac., Helleb., *Hepar*, HYOSC., IOD., IGNAT., IPECAC., Kali carb., Kreos., Laches., Lauroc., *Lycop.*, *Magn. carb.*, Magn. mur., Merc. viv., Merc. corr., *Natr. carb.*, NATR. MUR., Nitrum, Nitr. ac., Nux mosch., NUX VOM., Opium, *Petrol.*, *Phosphor.*, Phosph. ac., PULSAT., RHUS TOX., *Sabad.*, Scilla, *Secal.*, Sepia, *Spigel.*, *Spong.*, Staphis., *Stramon.*, SULPHUR, Thuya, *Valer.*, Veratr.

Chill; then **sensation of heat:** Menyanth., Sulphur.

— then **heat; of single spots:** Cyclam.

— — **face,** of the: Acon., *Ambra*, Cinchon., Cyclam., Kali carb., Kreos., *Nux vom.*, Opium, *Petrol.*, Stramon.

— — **head,** in the: Ipecac.

— — **with thirst:** *Acon.*, *Bellad.*, Borax, Cina, Droser., *Hepar*, Merc. viv., *Pulsat.*, *Rhus tox.*, Secal., Spigel., Sulphur.

— — **without thirst:** Amm. mur., Borax, Canthar., Cina, Coffea, Nux mosch., Phosph. ac., Rhus tox., *Spigel.*, Sulphur.

— — — and **without sweat:** Sepia.

— **with thirst,** then heat: Cina.

— — then **heat without thirst,** then sweat: Ignat.

— — then **heat with thirst,** then sweat: Corn. flor., Spong.

— **without thirst,** then heat with thirst: Petrol.

— — then **heat with,** then sweat without, then heat with thirst: Ant. crud.

— — then **heat without thirst:** Arsen., Cyclam., Droser., Helleb., Phosph. ac.

— then **heat, both with thirst:** Ant. crud.

— — then **chill with thirst:** Sulphur.

Chill; then heat, then sweat: Amm. carb., Amm. mur., Apis, ARSEN., Bellad., Bovist., *Bryon.*, Cact. grand., Capsic., Carb. an., Carb. veg., Caustic., Chamom., Cina, *Cinchon.*, Coccul., Corn. cir., Digit., Droser., *Eup. perf.*, *Eup. purp.*, Gelsem., *Graphit.*, Hepar, *Ignat.*, IPECAC., Kali carb., *Laches.*, Lycop.,

Magn. mur., Natr. carb., *Natr. mur.*, Nitr. ac., NUX VOM., Opium, Plumbum, PULSAT., *Rhus tox.*, *Sabad.*, Sabin., Sambuc., Sepia, *Spong.*, Staphis., *Sulphur*, Thuya, *Veratr.*

Chill; then heat, alternating with thirst, then **sweat:** Sabad.

— — then **sweat with thirst:** Rhus tox.

— — then **sweat without thirst:** Amm. mur., Nitr. ac.

— — then **sour sweat:** Lycop.

Chill; then **heat, with sweat:** *Acon.*, Ant. tart., BELLAD., Bryon., Capsic., Carb. veg., CHAMOM., Cina, *Cinchon.*, Corn. cir., Digit., Eup. perf., Graphit., Helleb., Hepar, Ignat., Kali carb., Mezer., Nitr. ac., *Nux vom.*, *Opium*, Phosphor., *Pulsat.*, RHUS TOX., *Sabad.*, Spigel., Sulphur.

— — **without sweat:** Graphit., Natr. mur.

— — **with sweat of the face:** Alum.

— — **with internal chill,** then heat and sweat: Phosphor.

— **with thirst,** then heat without thirst: *Hepar*, Nitrum.

— — — then **sweat:** Kali carb.

Chill; with simultaneous heat: ACON., Agn. cast., Alum., Amm. carb., Anac., Ant. tart., *Arnic.*, ARSEN., Baryt., *Bellad.*, Bovist., Bryon., CALC. CARB., Camphor., Canthar., Carb. veg., CHAMOM., Cina, Cinchon., *Coccul.*, COFFEA, Colchic., Coloc., *Digit.*, Euphorb., Graphit., *Helleb.*, IGNAT., Iod., Kali carb., Laches., Ledum, Lycop., *Merc. viv.*, *Mezer.*, Mosch., Natr. carb., NITR. AC., *Nux vom.*, Oleand., *Paris*, Petrol., Phosphor., Phosph. ac., Platin., PLUMBUM, *Pulsat.*, Ran. bulb., RHUS TOX., Sabad., Sambuc., *Scilla*, Selen., *Sepia*, Silic., *Spigel.*, Spong., *Sulphur*, THUYA, VERATR., *Zinc.*

— **with external heat:** Acon., Agn. cast., *Anac.*, *Arnic.*, *Arsen.*, *Bellad.*, Bryon., CALC. CARB., Cinchon., *Coccul.*, *Coffea*, Colchic., *Digit.*, *Helleb.*, IGNAT., Laches., *Lauroc.*, Lycop., *Menyanth.*, Merc. viv., Mezer., Nitrum, NUX VOM.,

Phosphor., Plumbum, *Ran. bulb.*, Rheum, *Scilla*, Selen., SEPIA, Silic., Sulphur, THUYA.

Chill: with flushes of heat: Arsen., Merc. viv., Platin., *Pulsat.*

— **with internal** heat: ACON., Arnic., ARSEN., Bellad., *Bryon.*, Calc. carb., *Chamom.*, Chelid., Cinchon., *Euphorb.*, Helleb., *Ignat.*, Iod., *Kali carb.*, Merc. viv., *Mezer.*, *Mosch.*, Nitr. ac., Nux vom., Oleand., Phosph. ac., *Pulsat.*, *Rhus tox.*, Sabad., *Scilla*, Secal., Spong., Stann., *Sulphur*, VERATR., *Zinc.*

— **with sensation** of heat: Oleand.

— **with internal** heat and thirst: Calc. carb., Kali carb.

— **with heat,** both internal: Petrol.

— **of single parts** with heat of others: Cinchon., *Ignat.*, Nux vom., *Rhus tox.*, Sabad.

— **with heat, without sweat:** Sulphur.

— — **with sweat:** Nux vom., *Veratr.*

— — then **sweat:** Graphit.

Chill; then sweat (without intervening heat): Amm. mur., *Bryon.*, Cact. grand., CAPSIC., *Carb. an.*, Carb. veg., CAUSTIC., Chamom., Chelid., *Clemat.*, Diadem., *Digit.*, Helleb., Hyosc., LYCOP., Merc. viv., Merc. corr., MEZER., Natr. mur., Natr. sulph., *Nitrum*, Nux vom., Opium, PETROL., Phosphor., Phosph. ac., *Rhus tox.*, Sabad., Sepia, Spigel., THUYA, *Veratr.*

— then **cold sweat:** Arsen., *Veratr.*

— then **sweat without heat** or thirst: Amm. mur., Bryon., Caustic.

— then **sweat,** then **heat:** Bellad.

— then **thirst:** Lycop.

— then **thirst,** then **sweat:** Thuya.

Chill alternating with heat: *Agn. cast.*, *Ambra*, Amm. carb., AMM. MUR., *Ant. tart.*, Arnic., ARSEN., *Asar.*,

Aurum, *Baryt.*, BELLAD., Borax, *Bryon.*, CALC. CARB., Canthar., Caustic., *Chamom.*, Chelid., CINCHON., *Coccul.*, Coffea, Coloc., Corn. cir., *Digit.*, Droser., Eup. perf., Graphit., HEPAR, *Hyosc.*, Iod., Kali carb., *Kreos.*, LACHES., Lachnanth., Lauroc., Ledum, *Lycop.*, MERC. VIV., Mosch., Natr. mur., Nitrum, Nitr. ac., NUX VOM., *Phosphor.*, *Phosph. ac.*, Rheum, Rhodod., RHUS TOX., Sabad., Sambuc., *Selen.*, Sepia, Silic., *Spigel.*, Stramon., Sulphur, Valer., *Veratr.*, *Zinc.*

Chill; alternating with heat, then **heat:** Veratr.

— — — then **sweat:** Bryon., *Kali carb.*, Spigel.

— **alternating with sweat:** Arsen., Calc. carb., *Euphorb.*, Ledum, Lycop., Nux vom., Pulsat., Sabad., Sulphur, Thuya, *Veratr.*

2. BEGINNING WITH HEAT.

Heat; then chill: Apis, Angust., *Bellad.*, *Bryon.*, Calad., CALC. CARB., Capsic., *Caustic.*, Cinchon., Dulcam., Eup. purp., *Helleb.*, Ignat., Lycop., Menyanth., Merc. viv., *Nitr. ac.*, NUX VOM., Petrol., Phosphor., Pulsat., SEPIA, STANN., *Staphis.*, *Sulphur*, Thuya.

— — then **heat,** then **sweat:** Rhus tox.

— then **coldness:** Calc. carb., Caustic., *Nux vom.*, Sepia, Sulphur.

— of the **face,** then **chill:** *Calc. carb.*, Lycop., Menyanth., Staphis., Sulphur.

— then **shivering:** *Angust.*, Capsic., Coccul., Helleb., Natr. mur., Pulsat., Rhus tox., *Sulphur.*

— of the **face,** then **shivering:** Sulphur.

— of the **head,** then **coldness,** then **heat:** Stramon.

— then **sweat:** *Amm. mur.*, Ant. crud., Ant. tart., ARSEN., Bellad., Borax, Bryon., Calc. carb., Carb. an., Carb. veg., CHAMOM., Cina, *Cinchon.*, COFFEA, Corn. cir., Graphit., Helleb., Hepar, *Ignat.*, *Ipecac.*, Kreos., Laches., Lobel. inf., Lycop., *Mangan.*, Nitr. ac., *Nux vom.*, Opium, Petrol., Pulsat., *Ran. scel.*, Rhodod., RHUS TOX., *Silic.*, Spong., Staphis., Strontia, Sulphur, VERATR.

Heat; then sweat, with sleep: Lobel. inf.

— then **cold sweat:** Capsic., *Veratr.*

— then **sweat,** then **thirst:** Calad.

— — then **heat:** Ant. crud.

Heat; with internal chill: Acon., *Anac.*, Arsen., *Bellad.*, Bryon., Calc. carb., Coffea, *Ignat.*, *Laches.*, Lauroc., Lycop., Menyanth., Merc. viv., Nitrum, *Nux vom.*, Phosphor., Sepia, Silic., Thuya.

— in the **head,** alternating with **chilliness** (in the legs): Sepia, Stramon.

— **and thirst,** alternating with **chill:** Calc. carb.

— **with external coldness:** Arnic., *Arsen.*, *Bellad.*, Bryon., *Calc. carb.*, Cinchon., Euphorb., Helleb., Iod., Merc. viv., *Mezer.*, Mosch., Phosphor., Phosph. ac., Pulsat., Rhus tox., *Sabad.*, Spong., Stann., *Veratr.*

— **with coldness** of single parts: Cinchon., Ignat., *Nux vom.*, Rhus tox.

Heat; with shivering: Acon., Arnic., Asar., *Bellad.*, Bryon., *Chamom.*, Coffea, *Helleb.*, Ignat., Lobel. inf., Merc. viv., Mosch., *Nux vom.*, Pulsat., *Rhus tox.*, Sepia, Spigel., Sulphur, *Zinc.*

— — **and thirst:** Capsic.

— — **without thirst:** *Helleb.*, Spigel.

— — then **sweat:** Capsic.

— alternating with **shivering:** Acon., *Bryon.*, *Coccul.*, *Ipecac.*, Laches., Mosch., Phosph. ac., *Platin.* (See shivering alternating with heat.)

Heat, with sweat: Acon., Alum., Amm. mur., *Bellad.*, Bryon., *Calc. carb.*, CAPSIC., *Chamom.*, Cina, Cinchon., *Conium*, Euphorb., HELLEB., *Hepar*, Ignat., *Ipecac.*, Lauroc., Lobel. inf., Merc. viv., NATR. CARB., Nitr. ac., *Nux vom.*, *Opium*, Paris, Phosphor., Plumbum, Psorin., Pulsat., RHUS

TOX., *Sabad.*, *Sarsap.*, Sepia, Spigel., Spong., STANN., *Staphis.*, STRAMON., Sulphur, SULPH. AC., Tarax., Thuya, *Valer.*, *Veratr.*, Viol. tr.

Heat; with sweat and thirst: Conium, Hepar, Merc. viv., Rhus tox.

— — **without thirst:** Amm. mur., Bellad., Bryon., Capsic., Hepar, Nux vom., Phosphor., Spigel., Stramon., Veratr.

— — **and thirst,** then **slight chilliness:** Stann.

— — then **chill:** Stann.

— — **with external coldness,** then **chill,** then **heat** with external coldness: Phosphor.

— alternating with **sweat:** *Amm. mur.*, Bellad., *Cinchon.*, Colchic., LEDUM, Natr. carb., Nux vom., *Sambuc.*, Sepia, Sulphur.

— **with thirst,** then **sweat:** Coffea, Lobel. inf.

3. BEGINNING WITH SHIVERING.

Shivering; then chill: Arsen., *Bryon.*, Ipecac., Laches.,

— — **without thirst:** Ipecac.

— — **then heat,** without sweat: Arsen.

— then **heat:** Angust., Apis, Asar., *Bellad.*, Bryon., Canthar., Carb. veg., Coccul., Conium, Cyclam., Graphit., *Ignat.*, Laches., Lauroc., Ledum, Mosch., Nux vom., *Sepia*, Silic., Staphis., *Sulphur.*

— — **with chill:** Bryon., Laches.

— — **with thirst:** Conium, Sulphur.

— then **sweat:** Bryon., Capsic., Caustic., *Clemat.*, Digit., Graphit., *Natr. mur.*, *Rhus tox.*

Shivering with heat: Acon., Anac., Arnic., Arsen., Asar., BELLAD., Bryon., Calc. carb., Capsic., *Chamom.*, Coffea, Droser., HELLEB., Ignat., Kali carb., Merc. viv., Mosch., *Nux vom.*, Pulsat., Rheum, *Rhus tox.*, Sepia, Spigel., Sulphur, *Zinc.*

Shivering; with heat of the face, without thirst: Anac., Arsen., Calc. carb., Droser., Kali carb.

— **with sweat:** Acon., *Rhus tox.*

Shivering alternating with heat: Acon., Amm. carb., ARSEN., Asar., *Bellad.*, Borax, Bryon., Calc. carb., Caustic., *Chamom.*, Chelid., Cinchon., *Coccul.*, Coffea, Coloc., Graphit., Hepar, Kali carb., Laches., MERC. VIV., Mosch., *Nux vom.*, Phosphor., Phosph. ac., *Platin.*, Rheum, Rhus tox., Sabad., *Sepia*, Silic., Spigel., Sulphur, Veratr.

4. BEGINNING WITH SWEAT.

Sweat, then chill: *Carb. veg.*, Corn. cir., Hepar, Nux vom.

— — then **sweat:** Nux vom.

— then **heat:** Capsic., *Nux vom.*

— alternating with **dryness of the skin:** *Apis.*

PART IV.

PATHOLOGICAL NAMES

OF THE

VARIOUS FEVERS.

Bilious fever: ACON., Alum., Ant. crud., Ant. tart., Arnic., *Arsen.*, Asaf., Asar., Aurum, *Baptis.*, BELLAD., *Bryon.*, Calc. carb., CHAMOM., Cinchon., Coccul., *Coffea*, COLOC., Corn. flor., Crocus, Cuprum, *Digit.*, *Eup. perf.*, *Gelsem.*, *Graphit.*, Hyosc., IGNAT., Ipecac., *Laches.*, Leptand., *Lycop.*, Magn. carb., Magn. mur., Merc. viv., Mezer., *Mur. ac.*, Natr. carb., Natr. mur., Nux mosch., NUX VOM., *Opium*, Petrol., *Phosphor.*, Phosph. ac., PLATIN., *Podophyl.*, *Pulsat.*,

Ran. bulb., Rhus tox., Sambuc., Secal., Selen., Seneg., Sepia, Silic., Spong., Stann., STAPHIS., Stramon., Strontia, Sulphur, Tarax., Veratr., Verbas., Zinc.

Catarrhal fever: Acon., Æsc. hip., Arsen., *Arum tr.*, Asar., *Baptis.*, *Bellad.*, BRYON., Camphor., Caustic., CHAMOM., Cinchon., Coccul., Coffea, Conium, *Dulcam.*, Eup. perf., Gelsem., Ignat., Ipecac., Mangan., Merc. viv., NUX VOM., Phosphor., *Pulsat.*, Rhus tox., Sabad., Scilla, Silic., Spigel., Stann., Sulphur, Veratr.

Cinchona fever: Amm. carb., Ant. tart., *Apis*, ARNIC., ARSEN., Asaf., *Bellad.*, Bryon., *Calc. carb.*, Capsic., CARB. VEG., Chamom., *Cina*, Cuprum, Cyclam., Digit., FERR., Helleb., IPECAC., *Laches.*, Mangan., Merc. viv., *Natr. mur.*, Nux mosch., Nux vom., Phosphor., *Phosph. ac.*, Plumbum, PULSAT., Sambuc., *Sepia*, Stann., Sulphur, Sulph. ac., *Veratr.*

Congestive (chills): Acon., Bellad., Chin. sulph., Gelsem., *Glonoin.*, Hyosc., Opium, Veratr.

Fever; overheating, from: ACON., Amm. carb., ANT. CRUD., Bellad., *Bryon.*, *Camphor.*, Capsic., *Carb. veg.*, Coffea, *Digit.*, Hepar, Ignat., Ipecac., KALI CARB., Mezer., Natr. mur., Nux mosch., Nux vom., Oleand., *Opium*, *Phosphor.*, Sepia, Silic., Staphis., THUYA, *Zinc.*

— **taking cold,** from: ACON., Agar., Alum., Amm. carb., Anac., *Ant. crud.*, Arnic., *Arsen.*, Aurum, Baryt., BELLAD., BRYON., *Calc. carb.*, Camphor., *Carb. veg.*, Caustic., CHAMOM., *Cinchon.*, Coccul., COFFEA, *Coloc.*, *Conium*, Crocus, Cuprum, *Cyclam.*, Digit., Droser., DULCAM., *Fluor. ac.*, *Graphit.*, *Hepar*, HYOSC., Ignat., *Ipecac.*, Kali carb., Ledum, *Lycop.*, Magn. carb., *Mangan.*, MERC. VIV., Natr. carb., *Natr. mur.*, *Nitr. ac.*, Nux mosch., NUX VOM., Opium, Petrol., PHOSPHOR., Phosph. ac., Platin., PULSAT., Ran. bulb., RHUS TOX., Ruta, Sabin., *Sambuc.*, Sarsap., Selen., *Sepia*, SILIC., SPIGEL., Stann., Staphis., Strontia, SULPHUR, Sulph. ac., Valer., *Veratr.*

— — **bathing,** from: *Ant. crud.*, Arsen., *Bellad.*, CALC.

CARB., Carb. veg., Caustic., *Ignat.*, Mangan., *Nitr. ac.*, Phosphor., RHUS TOX., Sarsap., *Sepia*, Sulphur.

Fever; taking cold, getting wet through, from: *Acon.*, ALUM., Amm. carb., Ant. tart., *Arnic.*, Arsen., *Bellad.*, Borax, BRYON., CALC. CARB., Camphor., Carb. veg., Caustic., *Colchic.*, *Dulcam.*, Euphorb., Fluor. ac., *Hepar*, *Hyosc.*, *Ipecac.*, *Kali carb.*, *Laches.*, *Lycop.*, Natr. mur., Nitr. ac., *Nux mosch.*, Phosphor., Plumbum, *Pulsat.*, RHUS TOX., *Sarsap.*, SEPIA, Sulphur, Veratr., Zinc.

— — — **sweating,** while: *Acon.*, Calc. carb., *Clemat.*, COLCHIC., *Dulcam.*, RHUS TOX., *Sepia.*

— — **getting the head wet:** *Baryt.*, BELLAD., Hepar, Hyosc., Ledum, Phosphor., *Pulsat.*, *Sepia.*

— — **getting the feet wet;** *Baryt.*, Bryon., Camphor., Chamom., *Colchic.*, Dulcam., Fluor. ac., *Laches.*, *Lycop.*, Merc. viv., *Natr. carb.*, PULSAT., *Rhus tox.*, *Sepia*, SILIC.

Gastric fever: Acon., Act. rac., *Ant. crud.*, *Ant. tart.*, Arsen., Asaf., *Asar.*, Aurum, Baptis., Bellad., *Bryon.*, Cact. grand., *Chamom.*, Cinchon., *Coccul.*, Coffea, Colchic., Coloc., Corn. cir., Cuprum, Cyclam., *Digit.*, *Eup. perf.*, Gelsem., Hydrast., Ignat., IPECAC., Magn. mur., Merc. viv., Mezer., *Mur. ac.*, Natr. carb., NUX VOM., Plumbum, Podophyl., PULSAT., Rheum, *Rhus tox.*, Scilla, Secal., Staphis., *Sulphur*, Tarax., *Veratr.*

Hectic fever: ARSEN., Asar., Baryt., Bellad., *Bryon.*, CALC. CARB., Carb. veg., *Cinchon.*, Coccul., Conium, Cuprum, Digit., Droser., Dulcam., Ferr., Gelsem., Graphit., Guaiac., Helleb., Hepar, Ignat., IOD., *Ipecac.*, KALI CARB., Laches., Ledum, LYCOP., Merc. viv., Merc. corr., Natr. carb., Natr. mur., Nitr. ac., *Nux vom.*, PHOSPHOR., *Phosph. ac.*, PULSAT., Sanguin., *Sepia*, *Silic.*, *Stann.*, Staphis., SULPHUR, Sulph. ac., *Thuya*, Veratr., Zinc.

Inflammatory fever: ACON., *Apis*, Arnic., *Arsen.*, Asar., Baryt., BELLAD., BRYON., Cact. grand., Calad., Calc. carb., Camphor., Cann. sat., *Canthar.*, Caustic., *Chamom.*, Cinchon., Coccul., Coffea, Colchic., Coloc., Conium, Digit., Droser., Dulcam., Gelsem., Hepar, *Hyosc.*, Ignat., Ipecac., Kali carb.,

Laches., Lauroc., *Lycop.*, MERC. VIV., Mezer., Natr. carb., Natr. mur., *Nitrum*, Nitr. ac., NUX VOM., Opium, PHOSPHOR., PULSAT., Rhus tox., Sabad., Scilla, Secal., Seneg., Sepia, *Silic.*, Spigel., Spong., Staphis., Stramon., Sulphur, Sulph. ac., Veratr.

Intermittent fever: Acon., Act. rac., Æsc. hip., Alum., Anac., Ant. crud., Ant. tart., *Apis*, Arnic., ARSEN., Asar., Baryt., *Bellad.*, Bovist., *Bryon.*, *Cact. grand.*, Calad., *Calc. carb.*, Camphor., Cann. sat., Canthar., CAPSIC., Carb. an., *Carb. veg.*, Caustic., Chamom., Chelid., Chin. sulph., Cicut., CINCHON., CIMEX., *Cina*, Cist. can., Clemat., Coccul., Coffea, Colchic., Corn. cir., Corn. flor., Crocus, *Cuprum*, Cyclam., DIADEM., Droser., Euphras., EUP. PERF., EUP. PURP., *Ferr.*, Fluor. ac., Gelsem., Graphit., Helleb., Hepar, Hydrast., Hydr. ac., Hyosc., *Ignat.*, Iod., IPECAC., Kali bichr., Kali carb., *Laches.*, Lachnanth., Leptand., Lobel. inf., Lycop., Magn. carb., Magn. mur., Mangan., Menyanth., Merc. viv., Mezer., Mosch., Natr. carb., *Natr. mur.*, Natr. sulph., Nitrum, Nitr. ac., Nux mosch., NUX VOM., Opium, *Petrol.*, Phosphor., Phosph. ac., Plumbum, Podophyl., Psorin., PULSAT., Ran. bulb., Ran. scel., Rheum, Rhodod., *Rhus tox.*, *Sabad.*, Sabin., Sambuc., Sanguin., Secal., Selen., *Sepia*, Silic., *Spigel.*, Spong., *Staphis.*, Stramon., SULPHUR, Sulph. ac., *Thuya*, Valer., *Veratr.*, Zinc.

— **infantile:** Arsen., Canthar., Cinchon., Cina, Laches., Natr. mur., Nux vom., Opium, Veratr.

— **quotidian:** *Acon.*, Alum., Apis, *Arnic.*, ARSEN., Bellad., *Bryon.*, *Cact. grand.*, Calc. carb., Camphor., CAPSIC., Carb. veg., Chamom., Chin. sulph., Cicut., Cina, Cinchon., Conium, *Cyclam.*, *Diadem.*, Droser., Eup. perf., Eup. purp., Ferr., Graphit., Hydrast., Hyosc., *Ignat.*, IPECAC., Kali carb., *Laches.*, Lobel. inf., Lycop., Menyanth., *Natr. mur.*, Nitrum, Nitr. ac., NUX VOM., Opium, Petrol., Podophyl., PULSAT., Rhus tox., Sabad., *Sambuc.*, Sepia, Spigel., Stann., Staphis., *Stramon.*, *Sulphur*, Thuya, Veratr.

— — **double:** *Arsen.*, *Bellad.*, Cinchon., Dulcam., *Graphit.*, Nux mosch., *Pulsat.*, Rhus tox., *Stramon.*, Sulphur.

Intermitent fever; tertian: Alum., Anac., *Ant. crud.*, Apis, Arnic., ARSEN., Baryt., *Bellad.*, *Bryon.*, *Calc. carb.*, CANTHAR., CAPSIC., Carb. veg., *Chamom.*, Cicut., Cina, Cinchon., Diadem., Droser., Dulcam., EUP. PERF., EUP. PURP., Ferr., Gelsem., Helleb., Hyosc., Ignat., IPECAC., *Laches.*, Lycop., Menyanth., Merc. viv., Mezer., *Natr. mur.*, Nux mosch., NUX VOM., Petrol., PULSAT., Podophyl., Ran. bulb., *Rhus tox.*, *Sabad.*, Sepia, Silic., Staphis., *Sulphur*, *Thuya*, *Veratr.*, Zinc.

— — **double:** Apis, ARSEN., Bellad., Cinchon., Dulcam., Eup. perf., Graphit., Nux mosch., *Pulsat.*, RHUS TOX., Stramon., Thuya, Veratr.

— **quartan:** Acon., Alum., *Anac.*, Apis, *Arnic.*, ARSEN., Bellad., Bryon., *Carb. veg.*, Cina, Cinchon., *Clemat.*, Eup. perf., *Hyosc.*, *Ignat.*, Iod., Ipecac., *Laches.*, LYCOP., Natr. carb., *Natr. mur.*, Nitr. ac., Nux mosch., *Nux vom.*, Petrol., Podophyl., PULSAT., Rhus tox., SABAD., Sepia, Sulphur, Thuya, *Veratr.*

Measles: ACON., *Ant. crud.*, *Apis*, Arsen., *Bellad.*, Bryon., Camphor., Carb. veg., Chamom., Cinchon., Coffea, Droser., *Euphras.*, *Gelsem.*, Hepar, Hyosc., Ignat., *Ipecac.*, KALI BICHR., Kali carb., Magn. carb., Nux vom., *Phosphor.*, PULSAT., *Rhus tox.*, Stramon., Sulphur, Veratr.

Milk fever: *Acon.*, Arnic., Arsen., *Bellad.*, Borax, *Bryon.*, CALC. CARB., Carb. veg., *Chamom.*, Cinchon., *Coffea*, Conium, Dulcam., Ignat., Kali carb., *Laches.*, Merc. viv., Nux vom., Opium, Phosphor., *Phosph. ac.*, PULSAT., Rhus tox., Scilla, SEPIA, *Silic.*, Staphis., Sulphur, Zinc.

Mucous fever: Alum., Arsen., *Asar.*, Bellad., Borax, Bryon., CALC. CARB., Chamom., Cina, *Cinchon.*, Digit., *Dulcam.*, Graphit., Hyosc., *Ignat.*, Ipecac., Lycop., *Merc. viv.*, Merc. corr., Mezer., *Nux vom.*, Paris, PHOSPHOR., PULSAT., Rheum, *Rhus tox.*, Selen., Seneg., Sepia, Spigel., Stann., SULPHUR, Sulph. ac., *Thuya*, Zinc.

Nervous fever: Acon., Argent., Arnic., *Arsen.*, *Bellad.*, BRYON., Camphor., Carb. veg., Chamom., Cinchon., Coccul.,

Cuprum, Helleb., *Hyosc.*, *Laches.*, Lachnanth., Lycop., *Merc. viv.*, Merc. corr., Mezer., MUR. AC., Natr. mur., Nitrum, Nux mosch., *Nux vom.*, *Opium*, Phosphor., *Phosph. ac.*, Pulsat., RHUS TOX., Stramon., *Sulphur*, Sulph. ac., Veratr.

Puerperal fever: ACON., Act. rac., Ant. crud., *Arnic.*, Arsen., BELLAD., BRYON., Calc. carb., Carb. an., CHAMOM., Cinchon., Coccul., Coffea, *Coloc.*, Conium, Crocus, Ferr., *Hyosc.*, Ipecac., Kali carb., Merc. viv., NUX VOM., Opium, Phosphor., *Platin.*, PULSAT., RHUS TOX., Sabin., *Secal.*, *Sepia*, Stramon., Sulphur, Veratr., Zinc.

Putrid fever: Arnic., *Arsen.*, Bellad., BRYON., Canthar., Carb. veg., *Cinchon.*, Digit., *Hyosc.*, Ipecac., *Merc. viv.*, Merc. corr., *Mur. ac.*, Nux mosch., *Nux vom.*, Opium, Phosphor., Phosph. ac., Pulsat., RHUS TOX., Sulphur.

Remittent fever; adynamic form: Arnic., Arsen., Bryon., Camphor., Carb. veg., Chin. sulph., Ferr., Gelsem., Hydr. ac., Laches., Phosph. ac., Podophyl., Rhus tox., Veratr.

— **comatose form:** Bellad., Gelsem., Hyosc., Laches., *Nux mosch.*, *Opium*, *Pulsat.*, STRAMON.

— **infantile:** Gelsem., Leptand., Podophyl., *Stramon.*

Rheumatic fever: ACON., *Act. rac.*, Ant. crud., Ant. tart., *Apis*, Arnic., *Arsen.*, Baptis., BELLAD., BRYON., Cact. grand., Calc. carb., Camphor., Cann. sat., Carb. veg., Caustic., CHAMOM., *Cinchon.*, Coffea, Colchic., Cuprum, Dulcam., Euphras., *Gelsem.*, Ignat., Ipecac., Laches., *Merc. viv.*, Mezer., *Nux vom.*, Phosphor., *Pulsat.*, Ran. bulb., Rhodod., RHUS TOX., Sabad., Scilla, Silic., Stann., Staphis., *Sulphur*, Thuya, Valer., Veratr.

Scarlatina (true, smooth): Amm. carb., Arum tr., Bellad., Calc. carb., Euphorb., Hyosc., Merc. viv., Thuya, Sulphur.

— **(common form):** *Acon.*, AMM. CARB., Amm. mur., *Apis*, Arnic., *Arsen.*, ARUM TR., Baryt., BELLAD., *Bryon.*, Calc. carb., Camphor., Carb. veg., Caustic., Chamom., Coffea, Colchic., *Crocus.*, Cuprum, Dulcam., Euphorb., Gelsem., Hepar, *Hyosc.*, Iod., Ipecac., Kali carb., Laches., Lycop., MERC. VIV.,

Mur. ac., Nitr. ac., Opium, Phosphor., Phosph. ac., Rhus tox., Silic., Stramon., *Sulphur*, Thuya, *Zinc.*

Slow fever: *Arsen.*, Bellad., Camphor., Cinchon., Coccul., Conium, Cuprum, Digit., Ferr., Helleb., Hyosc., Ignat., Iod., Merc. viv., Merc. corr., Nux vom., PHOSPHOR., *Phosph. ac.*, Sepia, Stann., Staphis., Veratr.

Spotted fever; (Cerebro Spinal Meningitis): Acon., *Act. rac. Apis*, ARGENT. NIT., *Arnic.*, Arum tr., Baptis., Bellad., Bryon., Chin. sulph., *Cicut.*, Crotal., *Cuprum*, *Eup. perf.*, Gelsem., Hyosc., Lycop., Opium, Pulsat.

Sweating sickness: Acon., ARSEN., Bryon., Calc. carb., Cinchon., SAMBUC., *Sepia*, Sulphur.

Teething fever: ACON., Agar., Bellad., Borax, Bryon., CALC. CARB., CHAMOM., Cicut., Coffea, Cuprum, Hepar, Hyosc., Ignat., Ipecac., Laches., Merc. viv., Merc. corr., Nitr. ac., *Nux vom.*, Pulsat., Rheum, Rhus tox., Secal., *Silic.*, Stramon., *Sulphur*, Thuya.

Traumatic fever: *Acon.*, Apis, *Arnic.*, Bryon., Carb. veg., Crocus, Euphras., Hepar, *Laches.*, Merc. viv., Natr. carb., *Nitr. ac.*, Phosphor., Phosph. ac., *Pulsat.*, *Rhus tox.*, *Staphis.*, Sulphur, *Sulph. ac.*

Typhus fever; (typhoid): *Act. rac.*, Ant. tart., *Apis*, *Arnic.*, ARSEN., Asar., BAPTIS., Bellad., BRYON., Calc. carb., *Carb. veg.*, *Cinchon.*, Coccul., Colchic., Corn. flor., Cuprum, Digit., Eup. perf., Fluor. ac,, *Gelsem.*, *Hyosc.*, Hydr. ac., Ignat., *Laches.*, Lachnanth., Leptand., LYCOP., Merc. viv., Merc. corr., Mosch., *Mur. ac.*, Nux mosch., Nitr. ac., Nux vom., Opium, Phosphor., *Phosph. ac.*, Podophyl., Psorin., Pulsat., RHUS TOX., Silic., Stramon., *Sulphur*, Sulph. ac., *Tarax*, Veratr., Zinc.

Variola: Act. rac., Amm. mur., Ant. crud., *Ant. tart.*, Apis, Arnic., Arsen., Baptis., Bellad., BRYON., Clemat., Camphor., Coccul., *Hydrast.*, (Hydr. ac.), Hyosc., *Merc. viv.*, Mur. ac., Phosphor., Pulsat., *Rhus tox.*, Silic., *Sulphur*, THUYA.

Worm fever: ACON., Ambra, Anac., Arsen., Asar., CALC. CARB., Cicut., CINA, CINCHON., Digit., Ferr.,

Gelsem., *Graphit.*, Hyosc., Ignat., Kali carb., Mar. ver., *Merc. viv.*, Natr. mur., Nux mosch., Nux vom., Petrol., Phosphor., *Platin.*, Pulsat., Ruta, SABAD., Sabin., SILIC., *Spigel.*, *Spong.*, Stramon., SULPHUR, Thuya, Valer.

Yellow fever: *Acon.*, Act. rac., Amm. carb., Ant. tart., *Apis*, Argent., *Arnic.*, ARSEN., BELLAD., Bryon., *Camphor.*, Canthar., Carb. veg., Chamom., Cinchon., Chamom., Coloc., Cuprum, Digit., Eup. perf., Gelsem., Helleb., Ipecac., LACHES., Merc. viv., Nitr. ac., NUX VOM., Phosphor., Plumbum, Pulsat., Rhus tox., Sabad., *Sepia*, Sulphur, Veratr.

CATALOGUE
OF WORKS ON
HOMŒOPATHY,
PUBLISHED BY
BOERICKE & TAFEL,

NEW YORK.

NOTICE.

Printed prices in our Catalogue are those at which books can generally be supplied by Pharmacies and Booksellers throughout the United States, who can readily procure for their customers any works not kept in stock. Where access to Bookstores or Pharmacies is not convenient, books will be sent by Mail post paid on receipt of price.—*But no risks are assumed on books thus ordered.*

A descriptive catalogue of medicine-cases and books, specially adapted for family use will be sent free on application.—Address: Boericke & Tafel, Homœopathic Pharmacy, 145 Grand St. New York.

All Homœopathic works published in England and Germany are constantly kept on hand, also a fair assortment of works in the French, Italian, and Spanish languages, complete catalogues of which will be sent free on application.

Address: BOERICKE & TAFEL,
NEW YORK.

Aconite, Monograph on, its Therapeutic and Physiological Effects, together with its Uses and Accurate Statements, derived from the Various Sources of Medical Literature, by A. Reil, M. D. Translated from the German by H. B. Millard, M. D. Prize Essay. 168 Pages. 8vo. 75 cts.

Annual Record of Homœopathic Literature 1870. Edited by C. G. Raue, M. D. 496 Pages. 8vo. $3.50.

☞ In the preparation of the Annual Record, Professor Raue has been assisted by an able corps of collaborators, and no labor or expense has been spared to have the whole a complete *digest of all the valuable information* scattered throughout the periodical literature of Homœopathy, during the year 1869. The Journals of the United States, England, Germany, France, Spain, and other countries, have furnished materials for this great work.

Annual Record of Homœopathic Literature, 1871. Edited by C. G. Raue, M. D. 255 Pages. 8vo. $2.50. N. B. The third Vol. will soon be in the printer's hands.

☞ The arrangement of the work is the same as that of last year. Dr. C. Hering has arranged the part on Materia Medica, Dr. T. F. Allen, the chapter on the eye, Dr. M. McFarlan, the surgical part, and the rest by Dr. C. G. Raue. There is no Appendix to this volume.

Apis Mellifica, or the Poison of the Honey Bee, considered as a Therapeutic Agent. By Dr. C. W. Wolff. 80 pages. 12mo. 25 Cents.

Baehr, Dr. B. The Science of Therapeutics, according to the Principles of Homœopathy, by B. BAEHR, M. D. Translated and enriched with numerous additions from Kafka and other sources. By C. J. Hempel, M. D. 2 vols. 1,387 pages. Royal 8vo. $10.00.

☞ This work is to take the place of the late Hartmann's Acute and Chronic Diseases, but in point of scientific value and practical usefulness, it is far superior to the former. Dr. Hempel has incorporated large sections from Kafka in the same, has also on suitable occasions introduced the new remedies and has made valuable additions from our Journals and his personal records.

Becker, Dr. A. C. Diseases of the Digestive Organs and Constipation, treated homœopathically. Second American from the third London Edition, with Additions. 128 pages. 12mo. 50 Cents.

Becker, Dr. A. C. Dentition according to some of the best and latest German Authorities. 82 pages. 12mo. 50 Cents.

Becker, Dr. A. C. Diseases of the Eye, treated homœopathically. From the German. 77 pages. 12mo. 50 Cents.

Bell, Dr. Jas. B. The Homœopathic Therapeutics of Diarrhœa, Dysentery, Cholera, Cholera morbus, Cholera infantum and all other loose evacuations of the Bowels. 168 pages. Bound in Muslin. 12mo. $1.25.
Interleaved with writing paper, half morocco. $2.25.

Berjeau, J. Ph. The Homœopathic Treatment of Syphilis, Gonorrhœa, Spermatorrhœa and Urinary Diseases. Revised with numerous additions. By J. H. P. Frost, M. D. 256 pages. 12mo. $1.50.

Boenninghausen, Dr. C. Essay on the Homœopathic Treatment of Intermittent Fever. Translated and edited by C. J. Hempel, M. D. 8vo. 50 Cents.

Boenninghausen, Dr. C. The Sides of the Body and Drug Affinities. Homœopathic Exercises. Translated and edited by J. C. Hempel, M.D. 12mo. 25 cts.

Boenninghausen, Dr. C. Therapeutic Pocket Book for Homœopathic Physicians, to be used at the bedside of the Patient and in Studying the Materia Medica Pura. 510 pages. 8vo. $3.00.

Breyfogle, Dr. W. L. Epitome of Homœopathic Medicines. 383 pages. 12mo. $1.50.
Interleaved with writing paper, half morocco. 18mo. $3.00.

☞ This work differs from other Epitomes, in treating of a larger number of remedies, and in the arrangement of its material in comparative form. The leading symptoms of all well-established provings are here arranged in as concise form as possible.

Bryant, Dr. J. A Pocket Manual or Repertory of Homœopathic Medicine, Alphabetically and Nosologically arranged; which may be used as the Physicians' Vade-Mecum, the Travellers' Medical Companion or the Family Physician, Containing the Principal Remedies for the most important Diseases, Symptoms. Sensations, Characteristics of Diseases, etc., with the Principal Pathogenetic Effects of the Medicines on the most important Organs and Functions of the Body, together with Diagnosis, Explanation of Technical Terms, Directions for the Selection and Exhibition of Remedies, Rules of Diet, etc. Compiled from the best Homœopathic Authorities. Third Edition. 352 pages. 18mo .$2.00.

Buchner, J. Morbus Brighti, translated by S. Lilienthal, M. D. $1.25

Burt, Dr. W. H. Characteristic Materia Medica. 460 pages. 12mo. $3.00.
Interleaved with writing paper, half morocco. $5.00.

☞ In this work the author gives the *characteristic symptoms* or key-notes of two hundred and three remedies, and has adopted the method of grouping those remedies which produce similar physico pathological and pathogenetic symptoms.

Caspari's Homœopathic Domestic Physician, edited by F. Hartmann, M. D., Author of the Acute and Chronic Diseases. Translated from the Eighth German Edition, and enriched by a Treatise on Anatomy and Physiology, by W. P. Esrey, M. D., with additions and a preface, by C. Hering, M. D. Containing also a Tabular Index of the Medicines and the Diseases, in which they are used, etc. With 30 illustrations. 475 pages. 8vo. $1.00.

Cockburn, Dr. S. Medical Reform; being an Examination into the Nature of the Prevailing System of Medicine, and an Exposition of some of its Chief Evils, with Allopathic Revelations. A Remedy for the Evil. 180 pages. 18mo. 50 cts.

Curtis, J. T., M. D. and **J. Lillie,** M. D. An Epitome of Homœopathic Practice, compiled chiefly from Jahr, Ruckert, Beauvais, Bœnninghausen, etc. 206 pages. 18mo. 75 Cents.

☞ This handy little volume contains the most prominent symptoms of 119 remedies, to which is added a well-arranged Repertory.

Douglas, Dr. J. S. Homœopathic Treatment of Intermittent Fevers. 108 pages. 18mo. 38 Cents.

Ellis, Dr. John. The Avoidable Causes of Disease, Insanity and Deformity. 12mo. $2.00.

Ellis, Dr. John. Family Homœopathy. 12mo. $1.50.

Franklin, Dr. E. C. The Science and Art of Surgery, embracing minor and operative Surgery, compiled from Standard Allopathic Authorities and adapted to Homœopathic Therapeutics, etc. Vol. I. 8vo. $8.00.

Goullon, Dr. H. On Scrofulous Diseases, translated by E. Tietze, M. D. (In Press.)

Gray & Hempel. Homœopathic Examiner. 2 Vols. 8vo. Bound $5.00.

Gross, Dr. H. Comparative Materia Medica, edited by C. Hering, M. D. Royal 8vo. Extra heavy tinted paper. $10.00.

☞ In this work the remedies are arranged alphabetically, so that in the left hand column will be found the remedy to be compared, and in the right hand column the remedies it is compared with, also in alphabetical order. The whole is enriched by numerous marginal annotations and remarks by the illustrious Editor.

Guernsey, Dr. H. N. The application of the Principles and Practice of Homœopathy to Obstetrics, and the Disorders peculiar to women and young children. With nearly one hundred illustrations. Second Edition. (In Press.)

Guernsey, Dr. E. Homœopathic Domestic Practice. With full descriptions, and the Dose in each single case. Containing also chapters on Anatomy, Physiology, Hygiene and an abridged Materia Medica. Ninth enlarged, revised and improved edition. 653 pages. 8vo. $2.50.

Guernsey, Dr. E. The Gentleman's Hand Book of Homœopathy, especially for Travellers and for Domestic Practice. 255 pages. 12mo. $1.00.

Hahnemann, Dr. S. The Lesser Writings of, collected and translated by R. E. Dudgeon, M. D. With a Preface and Notes by E. E. Marcy, M. D. With a steel engraving of Hahnemann, from the statue by Steinhauser. 784 pages. 8vo. $4.00.

☞ This valuable work contains a large number of Essays, of great interest to laymen as well as medical men, upon Diet, the Prevention of Diseases, Ventilation of Dwellings, etc. As many of these papers were written before the discovery of the Homœopathic Theory of cure, the reader will be enabled to peruse in this volume the ideas of a gigantic intellect when directed to subjects of general and practical interest.

Hahnemann, Dr. S. Materia Medica Pura, translated by C. J. Hempel, M. D. 808 pages. 8vo. $9.00.

☞ This famous work gives the pathogenesis of fifty-one remedies, and ought not to be missed in any Homœopathic Physician's library.

Hahnemann, Dr. S. The Chronic Diseases; their specific Nature and Homœopathic Treatment. Translated and edited by C. J. Hempel, M. D. With a Preface by C. Hering, M. D. 5 vols. 12mo. $10.00.

Hahnemann, Dr. S. Organon of Homœopathic Medicine. Fourth American Edition, with improvements and additions from the last German Edition, and Dr. C. Hering's Introductory Remarks. 229 pages. 8vo. $1.50.

Hale, Dr. E. M. Lecture on diseases of the heart. In three Parts. Part I. Functional Diseases of the Heart. Part II. Inflammatory Affections of the Heart. Part III. Organic Diseases of the Heart. 203 pages. 8vo. $2.00.

Hartmann, Dr. F. Diseases of Children and their Homœopathic Treatment, with Notes, and prepared for the use of the American and English professions, by C. J. Hempel, M. D. 509 pages. 12mo. $3.00.

☞ The present work on the diseases of children, is undoubtedly the best work which our school possesses on this interesting subject. In describing the pathognomic character of all the principal diseases, the author has not contented himself with furnishing notes from his own experience, but he has given the eminently interesting and scientific diagnosis of such pathologists as Schoenlein, Canstatt, Heim and others, thus imparting to his work a truly scientific character, which scarcely any similar work in our literature can boast of.

Helmuth, Dr. W. T. Surgery and its Adaptation to Homœopathic Practice. Illustrated with numerous Engravings on Wood. 651 pages. 8vo. $3.50.

Hempel, Dr. C. J. Homœopathic Domestic. in German. 12mo. 75 Cents.
" " in French. 12mo. 75 Cents.

Hempel, Dr. C. J. Organon of Specific Homœopathy, or an Inductive Exposition of the Principles of the Homœopathic Healing Art. 216 Pages. 8vo. $1.00.

Hempel, Dr. C. J. Homœopathy a Principle in Nature. Its Scientific Universality unfolded; its development and Philosophy explained and its Applicability to the Treatment of Diseases shown. 8vo. $1.00.

Hempel, Dr. C. J. Complete Repertory of the Homœopathic Materia Medica. 1224 pages. 8vo. $6.00.

☞ The object of this work is simply to make the finding of any symptom or group of symptoms which a Physician may be called upon to treat, a matter of perfect certainty; provided always such may exist among the results of our physiological provings. The classifications of the symptoms which has been adopted is more complete, and at the same time more simple and practical than anything of the kind ever published in our language.

Hempel, Dr. C. J. A New and Comprehensive System of Materia Medica and Therapeutics, arranged upon a Physiologico-Pathological Basis, for the use of Practitioners and students of Medicine. Second Edition revised and considerably enlarged. 2 Vols. 1896 pages. Royal 8vo. $12.00.

☞ The second Edition of this standard work contains, in the form of lectures, the pathogenesis of two hundred and twenty-seven remedies, and as these are interspersed with numerous therapeutic remarks, it is generally adapted to the study of Materia Medica.

Hempel, Dr. C. J. and **Dr. J. Beakley.** Homœopathic Theory and Practice; with the Homœopathic Treatment of Surgical Diseases, designed for Students and Practitioners of Medicine, and as a Guide for an intelligent Public generally. Fourth Edition. 1100 pages. 8vo. $3.50.

Henderson & Forbes. An Inquiry into the Homœopathic Practice of Medicine, by W. Henderson, M. D. Homœopathy, Allopathy and Young

Physic, by John Forbes, M. D. and Letter to Dr. John Forbes, by W. Henderson, M. D. 278 pages. 8vo. $1.00.

Hering, Dr. C. Homœopathic Domestic Physician. The only authorized English Edition, by the author himself thoroughly revised and reformed from the latest German Edition. 399 pages. 8vo. $2.50.

Hitchman, Dr. W. Consumption. its Nature, Prevention and Homœopathic Treatment, with illustrations of Homœopathic Practice. 184 pages. 12mo. 75 Cents.

Holcombe, Dr. W. C. Yellow Fever and its Homœopathic Treatment. 12mo. 38 Cents.

Homœopathic Cookery. Second Edition with Additions by the Lady of an American Homœopathic Physician, designed chiefly for the Use of such Persons as are under Homœopathic Treatment. 176 pages. 18mo. 50 Cents.

Hughes, Dr. R. Manual of Pharmacodynamics. 590 pages. 12mo. $2.00.

☞ This work gives in the form of letters the condensed pathogenesis of two-hundred remedies.

Hughes, Dr. R. Manual of Therapeutics. 540 pages. 12mo. $2.00.

☞ This work is a reprint from the English original, like its companion volume "on Pharmacodynamics" and is also intended "for Students and beginners."

Hull, Dr. A. G. Homœopathic Examiner, few copies only remain of this very valuable periodical, three vols. handsomely bound. $15.00.

Hull's Jahr. A New Manual of Homœopathic Practice. Edited with Annotations and Additions by F. G. Snelling, M. D., Sixth American Edition, with an Appendix of the New Remedies, by C. J. Hempel, M. D. 2 vols. 2076 pages. 8vo. $11.00.

☞ This is the most complete work on Materia Medica at present offered for sale. The *first volume* containing the Symptomatology, gives the complete Pathogenesis of 287 remedies, besides which a large number of new remedies were added by Dr. Hempel in the appendix. The second volume contains an admirably arranged *Repertory.* Each chapter is accompanied by copious clinical remarks and the concomitant symptoms of the chief remedies for the malady treated of, thus imparting a mass of information, rendering the work indispensable to every Student and Practitioner of Medicine.

Humphreys, Dr. F. Dysentery and its Homœopathic Treatment. Containing also a Repertory and numerous cases. 87 pages. 18mo. 50 Cents.

Humphreys, Dr. F. The Cholera and its Homœopathic Treatment. 72 pages. 18mo. 38 Cents.

Hydriatics, or Manual of the Water Cure, especially as practiced by Vincent Priesnitz in Græfenberg, compiled and translated from the writings of Dr. Chas. Munde, Dr. Oertel, Dr. B. Hirschel and other eye-witnesses and practitioners. By Francis Græter. 198 pages. 18mo. 50 Cents.

Jahr, Dr. G. H. G. Therapeutic Guide; the most important results of more than Forty Years' Practice, with personal observations regarding the truly reliable and practically verified curative indications in actual cases of disease. Translated with Notes and New Remedies. By C. J. Hempel, M. D. 364 pages. 8vo. $3.50.

Jahr, Dr. G. H. G. Clinical Guide or Pocket Repertory for the Treatment of Acute and Chronic Diseases. Translated by C. J. Hempel, M. D. Second American revised and enlarged Edition, from the third German Edition, enriched by the Addition of the New Remedies. By S. Lilienthal, M. D. 624 pages. 12mo. $3.00.

Jahr, Dr. G. H. G. The Homœopathic Treatment of Diseases of Females and Infants at the Breast. Translated from the French by C. J. Hempel, M. D. 422 pages. 8vo. $2.50.

☞ This work deserves the most careful attention on the part of Homœopathic Practitioners. The diseases to which the female organism is subject, are described with the most minute correctness, and the treatment is likewise indicated with a care that would seem to defy criticism. No one can fail to study this work with profit and pleasure.

Jahr, Dr. G. H. G. Diseases of the Skin; or Alphabetical Repertory of the Skin Symptoms and External Alterations of Substance, together with the Morbid Phenomena observed in the Glandular, Osseous, Mucous and Circulatory Symptoms, arranged with Pathological Remarks on Diseases of the Skin. Edited by C. J. Hempel, M. D 515 pages. 18mo. $1.50.

Jahr, Dr. G. H. G. New Manual of the Homœopathic Materia Medica, with Possart's Additions Arranged with reference to well authenticated Observations at the Sick bed, and accompanied by an alphabetical Repertory, to facilitate and secure the selection of a suitable remedy in any given case. Fifth Edition, revised and enlarged by the Author. SYMPTOMATOLOGY and REPERTORY. Translated and Edited by C. J. Hempel, M. D. 923 pages. 12mo. $4.50.

☞ In this work a condensed Pathogenesis is given of 226 remedies, 82 of which are additions by Possart, and are not contained in Jahr's former works. A well arranged Repertory of 225 pages completes the work, and renders it an admirable companion at the bedside.

Jahr, Dr. G. H. G. The Venereal Diseases, their Pathological Nature, correct Diagnosis, and Homœopathic Treatment. Prepared in accordance with the Author's own, as well as with the experience of other Physicians, and accompanied with critical Discussions. Translated, with numerous and important additions from the works of other authors, and from his own experience. By C. J. Hempel, M. D. 428 pages. 8vo. $4.00.

Index to the first eighteen volumes of the North American Journal of Homœopathy. 8vo. $2.00.

Johnson, Dr. J. D. Therapeutic Key; or Practical Guide for the Homœopathic Treatment of Acute Diseases. 179 pages. Bound in linen. 18mo. $1.25. Bound in flexible cover. $1.75.

Joslin, Dr. B. F. Principles of Homœopathy. In a Series of Lectures. 185 pages. 75 Cents.

Joslin, Dr. B. F. Homœopathic Treatment of Epidemic Cholera. Third Edition, with Additions. 252 pages. 12mo. $1.00.

☞ This work offers the advantage of a threefold arrangement of the principal medicines; viz.: 1st to the varieties of cholera; 2d, to its stages; and 3d, to its symptoms as arranged in repertories. These last will give the work a prominent value, in treating the more frequent complaints of summer.

Kreussler, Dr. E. The Homœopathic Treatment of Acute and Chronic Diseases. Translated from the German, with important Additions and Revisions, by C. I. Hempel, M. D. 190 Pages. 12mo. 75 Cents.

☞ The author is a practitioner of great experience and acknowledged talent. This work is distinguished by concise brevity and lucid simplicity in the description of the various diseases that usually come under the observation of physicians, and the remedies for the various symptoms are carefully indicated. Dr. Hempel has interspersed it with a number of highly useful and interesting notes which cannot fail to enhance the value of this work to American Physicians.

Laurie, Dr. J. Homœopathic Domestic. By A. Gerald Hull, M. D. Small Edition. 264 pages. 18mo. 60 Cents.

Laurie, Dr. J. Elements of Homœopathic Practice of Physic. An

Appendix to Laurie's Domestic, containing also all the Diseases of the Urinary and Genital Organs. 372 pages. 12mo. $1.25.

Laurie, Dr. J. The Parent's Guide. Containing the Diseases of Infancy and Childhood, and their Homœopathic Treatment. To which is added a Treatise on the Method of Rearing Children from their Earliest Infancy; comprising the essential branches of Moral and Physical Education, Edited, with Additions, by W. Williamson, M. D. 460 pages. 12mo. $1.00.

☞ All the diseases to which children are liable, are described in this volume with remarkable conciseness and accuracy, and their treatment is indicated in such plain and precise language that no intelligent parent can have any difficulty in conducting to a satisfactory termination the various diseases described in this work.

Laurie, Dr. J. The Homœopathic Domestic Medicine. First American from the twenty-first English edition. Edited and revised, with numerous important additions, and the introduction of the new remedies, by R. I. McClatchey, M. D. 1034 pages. 8vo. $5.00.

☞ The merits of "Laurie's Homœopathic Domestic Medicine" are best attested by the popularity of the work in Great Britain, where upwards of 21,000 copies have been sold to the most intelligent portion of the community, and in this country the work ran through three editions in the first year.

Lippe, Dr. A. Text Book of Materia Medica, 714 pages. 8vo. $6.00.

This work contains the characteristic and most prominent symptoms of two hundred and ten remedies. It has been introduced into our colleges as a Text Book and was very favorably received by the profession.

Lippe, Dr. A. Key to the Materia Medica, 144 pages. 8vo. 75 Cents

This is the first and only number of a series which were to contain a characteristic Materia Medica. The following remedies are treated of in this number: Aconitum nap., Arsemicum alb., Belladonna, Pulsatilla, Sepia, Sulphur, Phosphorus, Calcarea carb, Tilia europ., Agaricus musc Rhus tox.

Lord, I. S. P. On Intermittent Fever, and other Malarious Diseases. 341 Pages. 8vo. $3.00.

☞ In an introduction of forty-seven pages, the author lays down his theory, and substantiates his views by a record of two hundred and fifteen cases of ague, of all kinds, giving their treatment, and a running commentary thereon. To these a very copious double index—one to the remedies and the other to the spmptoms—serves as a concordance.

Lutze, Dr. A. Manual of Homœopathic Theory and Practice, Designed for the use of Physicians and families. Translated from the German with Additions by C. J. Hempel, M. D. From the 60th Thousand of the German Edition. 750 pages. 8vo. $2.50.

This work, from the pen of the late Dr. Arthur Lutze, has the largest circulation of any homœopathic work in Germany, no less than sixty thousand copies having been sold. The Introduction, occupying over fifty pages, contains the question of dose and rules for examining the patient and diet; the next sixty pages, contain a condensed pathogenesis of the remedies, treated of in the work; the description and treatment of diseases occupy four hundred and eighteen pages, and the whole concludes with one hundred and seventy-three pages of Repertory and a copious Index; thus forming a concise and complete work on Theory and Practice.

Madden, Uterine Diseases, with an Appendix, containing Abstracts of 180 Cases of Uterine Diseases and their Treatment, together with analytical Tables of Results, Ages, Symptoms, Dose, etc., to which is added a Clinical Record of interesting cases, treated in the Manchester Homœopathic Hospital. 111 pages. 8vo. 50 Cents.

Malan, H. Family Guide to the Administration of homœopathic Remedies. 112 pages. 24mo. 30 Cents.

Malan, H. Family Guide, in Spanish 12mo. 75 Cents.

Marcy, Dr. E. E. Homœopathy and Allopathy. Reply to an Examination of the Doctrines and Evidences of Homœopathy, by Worthington Hooker, M. D. 144 pages. 12mo. 50 Cents.

Marcy, Dr. E. E. and F. W. Hunt, M. D. The Homœopathic Theory and Practice of Medicine. 2 vols. 1896 pages. 8vo. $12.00.

☞ Of this work over three thousand copies are in circulation and the demand still continues. It is used as a Text Book in all our Homœopathic Colleges ever since it was published, and is especially recommended to Students of Medicine.

Metcalf, Dr. Jas. W. Homœopathic Provings. Containing the Vienna Provings of Colocynth and Thuja-occidentalis, and the Symptoms of Æthusa-cynapium, Alcohol-sulphuris, Amphisbæna-vermicularis, Anagallis-arvensis, Apis-mellifica, Aristolochia-milhomens, Arsenicum-metallicum, Artemesia-vulgaris, Asterias-rubens, Cinnabaris, Turpethum, Coccus-cacti. 417 pages. 8vo. Bound. $1.50.

Millard, Dr. H. B. The Climate and Statistics of Consumption. Read before the American Geographical and Statistical Society. With extensive additions by the Author. 108 pages. 12mo. 75 Cents.

Morgan, Dr. W. The Homœopathic Treatment of Indigestion, Constipation Hæmorrhoids. Edited with notes and annotations, by A. E. Small, M. D. 166 pages. 12mo. 75 Cents.

☞ Diseases resulting from irregularity or debility of the digestive organs are so frequent in their occurrence, that scarcely a family can be found, in which one or more of its members are not sufferers thereby. The present work gives in a concise manner the hygienic measures as well as the medical treatment that may be observed, calculated not only to obviate the necessity of recourse to dangerous palliatives, but to promote a complete restoration of health.

Morgan, Dr. W. The Text Book for Domestic Practice; being plain and concise directions for the administration of Homœopathic Medicines in single ailments. 191 pages. 24mo. 60 Cents.

Munde, Dr. Chas. Hydriatic Treatment of Scarlet Fever in its different Forms, or how to save, through a Systematic Application of the Water Cure many Thousand Lives and Healths which now annually perish. Being the Result of twenty-one years' Exp rience, and Cure of Several hundred Cases of Eruptive Fevers. Fourth Edition. 92 pages. 12mo. 50 Cents.

Mure, Dr. B. Materia Medica, or Provings of the Principal Animal and Vegetable Poisons of the Brazilian Empire, and their Application in the Treatment of Disease. Translated from the French, and arranged according to Hahnemann's method by C. J. Hempel, M. D. 220 pages. 12mo. $1.00.

☞ This volume, from the pen of the celebrated Dr. Mure, of Rio Janeiro, contains the pathogenesis of thirty-two remedies, a number of which are used in general practice ever since the appearance of the work. A faithful wood-cut of the plant or animal treated accompanies each pathogenesis.

Neidhard, Dr. C. On the Efficacy of Crotalus-horridus in Yellow Fever; also in Malignant, Bilious and Remittent Fevers. With an Account of Humboldt's Prophylactic Inoculation of the Venom of a Serpent, at Havana, Cuba. 82 pages. 8vo. $1.00.

Neidhard, Dr. C. Diphtheria, as it prevailed in the United States from 1860 to 1866, preceded by an Historical Account of its Phenomena, its Nature and Homœopathic Treatment. 176 pages. 8vo. $1.75.

☞ This treatise is the result of the Author's researches, and experience gained by attending about one hundred and eighty malignant or severe cases of Diphtheria and Dyphtheritic croup, and at least four hundred and twenty slighter cases of the disease.

New Provings of Cistus Canadensis, Cobaltum, Zingiber and Mercurius Proto-Iodatus. 96 pages. 8vo. 75 Cents.

North American Journal of Homœopathy. Published Quarterly on the first Days of August, November, February, and May. Edited by S. Lilienthal, M. D. Vol. 1, New Series commenced in August 1869. Subscription Price per volume in advance, $4.00. Complete Sets of the first eighteen volumes, in half Morocco Binding, including index to the same. $75.00. Index to the first 18 volumes, $2.00.

Peters, Dr. J. C. A Complete Treatise on Headaches and Diseases of the Head. 1. The Nature and Treatment of Headaches; 2. The Nature and Treatment of Apoplexy; 3. The Nature and Treatment of Mental Derangement; 4. The Nature and Treatment of Irritation, Congestion, and Inflamation of the Brain and its Membranes. Based on Th. J. Rückert's "Clinical Experience in Homœopathy." 586 pages. 8vo. $3.00.

Peters, Dr. J. C. A Treatise on Apoplexy, with an Appendix on Softening of the Brain, and Paralysis. Based on Th. J. Rückert's "Clinical Experience in Homœopathy." 164 pages. 8vo. $1.00.

Peters, Dr. J. C. The Diseases of Females and Married Females. Second Edition. Two Parts in one volume. 356 pages. 8vo. $1.50.

Peters, Dr. J. C. The Diseases of Married Females. Disorders of Pregnancy, Parturition, and Lactation. 196 pages. 8vo. $1.00.

Peters, Dr. J. C. A Treatise on the Principal Diseases of the Eyes, including Diseases of the Eyelids, Conjunctiva, Correa, Sclerotica, Crystalline Lens, Choroid, Retina and Optic Nerve. Based on Th. J. Rückert's "Clinical Experience in Homœopathy." 291 pages. 8vo. $1.50.

Peters, Dr. J. C. A Treatise on the Internal Diseases of the Eyes, including Diseases of the Iris, Crystalline Lens, Choroid, Retina, and Optic Nerve. Based on Th. J. Rückert's "Clinical Experience in Homœopathy." 123 pages. 8vo. $1.00.

Peters, Dr. J. C. A Treatise on the Inflammatory and Organic Diseases of the Brain. Based on Th. J. Rückert's "Clinical Experiences in Homœopathy." 156 pages. 8vo. $1.00.

Peters, Dr. J. C. A Treatise on Nervous Derangements and Mental Disorders. Based on Th. J. Rückert's "Clinical Experiences in Homœopathy." 104 pages. 8vo. $1.00.

Physician's Visiting List, The Homœopathic. By R. Faulkner, M. D. with a Repertory by W. J. Blakely, M. D. Morocco Gilt Edge. 12mo. $1.50.

☞ This visiting list differs materially from any hitherto published, and has been arranged with a view of affording the physician a book much less cumbersome, than those at present in use, and yet containing everything necessary in a work of this kind. This has been accomplished by increasing the length, and by the omission of a large number of pages usually devoted to subjects entirely foreign, and of which but little use is made by the physician.

Practical Guide to the Treatment of the Common Disorders with Homœopathic Remedies. With Instructions as to Diet and Hygienic Recommendations. 64 pages. 64mo. 20 Cents.

Philadelphia Journal of Homœopathy, edited by W. A. Gardiner, M. D., assisted by the following contributors: Drs. B. F. Joslin, A. H. Okie, H. C. Preston, I. P. Dake, P. P. Wells, W. E. Payne, C. Dunham, Jas. Kitchen, W. S. Helmuth, A. E. Small, S. R. Dubbs. 4 volumes. Bound. 8vo. $8.00.

Rapou, Dr. A. Treatise on Typhoid Fever and its Homœopathic Treatment. Translated from the French by A. A. Granville. 96 pages. 12mo. 50 Cents.

☞ Dr. Rapou has earned his title to instruct us on the subject he has chosen, at the bedside of from seventy to eighty patients attacked with Typhoid Fever, in all degrees of severity of whom he has lost not a single case.

Rau, Dr. G. L. Organon of the Specific Healing Art of Homœopathy. By C. J. Hempel, M. D. 200 pages. 8vo. $1.25.

Raue, Dr. C. G. Special Pathology and Diagnosis, with Therapeutic Hints. 644 pages. Extra 8vo. $5.00.

☞ This standard work is used as a Text Book in all our colleges, and is found in almost every physician's library. An especially commendable feature is, that it contains the application of nearly all the *new remedies* contained in Dr. Hale's work on Materia Medica.

Raue, Dr. C. G. Annual Record of Homœopathic Literature, 1870. 496 pages. 8vo. $3.50.

Raue, Dr. C. G. Annual Record of Homœopathic Literature, 1871. 8vo. $2.50.

Reil, Dr. A. Monograph on Aconite, its Therapeutic and Physiological Effects, together with its Uses and Accurate Statements, derived from the various sources of Medical Literature. Translated from the German by H. B. Millard, M. D. Prize Essay. 168 pages. 8vo. 75 Cents.

☞ Few remedies in the Materia Medica enjoy a higher and more deserved reputation for usefulness than that which is the subject of this Monograph, or have received more consideration from writers eminent in medicine, of every age and school. The Essay of Dr. Reil, containing the most recent facts and experience in relation to the subject, and completely exhausting, as it does, everything of interest connected with it, may be justly regarded as the most thorough and complete treatise upon Aconite ever yet presented.

Rokitansky's Pathological Anatomy. The Abnormal Conditions of the Organs of Respiration. Translated from the German, with Additions on Diagnosis, from Schönlein, Skoda and others, by J. C. Peters, M. D. 164 pages. 8vo. 75 Cents.

☞ Rokitansky's book is what it professes to be; it is morbid anatomy in its densest and most compact form, scarcely ever alleviated by cases, histories or hypotheses; it is just such a work as might be expected from its author, who is said to have written in it the results of his experience gained in the careful examination of over 12,000 bodies, and who is possessed of a truly marvelous power of observing and amassing facts.

Rueckert, Dr. E. F. Therapeutics; or Successful Homœopathic Cures, collected from the best Homœopathic Periodicals. Translated and Edited by C. J. Hempel, M. D. 496 pages. 8vo. $4.00.

☞ We possess a rich treasure of successful cures, all of which are of great importance to the practitioner. Those cases which have been affected by one single, or at most two or three remedies appear to be the most instructive, and the present collection is chiefly composed of such cases. The author has intermixed them with practical remarks and he constantly indicated the source whence the information has been derived.

Ruoff's Repertory of Homœopathic Medicine, Nosologically arranged. Translated from the German by A. H. Okie, M. D. With Additions and Improvements, by G. Humphrey, M. D. 251 pages. 12mo. $1.50.

☞ As a book of reference for the practitioner, the present work far excels every other work, presenting him at a single glance, what he might otherwise seek for amidst a confused mass of records and never find. The indefatigable author has drawn his matter from the infallible results of experience, leaving out all guess work and hypothesis.

Rush, Dr. John. Veterinary Surgeon. The Handbook to Veterinary Homœopathy, or the Homœopathic Treatment of Horses, Cattle, Sheep, Dogs and Swine. From the London Edition. With numerous Additions from the 7th German Edition of Dr. F. E. Günther's "Homœopathic Veterinary." Translated by J. F. Sheek, M. D. 150 pages. 24mo. 50 Cents.

Schaefer, J. C. New Manual of Homœopathic Veterinary Medicine, an easy and comprehensive arrangement of Diseases, adapted to the use of every owner of Domestic Animals, and especially designed for the Farmer, living out of the reach of medical advice, and showing him the way of treating his sick Horses, Cattle, Sheep, Swine and Dogs, in the most simple, expeditious, safe and cheap manner. Translated from the German, with numerous Additions from other Veterinary Manuals by C. J. Hempel, M. D. 321 pages. 8vo. $2.00.

Sharp, W. Tracts on Homœopathy. 12 Numbers. 50 Cents. Bound in muslin. 12mo. 75 Cents.

Small, Dr. A. E. Manual of Homœopathic Practice, for the use of Families and Private Individuals. Fourteenth Enlarged Edition. 831 pages. 8vo. $3.00.

Small, Dr. A. E. Manual of Homœopathic Practice. Translated into German, by C. J. Hempel, M. D. Eleventh Edition. 643 pages. 8vo. $3.00.

Small, Dr. A. E. The Pocket Manual of Homœopathic Practice. Abridged from the "Manual of Homœopathic Practice," by J. F. Sheek, M. D. 126 pages. 36mo. 40 Cents.

Small, Dr. A. E. Diseases of the Nervous System, to which is added a Treatise on the Diseases of the Skin, by Dr. C. E. Toothacker. 216 pages. 8vo. $1.00.

☞ This treatise is from the pen of the distinguished author of the well known and highly popular work entitled "Small's Domestic Practice;" it contains an elaborate description of the various diseases of the nervous system, together with a full statement of the remedies which have been used with beneficial effect in the treatment of these disorders.

Stapf, Dr. E. Additions to the Materia Medica Pura. Translated by C. J. Hempel, M. D. 292 pages. 8vo. $1.50.

☞ This work is an indispensable appendix to Hahneman's Materia Medica Pura. Every remedy is accompanied with extensive and most interesting clinical remarks and a variety of cases illustrative of its therapeutical uses.

Tarbell, Dr. J. A. Sources of Health and the Prevention of Disease, or Mental and Physical Hygiene. 170 pages. 12mo. 50 Cents.

Tessier, Dr. J. P. Clinical Researches concerning the Homœopathic Treatment of Asiatic Cholera, Translated by C. J. Hempel, M. D. 109 pages. 8vo. 75 Cents.

Tessier, Dr. J. P. Clinical Remarks concerning the Homœopathic Treatment of Pneumonia, preceded by retrospective views of the Allopathic Materia Medica, and an explanation of the Homœopathic Law of Cure. Translated by C. J. Hempel. 131 pages. 8vo. 75 Cents.

Therapeutic Guide, Forty Years' Practice. By G. H. G. Jahr. 8vo. $3.50,

Therapeutics, The Science and Art of, B. Baehr. 2 vols. Royal 8vo. $10.00.

Williamson, Dr. W. Diseases of Females and Children and their Homœopathic Treatment. Third Enlarged Edition. 256 pages. 12mo. $1.00.

☞ This work contains a short treatise on the Homœopathic Treatment of the Diseases of Females and Children, the conduct to be observed during pregnancy, labor and confinement, and directions for the management of new-born infants.

Wolf, Dr. C. W. Apis-Mellifica; or, the Poison of the Honey Bee, Considered as a Therapeutic Agent. 80 pages. 12mo. 25 Cents.

☞ This is the most elaborate treatise upon the above drug in print as the author, (one of our most skillful physicians) spared no pains in making it an excellent exponent of Apis mellifica and its medical virtues.

www.ingramcontent.com/pod-product-compliance
Lightning Source LLC
LaVergne TN
LVHW010245110826
845151LV00004B/1394

* 9 7 8 1 4 2 5 5 2 4 0 9 8 *